Upper Cervical Syndrome:

Chiropractic Diagnosis and Treatment

Upper Cervical Syndrome:

Chiropractic Diagnosis and Treatment

Edited by

Howard Vernon, D.C., F.C.C.S. (C)
Director of Research
Canadian Memorial Chiropractic College
Toronto, Ontario, Canada

SANS TACHE

WILLIAMS & WILKINS
Baltimore • Hong Kong • London • Sydney

Editor: Timothy S. Satterfield
Associate Editor: Victoria M. Vaughn
Copy Editor: Susan Vaupel
Design: Saturn Graphics
Illustration Planning: Wayne Hubbel
Production: Charles E. Zeller

428 East Preston Street
Baltimore, MD 21202, U.S.A.

Accurate indications, adverse reactions, and dosage schedules for drugs are provided in this book, but it is possible that they may change. The reader is urged to review the package information data of the manufacturers of the medications mentioned.

Printed in the United States of America

Library of Congress Cataloging-in-Publication Data

Upper cervical syndrome : chiropractic diagnosis and treatment /
edited by Howard Vernon.
p. cm.
Much of the material in this text was previously presented at the Upper Cervical Spine Conference. Canadian Memorial Chiropractic College, Jan. 25–26, 1986.
Includes bibliographies and index.
ISBN 0-683-08591-3
1. Cervical syndrome—Treatment—Congresses. 2. Spinal adjustment—Congresses. 3. Manipulation (Therapeutics)—Congresses. I. Vernon, Howard. II. Upper Cervical Spine Conference (1986 : Canadian Memorial Chiropractic College)
[DNLM: 1. Cervical Vertebrae—anatomy & histology—congresses. 2. Cervical Vertebrae—physiopathology—congresses. 3. Chiropractic—methods—congresses. WE 725 U68 1986]
RC422.C4U66 1988
617'.56—dc19
DNLM/DLC
for Library of Congress
88-123
CIP

88 89 90 91 92
1 2 3 4 5 6 7 8 9 10

Foreword

It gives me great pleasure to accept the honor of being asked to write a foreword to this excellent book.

This is especially a privilege because several of the authors have become personal friends of mine through our work together as chiropractors, anatomists, and an orthopedic surgeon. These are writers for whose work I have the highest regard. Most of them come from the Canadian Memorial Chiropractic College in Toronto, whose reputation is as high as any in the world, but one author joins them from the other side of the Pacific in Melbourne, "ex terra ad terram."

Dr. Howard Vernon, Director of Research at the College in Toronto, is to be congratulated on his vision of the importance of this syndrome, and for the hard work that has translated that vision into practice—a book that will be of great practical value for chiropractors, osteopaths, physiotherapists, and many physicians.

Dealing with this important subject, one neglected by members of my profession for far too long, this text is clearly and concisely written, well illustrated, and comprehensive.

A foreword need say no more. Let the reader see for him- or herself. Those of you who come to read will stay to praise. I commend this book wholeheartedly and wish it, as it deserves, the widest possible circulation.

William H. Kirkaldy-Willis, M.D., F.R.C.S.
Emeritus Professor of Orthopaedics
University Hospital
Saskatoon, Saskatchewan
Canada

Preface

In only the second generation after the initial development of chiropractic by D.D. Palmer, there arose a striving for philosophic purity, for a crystalization of the fundamental concepts, that distinguished the young chiropractic profession. By the early 1930s, B.J. Palmer had found this in the singular idea that the whole of innate intelligence expression could be interfered with at one central focus. Whereas according to D.D. Palmer, the power to affect health and disease was distributed equally and segmentally to all parts of the spine, for B.J. Palmer, purity lay in the reduction of spine and innate to a single spinal focus. Thus was the upper cervical spine elevated to an almost mythical status, and thus was H.I.O. Technique born. This singularity of philosophy and practice came to occupy epic proportions in the development of modern chiropractic.

The modern chiropractor happily can accept B.J. Palmer's legacy of enthusiasm for the clinical importance of this region of the spine, even as he or she eschews the obsessiveness and dogmatism that unfortunately arose from his vision and that of his colleagues. Today we understand the upper cervical spine to have immense importance in the physiology and pathology of the human organism. Structurally, it assumes the characteristics of the most complex junctional unit of the human vertebral column that enhances craniocervical movement, while at the same time preserving its equilibratory stability.

Functionally, no other region of the spine shares its potential to influence human form and activity. The region from C0 to C2 is a self-contained organ of balance, providing crucial information subserving balance, eye movements and cranial position. In addition, this region exerts profound influences on all of the caudal muscular structures and is therefore a fundamental determinant of posture, gait, and all dynamic activity.

In this book, we explore the structure and function of this craniovertebral complex. Our fundamental perspective is chiropractic. I use that word as an adjective, and in so doing, I describe a unique perspective on human physiology that emphasizes the influence of structure, or form, on function. It is a perspective that constantly appreciates the presence of the nervous system operating within the form and function of all regions of the body; it is a perspective that appreciates the interdependence and wholistic integration of the parts of the body, both by direct structural linkages and by the indirect mediation of the nervous system; and finally, it is a perspective that is as equally comfortable with the purely mechanical as it is with the purely neurological.

This text is the product of the efforts of an academic collective at the Canadian Memorial Chiropractic College. It is no accident of fate, although it is a very fortunate circumstance for our students, that the contributors to this text share a consensual perspective on chiropractic matters. This intellectual unity has allowed each of us to deal with our assigned topics while being fully confident of the tone, approach, and scope of the other authors' efforts. In the truest sense, this book is a team effort.

Much of the material in this text was presented at the Upper Cervical Spine Conference, at the Canadian Memorial Chiropractic College, January 25–26, 1986. Even so, the ultimate goal of this team of authors was a text that aspired to the highest academic standards and expressed the unique approach to the chiropractic clinical paradigm as taught at CMCC. As editor of this enterprise, I was very fortunate to have authors of the highest scholastic caliber, whose area of expertise is the upper cervical spine. Each of them eagerly agreed to participate in this project.

This text, then, explores the chiropractic perspective on the upper cervical spine. Necessarily, we place less emphasis on pathological afflictions and congenital anomalies of the region, which are the bailiwick of the medical specialist, and their profound but admittedly rare impact, especially on the nervous system. Rather, our focus is on functional derangements of the vertebral column and their effect, via the intact but disturbed nervous system, on health.

This book is not fundamentally about the upper cervical techniques devised and practiced by numerous chiropractors. While we do have an historical look at the development of some of these techniques, our main purpose is to explore the fundamental chiropractic physiological and clinical bases for any of the manipulative treatments of the upper cervical spine.

We are aware that by concentrating on the upper cervical spine, we may appear to be ignoring the role of other contiguous or distal spinal structures. We do try, however, to walk the thin line between specialized concentration on our topic area and fallacious exaggeration or tunnel vision.

B.J. Palmer's vision was a lure of great treasure with the promise of greater understanding of human health and disease. But it was also a trap in which physiological reality was distorted beyond all reasonable limits to satisfy the need for philosophical purity. We hope, in the offerings of this book, to travel cautiously in search of the promise; we leave the study of the trap to historians.

Howard Vernon D.C., F.C.C.S. (C)
Editor

Acknowledgments

I gratefully acknowledge some important contributions to the creation of this text. First, I thank all of the contributors—their chapters are labors of love, and the time they took from their busy teaching and practice schedules is much appreciated. Second, thanks go to the Canadian Memorial Chiropractic College for its support, material and academic, and specifically to Dr. Terry Hill, Director of Postgraduate Studies, and his staff for their assistance in convening the Upper Cervical Spine Conference in 1986. Veronica Nass did excellent work typing most of the manuscripts and the word processing of Sheila Talaga was invaluable, as was the photo work of Dan McGinty and the illustrations prepared by Lydia Kibiak and Marilyn Staines. Thanks to the College of Chiropractic Clinical Sciences for a generous grant in support of this text. Tim Satterfield, Vicki Vaughn, Sue Vaupel, Wayne Hubbel, and Chuck Zeller deserve my gratitude. Finally, I thank my family and those of my co-contributors for their support and encouragement. I would personally like to dedicate this text to my father—he would have loved to have read it.

Howard Vernon, D.C., F.C.C.S.(C)

Contributors

Lu Barbuto, D.C., F.C.C.S.(C)
Assistant Professor
Division of Clinical Sciences
Canadian Memorial Chiropractic College
Toronto, Ontario, Canada

David J. Brunarski, D.C., F.C.C.S.(C)
Division of Clinical Training
Canadian Memorial Chiropractic College
Toronto, Ontario, Canada

J. David Cassidy, M.Sc., D.C., F.C.C.S.(C)
Research Fellow
Department of Orthopedics
University Hospital
Saskatoon, Saskatchewan, Canada

John Duckworth, M.B., Ch.B., M.D.
Chairman, Faculty of Anatomy
Canadian Memorial Chiropractic College
Toronto, Ontario, Canada

Don E. Fitz-Ritson, B.A., D.C.
Assistant Professor
Department of Chiropractic Sciences
Canadian Memorial Chiropractic College
Toronto, Ontario, Canada

Bruce Fligg, D.C.
Director, Division of Chiropractic Sciences
Canadian Memorial Chiropractic College
Toronto, Ontario, Canada

Allan Gotlib, B.S., D.C.
Assistant Professor
Department of Chiropractic Sciences
Canadian Memorial Chiropractic College
Toronto, Ontario, Canada

Adrian Grice, D.C, F.C.C.S.(C)
Professor
Canadian Memorial Chiropractic College
Toronto, Ontario, Canada

Donald J. Henderson, B.Sc., D.C., F.C.C.S.(C), D.A.C.B.R., F.C.C.R., F.I.C.C.
President
Canadian College of Chiropractic Sciences
Toronto, Ontario, Canada

Marilyn Staines, M.A., D.C.
Department of Radiology
Canadian Memorial Chiropractic College
Toronto, Ontario, Canada

Zoltan Szaraz, D.C.
Assistant Director
Division of Chiropractic Sciences
Canadian Memorial Chiropractic College
Toronto, Ontario, Canada

Allen Terrett, Dip. App. Sci. (Hum. Biol.), B. App. Sci (Chir.), (P.I.T.), Dip. Tert. Ed. (H.I.E.) F.A.C.C.S.
Department of Diagnostic Sciences
Phillip Institute of Technology
Melbourne, Australia

Haymo Thiel, D.C.
Senior Clinical Resident
Canadian Memorial Chiropractic College
Toronto, Ontario, Canada

Howard Vernon, D.C., F.C.C.S.(C)
Director of Research
Canadian Memorial Chiropractic College
Toronto, Ontario, Canada

Contents

1 Normal Anatomy and Physiology Section

1 Anatomy of the Suboccipital Region

John Duckworth, M.B., Ch.B., M.D.

The importance of the suboccipital region derives from the fact that the slender cervical part of the vertebral column must support the weight of the head. There is a greater range of movement between the head and the first two cervical vertebrae than in any other region of the column. As well, this area must allow for the transfer of forces applied to the head onto the vertebral column and still maintain its integrity.

OSTEOLOGY OF THE SUBOCCIPITAL REGION

The bones involved in this region are the external aspect of the occipital bone, the mastoid part of the temporal bone, and the upper cervical vertebrae (Fig. 1.1).

Occipital Bone

The chief features to be noted on the occipital bone are the external occipital protuberance, the superior nuchal line passing laterally from it to the posterior aspect of the mastoid processes of the temporal bone, and the external occipital crest passing forward from it in the median plane to the posterior aspect of the foramen magnum.

The inferior nuchal lines (Fig. 1.2) curve laterally from the midpoint on the external occipital crest to the posterior part of the jugular processes of the occipital bones. These processes are homologous with the tips of the transverse processes of a cervical vertebra and represent the inferior aspects of the transverse processes of the proatlas vertebra.

Occasionally the tip is enlarged to form a paramastoid process that projects inferiorly and may articulate with the superior aspect of the tip of the transverse process of the atlas or first cervical vertebra.

The occipital condyles (Fig. 1.2) lie anterolateral to the foramen magnum. Their articular surfaces are convex from front to back, and from side to side, and face inferolaterally. Their long axes are directed forward and medially.

Immediately posterior to the occipital condyles lie the openings of the posterior condylar canals, which are not always present. They transmit a vein which connects the lower end of the sigmoid sinus with the vertebral veins.

One centimeter superior to the superior nuchal lines lie the supreme nuchal lines, which give attachment to the posterior bellies of the occipitofrontales muscles. Between the superior nuchal lines and the supreme nuchal lines lies a sheet of connective tissue, which is traversed by the greater occipital nerves and the occipital arteries as they pass forward and upward to enter the scalp, 2.5 cm lateral to the external occipital protuberance. Occasionally these nerves are entrapped in this fascia, causing numbness over the back of the scalp and occipital headaches.

Cervical Vertebrae

The first two cervical vertebrae (C1 and C2) are considerably different from the typical cervical vertebrae (C3–C5) due to modifications associated with the support and movements of the head on the vertebral column (Figs. 1.3–1.6).

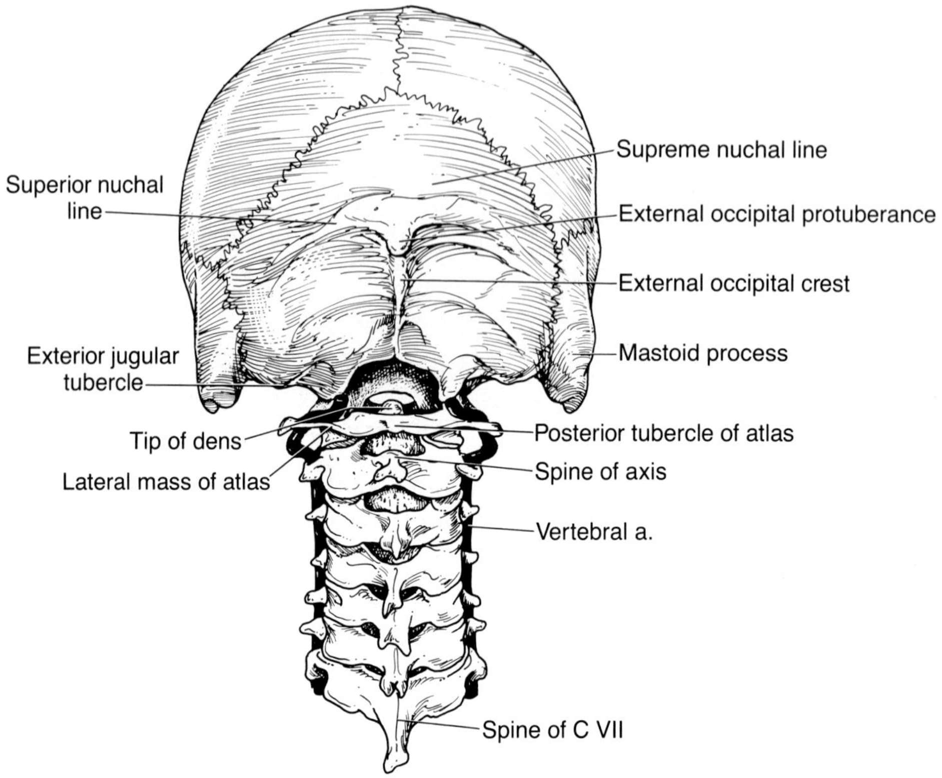

Figure 1.1. Suboccipital skeleton.

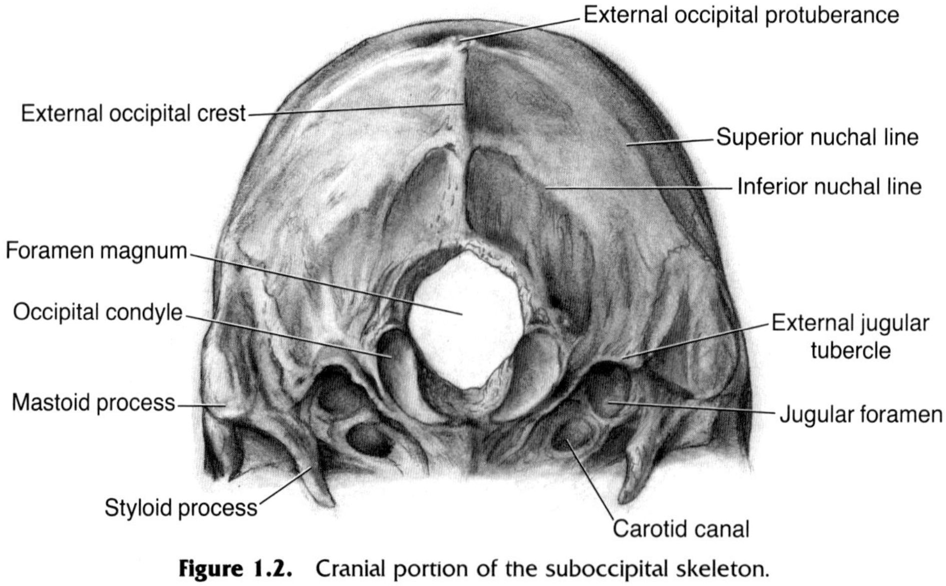

Figure 1.2. Cranial portion of the suboccipital skeleton.

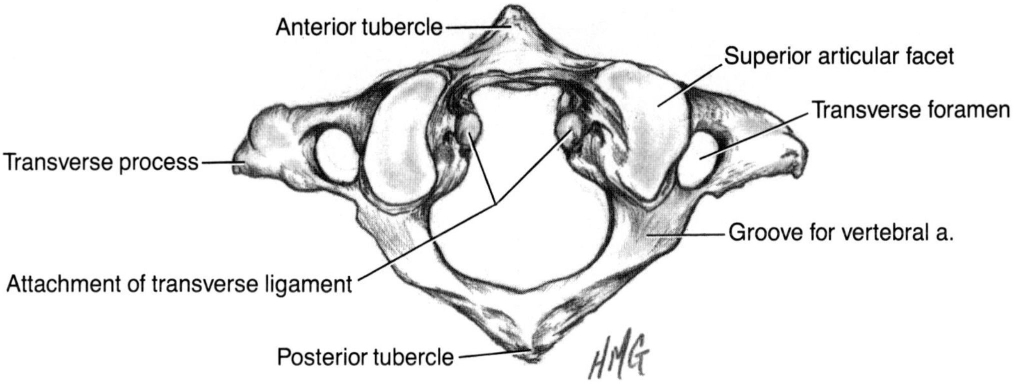

Figure 1.3. Atlas, superior view.

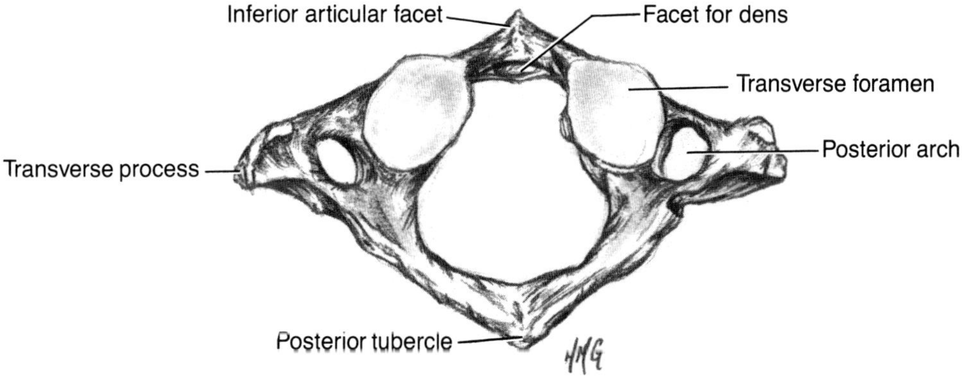

Figure 1.4. Atlas, inferior view.

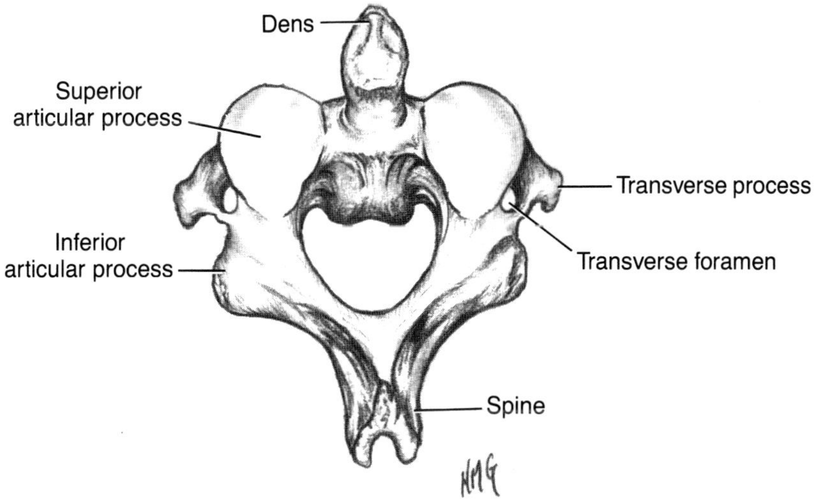

Figure 1.5. Axis, superior view.

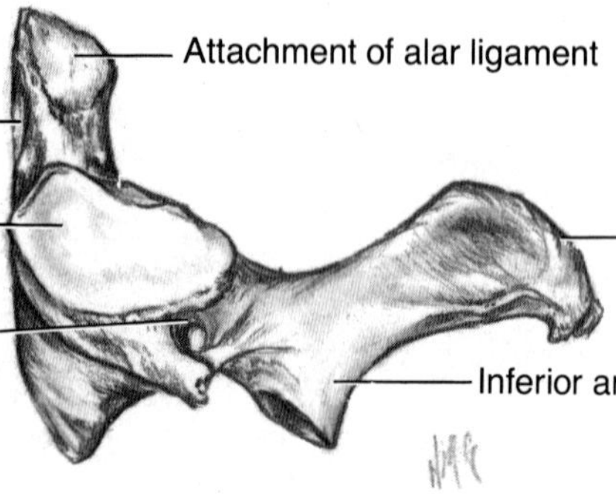

Figure 1.6. Axis, lateral view.

The first cervical vertebra or atlas has no central part to its body. This part is fused to the superior part of the body of the second cervical vertebra or axis to form the dens, which acts as a pivot around which the atlas and skull can rotate during side-to-side rotation of the head.

The pedicles of the atlas are enlarged to form the lateral masses. They are united anteriorly by the anterior arch, a formation which is not found in any other human vertebra. On the superior aspects of the lateral masses lie the concave articular facets for articulation with the occipital condyles of the skull. They face superomedially and are closer together anteriorly than posteriorly, in conformity with the occipital condyles of the skull (Fig. 1.3).

On the inferior aspects of the lateral masses lie the almost circular facets for articulation with the superior facets on the axis or second cervical vertebra. They are almost flat and face inferomedially. Posteriorly, the lateral masses are united by the two halves of the posterior arch, which meet in the median plane at a small posterior tubercle. (Fig. 1.4). On the superior aspect of each half of the posterior arch lies a deep groove in which lie the first cervical nerve and the vertebral artery. This groove is sometimes ossified over laterally to form a pons lateralis, or posteriorly to form a pons posterior (Fig. 1.3).

The transverse processes of the atlas are long and have no anterior tubercles. They can be palpated in the side of the neck between the tips of the mastoid processes and the angles of the mandible. Passing through the processes are the transverse foramina, which transmit the vertebral arteries and vertebral veins, on their way to the grooves on the superior aspect of the posterior arch.

In the second cervical vertebra, the central part of the body of the atlas is fused to the superior aspect of its body to form the dens, around which the skull and atlas can rotate. In addition, the superior parts of its pedicles are enlarged to form the articular surfaces for the corresponding facets on the inferior aspects of the lateral masses of the atlas. These facets are almost circular, convex, and face superolaterally (Fig. 1.5).

The spine is larger than on the other cervical vertebrae, and its posterior aspect is V-shaped, with open end facing inferiorly. The transverse processes have both anterior and posterior tubercles and are pierced by the transverse foramina, which unlike the other transverse foramina, make right angle bends in the transverse processes to emerge from their lateral aspects between the anterior and posterior tubercles. This is because the transverse foramina in the atlas are placed further laterally than those in the axis and because the vertebral arteries must loop laterally to allow for the wide range of movement between the atlas and axis during rotation of the head from side to side (Fig. 1.11).

The inferior articular processes lie at the junction of the laminae and pedicles and thus lie posterior to the emerging spinal nerves, unlike the articular facets between the skull and atlas and the atlas and axis, which lie anterior to the emerging nerves (Fig. 1.6). The inferior articular facets are flat and face anteroinferiorly.

The typical cervical vertebrae are the third, fourth, and fifth, all of which have similar features. Their bodies are broader transversely than anteroposteriorly. The superior surfaces of the bodies are concave, while their inferior surfaces are convex. The posterolateral edges of the bodies curve superiorly to articulate with corresponding areas on the inferior aspects of the bodies above, to form the small uncovertebral joints, or joints of von Luschka.

The laminae are more slender than those on the second cervical vertebra, and the spines are bifid. Their superior articular processes have flat articular facets, which face posterosuperiorly, while the inferior articular facets face anteroinferiorly.

The transverse processes have anterior and posterior tubercles, and their transverse foramina run inferosuperiorly, transmitting the vertebral arteries and a pair of vertebral veins. The costotransverse bars are bowed inferiorly and increase in size downward to accommodate the increasing size of the roots of the brachial plexus, which emerge immediately posterior to the vertebral arteries to pass laterally between the scalenus anterior and the scalenus medius muscles.

The sixth cervical vertebra differs from a typical cervical vertebra in having a long, straight spine, to which is attached the lower end of the ligamentum nuchae.

The seventh cervical vertebra has an even longer spine than the sixth, which forms a prominence on the back of the neck and marks the end of the ligamentum nuchae. Its transverse foramina do not transmit the vertebral arteries.

Occasionally the costal elements of the transverse processes are enlarged to form a partial or complete cervical rib, which may compress the T1 root of the brachial plexus, or the subclavian artery as it arches over it.

ARTHROLOGY OF THE SUBOCCIPITAL REGION

Atlantooccipital Joints

The atlantooccipital joints are formed by the articulation of the cartilage-covered surfaces of the occipital condyles with the kidney-shaped articular surfaces on the superior aspects of the lateral masses of the atlas (Figs. 1.2 and 1.3).

The occipital condyles are convex anteroposteriorly and, to a lesser extent, from side to side. They face inferolaterally and are closer to the median plane anteriorly than posteriorly.

The superior articular surfaces on the atlas are concave and are closer to the median plane anteriorly than posteriorly to match those on the occipital condyles.

The cartilage-covered surfaces are enclosed by a synovial capsule, which is supported by a fibrous capsule. This capsule is supplied by pain and proprioceptive nerves, which it receives via a communicating branch from the second cervical, or greater occipital nerve.

Atlantoaxial Joints

The axis articulates with the atlas by means of paired lateral atlantoaxial joints and a median atlantoaxial joint (Fig. 1.6).

The lateral atlantoaxial joints are formed by the articulation of the inferior articular surfaces on the lateral masses of the atlas with the articular surfaces on the superior aspect of the pedicles of the axis. The articular surfaces on the atlas are flat or very slightly concave and face inferomedially, while those on the axis are convex and face superolaterally.

The articular surfaces are enclosed by a synovial capsule, which is supported by a fibroelastic capsule, which is sufficiently lax to allow considerable overriding of the articular surfaces during rotation of the atlas on the axis.

These joints receive their nerve supply from the posterior rami of the second cervical nerve.

The median atlantoaxial joint is formed by the articulation of a concave, circular articular surface on the middle of the posterior surface of the anterior arch of the atlas, with a convex articular surface on the anterior aspect of the odontoid process. The cartilage-covered surfaces are enclosed by a synovial capsule, supported by a fibrous capsule (Fig. 1.6).

Another joint exists between the posterior aspect of the neck of the odontoid process and the anterior aspect of the transverse ligament of the atlas. This cavity may communicate with the cavity of the anterior joint.

The atlantooccipital and atlantoaxial joints are supported by the ligaments described below.

Transverse Ligament of the Atlas: (Fig. 1.7). This ligament is attached to a small tubercle on the medial side of each lateral mass of the atlas and arches across the posterior aspect of the neck of the odontoid process. It secures the odontoid process against the anterior arch of the atlas. Extensions from the transverse ligament pass superiorly to the basioccipital bone just inside the foramen magnum, and inferiorly to the posterior aspect of the body of the axis.

Alar Ligaments: (Fig. 1.7). These ligaments pass from the lateral aspect of the superior end of the odontoid process to the medial aspect of the occipital condyles. They secure the odontoid process between the lateral masses of the atlas. They are tight when the head is flexed and turned to either side.

Posterior Longitudinal Ligament: (Fig. 1.7). The upward extension of this ligament, the membrana tectoria, lies posterior to the transverse ligament and its extensions and is attached to the posterior aspect of the body of the axis and to the internal aspect of the basioccipital bone just superior to the superior band of the transverse ligament.

Posterior Atlantooccipital Membrane. This fibroelastic membrane is attached to the posterior rim of the foramen magnum and to the superior aspect of the posterior arch of the atlas. Immediately posterior to the occipital condyles, it is pierced by the vertebral arteries and the first cervical nerves.

Anterior Atlantooccipital Membrane. This fibroelastic membrane is attached to the anterior rim of the foramen magnum and to the superior aspect of the anterior arch of the atlas.

Ligamentum Nuchae. This ligament is attached to the external occipital crest, to the posterior tubercle of the atlas, and to the spines of all of the cervical vertebrae. It helps stabilize the skull on the cervical spine.

Apical Ligament: (Fig. 1.7). This ligament which is formed from the remains of the notochord, is attached to the apex of the odontoid process and to the midpoint on the anterior rim of the foramen magnum. Occasionally, a small ossicle is found in this ligament, which represents the centrum of the proatlas vertebra.

The movements occurring at the suboccipital joints are as follows.

Atlantooccipital Joints. The principal movements occurring at these joints are flexion and extension. A small amount of lateral bending can also occur.

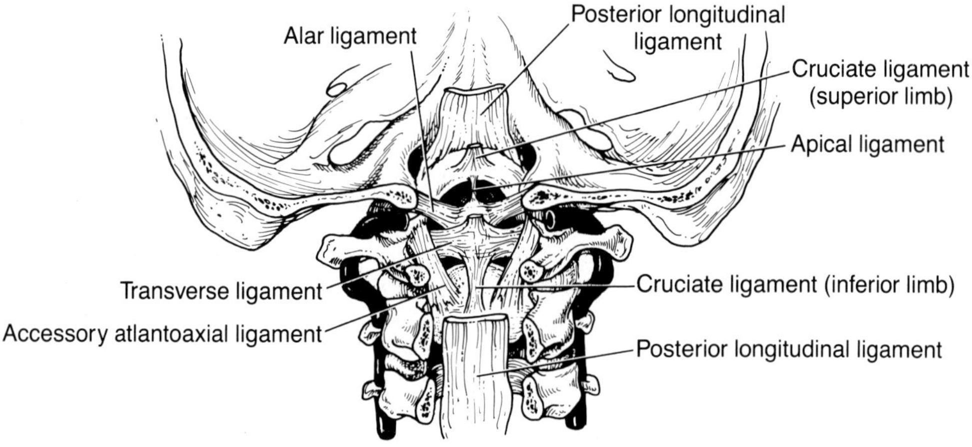

Figure 1.7. Upper cervical ligaments, posteroanterior view.

Atlantoaxial Joints. The principal movements occurring at these joints are rotation of the skull and atlas on the axis. Because the facets on the lateral atlantoaxial joints are slightly convex, there is a slight ascent of the atlas as the head is rotated to either side.

Zygapophyseal Joints of C2–C7. The flat articular surfaces lie on the superior and inferior aspects of the articular processes, which are situated where the pedicles and laminae join. The superior pairs face posterosuperiorly, while the inferior pairs face anteroinferiorly. Their articular capsules allow some overriding during flexion, extension, and lateral bending and have an abundant nerve supply.

The small uncovertebral joints, or joints of von Luschka, lie between the posterolateral aspects of the vertebral bodies immediately anterior to the emerging anterior rami of the spinal nerves.

MUSCLES OF THE SUBOCCIPITAL REGION

Muscles Acting Only on the Atlantooccipital Joints (Figs. 1.8 and 1.10)

Obliquus Superior. This muscle arises from the tip of the transverse process of the atlas and inserts into the lateral part of the area between the superior and inferior nuchal lines. Its direction is posterior and slightly superior, so that its action is to bend the head to its own side and to extend the head at the atlantooccipital joint.

Rectus Capitis Posterior Minor. This muscle arises from the posterior tubercle of the atlas and inserts into the medial part of the area between the inferior nuchal line and the foramen magnum. It extends the head at the atlantooccipital joints.

Rectus Capitis Lateralis. This muscle arises from the superior aspect of the transverse process of the atlas and, passing upward and slightly laterally, inserts into the inferior aspect of the jugular process of the occipital bone. It bends the head to its own side at the atlantooccipital joints. Directly anterior to this muscle lies the spinal accessory nerve and the internal jugular vein.

Rectus Capitis Anterior. This muscle arises from the articular surface of the lateral mass of the atlas and, passing upward and medially, directly in front of the atlantooccipital joint, inserts into the base of the occipital bone, posterolateral to the pharyngeal tubercle.

All of these muscles are supplied with motor fibers from the first cervical nerve and proprioceptive and pain fibers via a communicating branch from the second cervical nerve.

Muscle Acting Only on the Atlantoaxial Joint

Obliquus Inferior (Fig. 1.8). This muscle arises from the tip of the second cervical spine between the origin of the rectus capitis posterior major above and the insertion of semispinalis capitis below and passes laterally and upward to insert into the posterior aspect of the tip of the transverse process of the atlas. It is supplied with motor fibers from the first cervical nerve and sensory fibers from the second cervical nerve.

Muscles Acting on the Craniocervical Joints (Fig. 1.9)

Trapezius. This muscle arises from the medial third of the superior nuchal line, the posterior border of the ligamentum nuchae, and all of the thoracic spines and is inserted into the medial third of the clavicle, the medial border of the acromial process, the superior border of the spine of the scapula, and the inferior border of the spine of the scapula as far as the tubercle. It is supplied by the spinal part of the accessory nerve and the ventral rami of the third and fourth cervical nerves. Its action on the craniovertebral joints occurs when the shoulder is fixed. The upper fibers of trapezius can then draw the head to its own side. If both muscles contract together, it can extend the head. Its chief function is to aid in supporting the upper limb on the trunk.

Splenius Capitis. This muscle runs obliquely and arises from the lower half of the ligamentum nuchae, the seventh cervical spine, and the upper six thoracic spines.

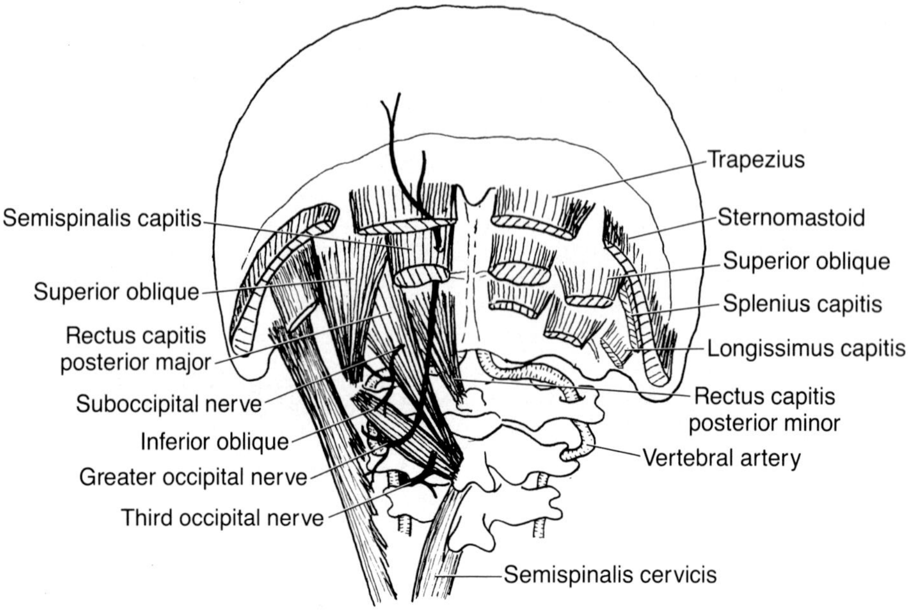

Figure 1.8. Suboccipital muscles and nerves.

It inserts into the posterior aspect of the mastoid process, deep to the sternomastoid, and superficial to the longissimus capitis. It is supplied by the posterior rami of the fourth through eighth cervical nerves. When both muscles contract, it will extend the head and neck. If only one muscle contracts, it will bend the head and neck to its own side and turn the face to that side.

Semispinalis Capitis. This muscle arises from the posterior aspect of the transverse processes of the upper six cervical vertebrae and inserts into the medial part of the area between the superior and inferior nuchal lines. It is supplied by the dorsal rami

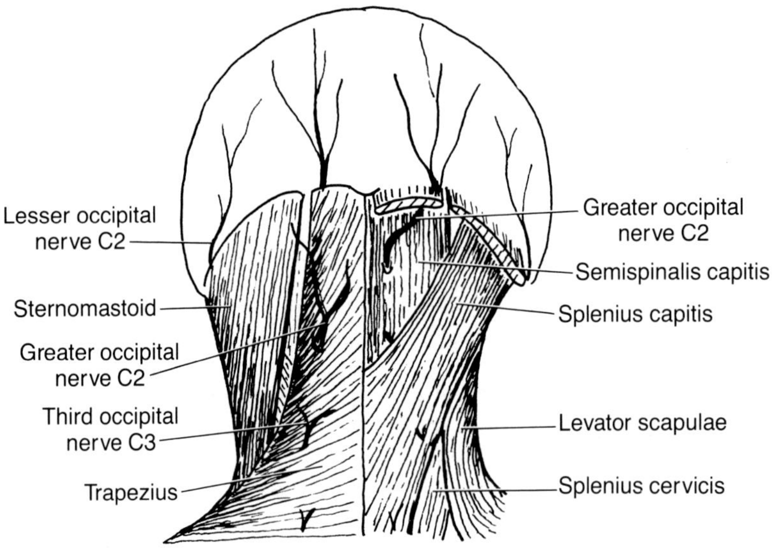

Figure 1.9. Superficial and intermediate musculature. Cutaneous nerves of the upper cervical spine.

of C2–C5. This muscle is the most powerful extensor of the head and upper cervical region. When one muscle contracts alone, it will extend the head and turn the face to the opposite side.

Longissimus Capitis. This muscle arises from the posterior aspect of the upper six cervical transverse processes lateral to the semispinalis capitis and inserts into the posterior aspect of the mastoid process deep to the splenius capitis. It extends the head and turns the face to the same side. When both muscles contract, they extend the head.

Longus Capitis (Fig. 10). This muscle arises from the anterior tubercles of the upper six cervical transverse processes and is inserted into the basal part of the occipital bone, just lateral to the pharyngeal tubercle. It flexes the head and neck. It is supplied by the anterior rami of C1–C4.

Sternocleidomastoid. This muscle arises by a tendon from the anterior aspect of the manubrium sterni and by muscle fibers from the medial one-third of the upper border of the clavicle. It inserts into the posterior part of the mastoid process and the lateral two-thirds of the superior nuchal line. It extends the head and turns the face to the opposite side. It is supplied by the spinal part of the accessory nerve and by the anterior ramus of the second cervical nerve.

NERVE SUPPLY OF THE SUBOCCIPITAL REGION (SEE FIG. 9)

Sensory Nerve Supply

Greater Occipital Nerve (Figs. 1.8 and 1.9) This nerve is formed by the posterior ramus of C2. It arises from the ganglion that lies between the posterior arch of the atlas and the lamina of C2 and, curving around the inferior border of the inferior oblique muscle, ascends superomedially through the semispinalis capitis muscle. It emerges through the posterior aspect of this muscle one-quarter inch lateral to the ligamentum nuchae and 1 inch below the superior nuchal line, and passes superiorly between the origin of trapezius and the insertion of sternomastoid to enter the scalp, where it supplies the skin as far as the vertex. It is the largest posterior ramus in the body and is the nerve most frequently involved in sensory disorders in this region.

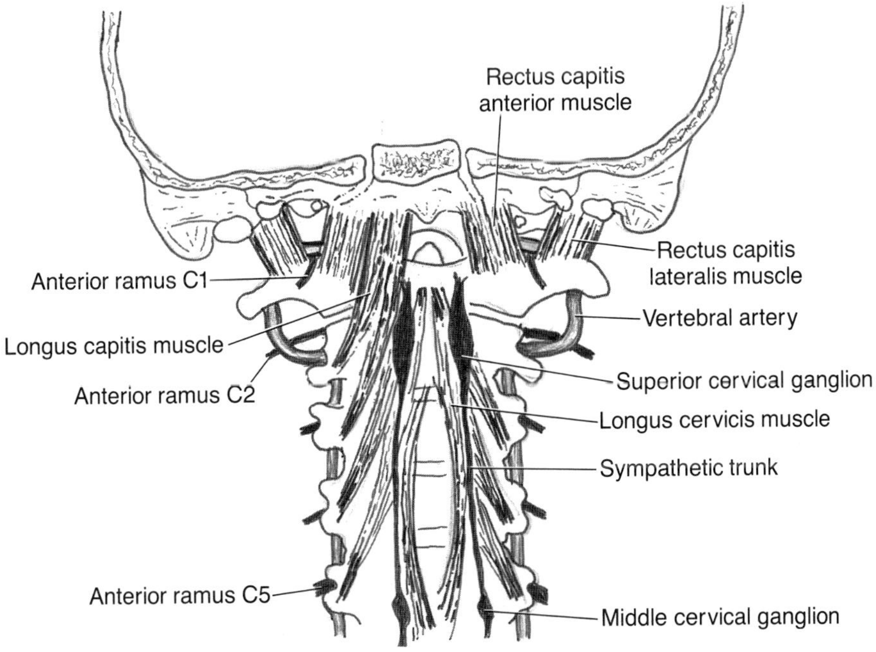

Figure 1.10. Prevertebral muscles.

Third Occipital Nerve (Figs. 1.8 and 1.9). This nerve is formed by the posterior ramus of C3. It passes posteriorly immediately inferior to the articular process of the axis and lateral to the insertion of the semispinalis cervicis. It then passes through the semispinalis capitis and trapezius to supply the skin of the upper half of the back of the neck and head.

Lesser Occipital Nerve (Fig. 1.9). This nerve is formed by the articular ramus of C2. It emerges at the posterior border of the sternomastoid, immediately inferior to the spinal accessory nerve, and ascends along the posterior border of the external occipital protuberance and the mastoid process as far as the vertex.

Motor Nerve Supply

Suboccipital or First Cervical Nerve (Fig. 1.8). This nerve emerges in the groove on the superior aspect of the posterior arch of the atlas, inferior to the vertebral artery. Its anterior ramus passes medial to the vertebral artery and between the rectus capitis anterior and rectus capitis lateralis, where it supplies these muscles and longus capitis, before joining the hypoglossal nerve. It travels with this nerve to supply the genioglossus and the external muscles of the larynx. The posterior ramus passes posteriorly in the posterior triangle of the neck to supply the inferior superior oblique, rectus capitis posterior major, rectus capitis posterior minor, and semispinalis capitis.

Greater Occipital Nerve. This nerve, described above, supplies semispinalis capitis.

Remaining Posterior Rami. These pass posteriorly immediately inferior to the articular processes to supply the ligaments and muscles at their levels.

BLOOD SUPPLY OF THE SUBOCCIPITAL REGION

Occipital Arteries (Fig. 1.11)

The occipital arteries arise from the external carotid arteries at the lower borders of the posterior bellies of the digastric muscles. They run posterosuperiorly, just medial to the digastric muscles, grooving the skull medial to the mastoid process. They continue posterosuperiorly deep to the attachments of the splenius capitis and sternomastoid muscles. Finally, they turn superiorly between the origin of the trapezius and the insertion of the sternomastoid, where they lie in company with the greater occipital nerve and spread out toward the vertex of the scalp.

Deep Cervical Arteries

These arteries arise from the costocervical trunks of the subclavian arteries at the level of the upper border of the first ribs. They pass posteriorly between the upper border of the first rib and the transverse process of the seventh cervical vertebra and ascend in the back of the neck, between semispinalis cervicis and semispinalis capitis, to the back of the skull, where they anastomose with the occipital arteries and the vertebral arteries.

Vertebral Arteries

The right vertebral artery arises from the right subclavian artery close to its origin from the brachiocephalic artery. The left vertebral artery arises from either the left subclavian artery or directly from the arch of the aorta.

Both vertebral arteries ascend in front of the transverse processes of the seventh cervical vertebra and then ascend through the transverse foramina of the sixth to the second cervical vertebrae. In the transverse foramina of the second cervical vertebra, the arteries make a right-angle bend to emerge from the lateral aspect of the transverse process. They then loop laterally and superiorly to pass through the transverse foramina of the first cervical vertebra before turning medially in a deep groove on the superior aspect of the posterior arch of the atlas. At the medial end of this groove they pierce the posterior atlantooccipital membrane, dura, and arachnoid to enter the subarachnoid space, in which they ascend through the foramen magnum to meet at the lower border of the pons, where they unite to form the basilar artery.

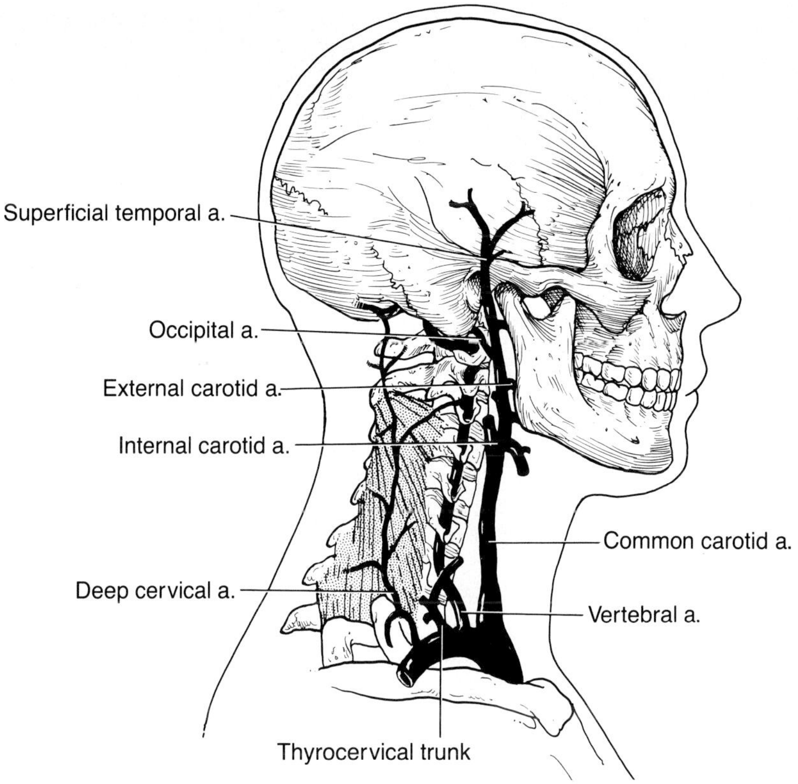

Figure 1.11. Blood supply of the suboccipital region.

CLINICAL ANATOMY OF THE SUBOCCIPITAL REGION

Skeletal Abnormalities

Incorporation of the Atlas into the Skull (Figs. 1.12 and 1.13)

The atlas may be completely or partially incorporated into the skull, and this incorporation may be symmetrical or asymmetrical. When it is symmetrical, the patient cannot flex his head at the atlantooccipital joints but can turn his head from side to side. When it is asymmetrical, it may result

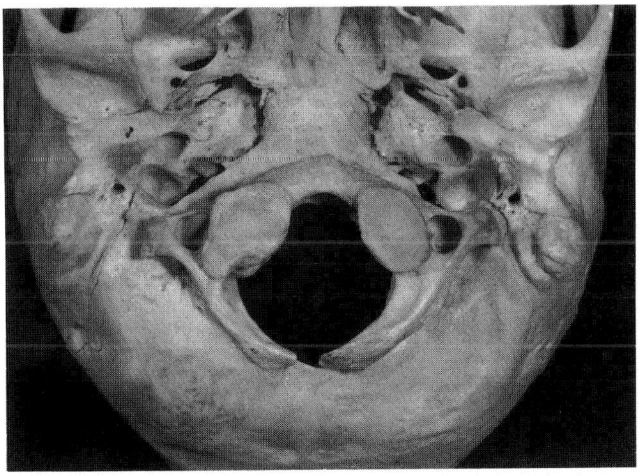

Figure 1.12. Incorporation of atlas into the skull, inferior view.

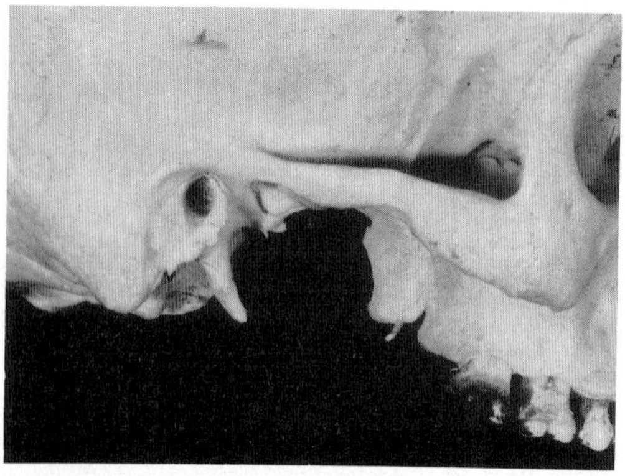

Figure 1.13. Incorporation of atlas into the skull, lateral view.

in congenital wryneck, as well as inability to flex the head at the atlantooccipital joints.

Basilar Invagination (Figs. 1.14 and 1.15)

In this condition, the margins of the foramen magnum are invaginated into the posterior cranial fossa. It may result from imperfect ossification of the occipital bone due to osteomalacia, rickets, Paget's disease, or congenital hypoplasia. It may cause vertebral artery compression just posterior to the occipital condyles, leading to dizziness, dimness of vision, and incoordination.

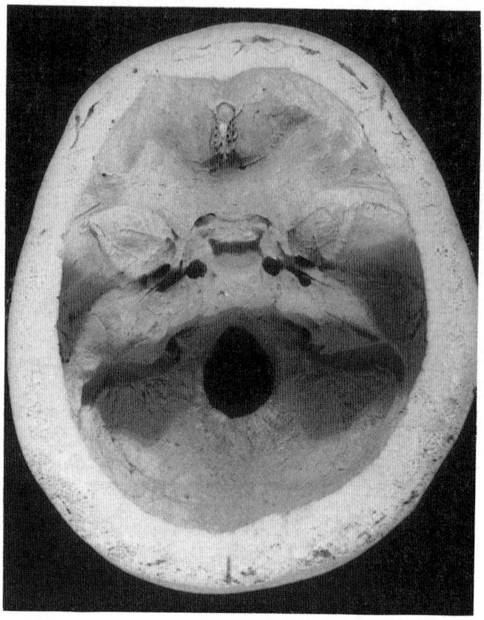

Figure 1.15. Basilar invagination in Paget's disease.

Paramastoid Process (Figs. 1.16 and 1.17)

This process projects inferiorly from the jugular process of the occipital bone toward the superior aspect of the tip of the transverse process of the atlas, with which it

Figure 1.14. Basilar invagination.

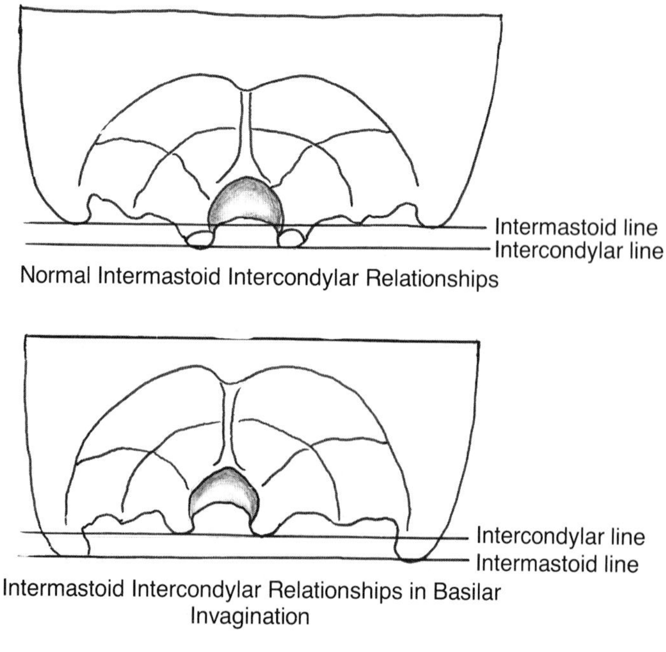

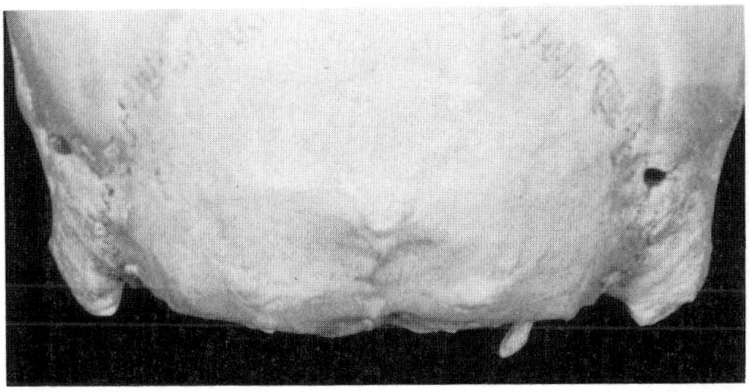

Figure 1.16. Paramastoid process, inferior view.

sometimes forms a pseudoarthrosis. It causes pain on lateral flexion of the head at the atlantooccipital joint, on the affected side, and greatly limits or abolishes lateral flexion.

Anomalies of the Atlas (Fig. 1.18)

There are three types of these anomalies. The posterior arch of the atlas ossifies from centers in the lateral masses, which extend posteriorly to form each half of the arch. Arrest in this development will give rise to various degrees of spina bifida.

The anterior arch of the atlas normally ossifies from a center that appears in its cartilaginous precursor in the median plane. Sometimes, however, it may ossify from the centers forming the lateral masses. Imperfect ossification can thus result either in a separate median ossicle or in two short processes that extend forward and medially from each lateral mass.

Condylar hypoplasia results from imperfect development of the lateral masses of the atlas. It may be unilateral or bilateral. This may result in impingement of the tip of the odontoid process on the anterior margin of the foramen magnum, where it forms a pseudoarthrosis. If the condition is unilateral, it may result in congenital wryneck, because in this condition there is less space between the occipital condyle and the lateral mass on the affected side. It may also result in compression of the vertebral artery posterior to the condyle.

Anomalies of the Axis (Fig. 1.19)

The dens is ossified from three centers—one for the tip and one in each half of the shaft. Failure of the ossification in the tip results in the dens ending in a bifid tip. Failure of the lateral parts to ossify may result in the absence of the dens, or in a little median ossicle at the anterior margin of the foramen magnum. If the dens fails to fuse with the body of the axis, it may simulate a fracture of the dens.

The rest of the axis ossifies from one center for the body and one center for each pedicle, transverse process, and corresponding half of the arch. A secondary cen-

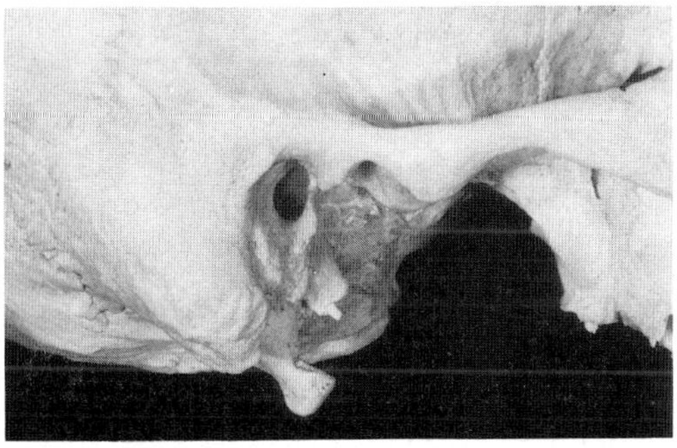

Figure 1.17. Paramastoid process, lateral view.

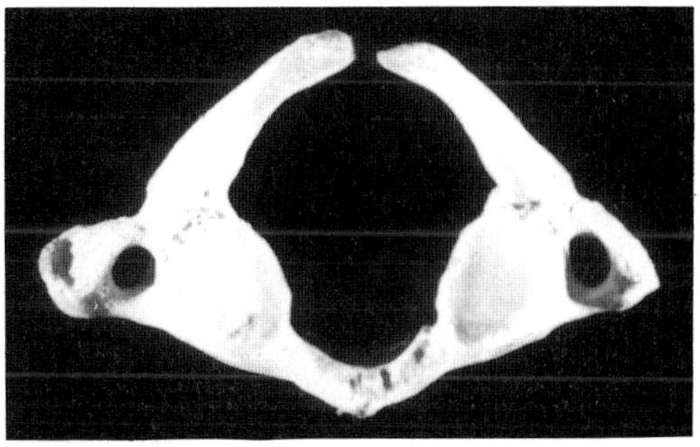

Figure 1.18. Spina bifida, atlas.

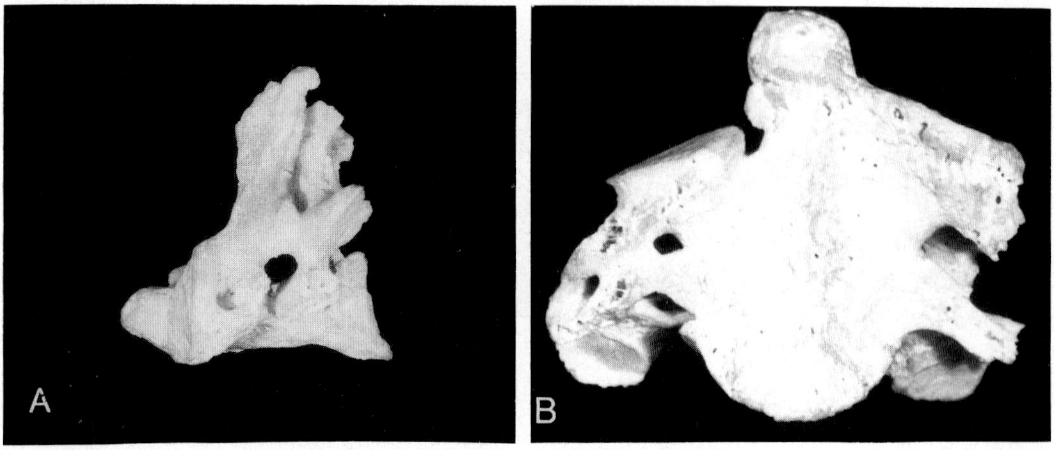

Figure 1.19. Anomalies of the axis. *A,* congenital fusion C2–C3. *B,* congenital fusion C2–C3 with assymetrical development of C2 superior articular processes.

ter appears in the epiphyseal plate on the inferior aspect of the body at puberty.

Anomalies therefore, can, arise from a failure of one or more of these elements.

Cervical Fusions (Fig. 1.20)

Fusion of the axis with the third cervical vertebra is the commonest fusion in this region. It may be congenital or acquired. In the congenital type, the fusion may be asymmetrical and cause compression of the vertebral artery on one or both sides (see Fig. 1.21).

Pathological Abnormalities

Ankylosing Spondylitis

This condition is common in older people but may commence in younger people as well. It results in calcification extending into the ligaments of the vertebral column, leading to gradual immobilization of the spine.

Rheumatoid Arthritis

In this condition, there is a destruction of the cartilage of the joints and disintegration

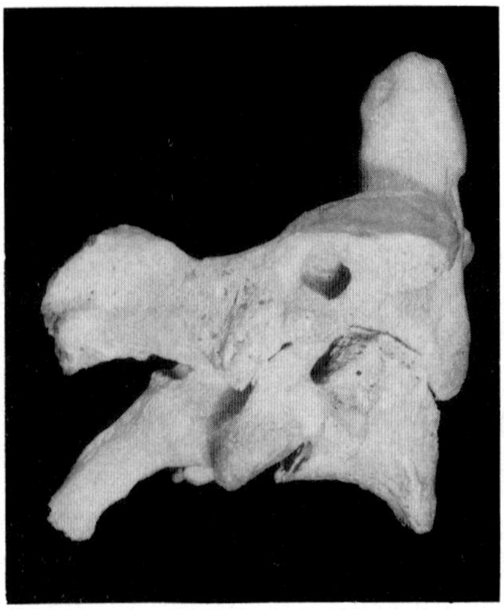

Figure 1.20. Osteoarthritic fusion C2–C3. Lateral views.

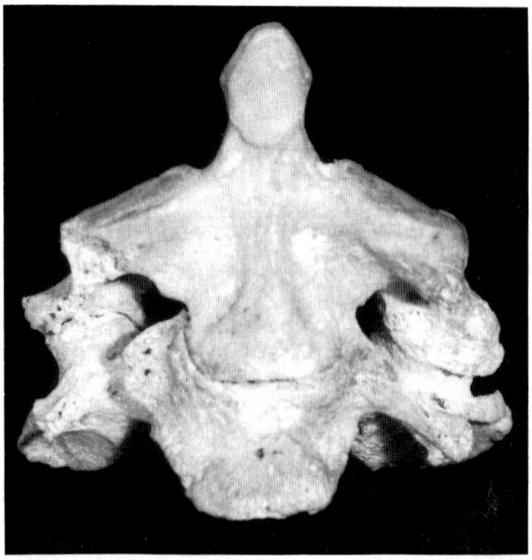

Figure 1.21. Osteoarthritic fusion of C2–C3, anterior view.

of the joint ligaments. This leads to laxity of the ligaments and a tendency toward subluxations. These subluxations may result in compression of the spinal cord or anterior or posterior spinal arteries, resulting in paralysis according to the area compressed.

Grisel's Torticollis

This condition is usually associated with nasopharyngeal infections involving the retropharyngeal space and results in the pharynx being displaced forward and a ladder-like deformity of the cervical vertebrae starting at the atlas and increasing inferiorly.

Tuberculous Disease of the Cervical Spine

In this condition, there are varying degrees of bone destruction. This may proceed to abscess formation with displacement of the prevertebral fascia forward. It then usually extends laterally pointing to the posterior triangle of the neck.

TRAUMA

Injuries to the suboccipital region of the neck are common, usually resulting from motor vehicle, diving, and industrial accidents.

Hyperextension Injuries

These may result in: *(a)* hemorrhage into the prevertebral muscles from overstretching; *(b)* fracture of the odontoid process; or *(c)* bruising of the posterior root ganglion of the second cervical or greater occipital nerve (Fig. 1.22).

(This injury occurs when the head is hyperextended while it is turned to the right or left and is due to the compression of the ganglion between the inferior aspect of the posterior arch of the atlas and the superior aspect of the lamina of the axis. Compressor occurs on the side opposite to which the face is turned.)

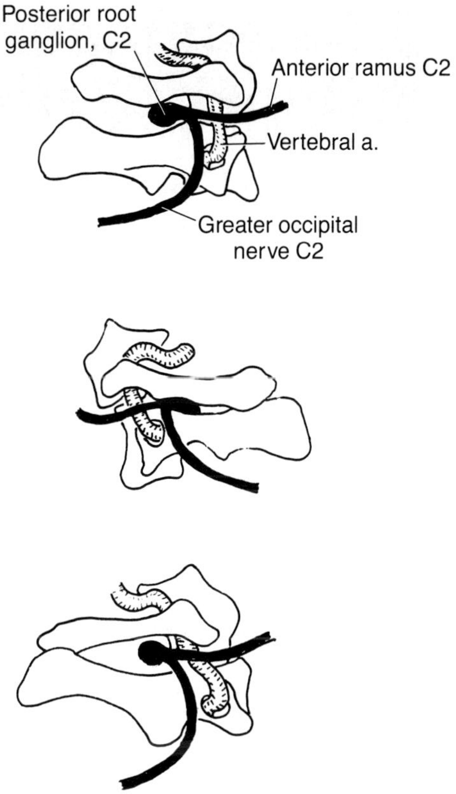

Figure 1.22. Hyperextension injury—compression of C2 dorsal root ganglion. *Top,* Normal. *Middle,* Left lateral view of atlas in left rotation and extension. *Lower,* Right lateral view of atlas in left rotation and extension.

Hyperflexion Injuries

These may take the form of a rupture of the transverse ligament or of the alar ligaments.

Rotational Injuries

These may involve dislocation of the atlantooccipital joints or of the atlanto-axial joints.

Axial Injuries

Forces applied in the long axis of the vertebral column either via the top of the head or via the vertebral column below may lead to fracture of the base of the skull around the foramen magnum or compression fracture of one or both lateral masses of the atlas.

2 Radiographic Evaluation of the Upper Cervical Spine

Donald J. Henderson, B.Sc., D.C., F.C.C.S., D.A.C.B.R., F.C.C.R., F.I.C.C.

Marilyn Staines, M.A., D.C.

Radiography is one of the few objective diagnostic tools providing the practitioner of manipulation with information that cannot be gained in any other way. Visualization of the area under study, even if negative for structural and functional pathology, can help the practitioner arrive at a clinical decision. Like all other diagnostic procedures, however, it is not absolute and it is only one of the components of the total clinical information on the patient's health. Its significance to patient management depends on the interpretive skills of the examiner (in light of data collected from the history/examination) and on the technical precision used in processing the diagnostic image—the radiograph.

Health professionals agree that radiographic screening should be performed before spinal manipulation is contemplated(1–7). There are many pathological processes that can weaken or destabilize the supportive elements of bone and joint. Where manual correction of articular dysfunction is necessary, it is judicious to evaluate the integrity of the tissues.

As a research modality, radiography can provide a better understanding of the role of manipulation in neuromusculoskeletal disorders. However, the risk versus benefit of radiation exposure must be considered from both a clinical and ethical standpoint.

In this chapter, we review the technical and roentgenometric aspects of the radiologic examination as well as the structural and functional conditions affecting the upper cervical complex.

RADIOGRAPHIC PROJECTIONS

The minimal number of views for any spinal area is two projections at right angles to one another. To evaluate the cervical spine, however, at least three views are necessary:

1. anterior-posterior lower cervical spine (C2–T2);
2. anterior-posterior open-mouth view (occiput C1–C2);
3. lateral view, which should extend from the sella turcica to the C7–T1 interspace.

A swimmer's view may be required to complement the lateral view for visualization of the lower cervical vertebrae if obscured by the increased tissue density of the shoulders.

These views give us a three-dimensional perspective of the area under study. A full examination may reveal the need for additional projections (Figs. 2.1 and 2.2; also Table 2.1.) The clinician is advised to consult a text or manual on radiographic positioning for a detailed description(8–14).

FUNCTIONAL ROENTGENOLOGY

The clinician can assess objectively the quality and quantity of intersegmental movement through stress radiography. An understanding of what constitutes normal structural anatomy and the functional limits possible within this anatomical framework

Table 2.1
Radiographic Projections of the Cervical Spine

Projection	Purpose/Area Visualized/Points of Interest
Static assessment	
Anteroposterior lower cervical spine	Visualize lower 5 cervical and upper 2 or 3 thoracic vertebrae. Visualize TVPs, interpediculate spaces, cervical ribs. Central ray may be angled 15° cephalad to better demonstrate intervertebral spacing, C2 and C3.
Anteroposterior open mouth view (see Fig. 2.1)	Structures shown to best advantage are the lateral masses and TVPs of atlas, axis including entire odontoid process, and paraatlantal joint spaces.
Base-posterior (semiaxial view of atlas) (see Fig. 2.2)	AP projection, central ray perpendicular to film. Patient's head extended so that chin and mastoid tips are perpendicular to the film. Odontoid process, shadow of foramen magnum, and atlantal ring demonstrated. This view is helpful in revealing occult fractures of the atlas and odontoid as well as rotational subluxations of atlas.
AP moving jaw (Ottonello portion)	Allows visualization of entire lower cervical spine and upper two cervical segments. Although detail may be slightly compromised, the entire cervical column may be seen. Requires rapid opened and closed movement of the jaw during the exposure.
Lateral cervical spine	Seen to advantage are the prevertebral, vertebral, and intervertebral disc structures, spinal canal, and posterior spinal elements. Shoulder depression with weights may well enhance detail of C6 and C7 segments. Periodontal structures, spacing, and segment alignment shown.
Oblique projections (PA or AP)	Demonstrates intervertebral foramen, pedicles, Luschka joints, and articular processes. Foramena are largest at the C2-3 level diminishing in size to C5–6 level.
Pillar View (vertebral arch projections)	AP projection with 20–30° caudal angulation of the tube. Head should be extended by a similar angle to eliminate mandibular projection over the lower cervical spine. The articular processes, apophysial joints, laminale, and spinous processes are well seen.
Oblique pillar views	Similar positioning to the pillar view, the head is rotated maximally to the side opposite the side of interest. Fracture or impaction of lateral articular mass may be better visualized.
Swimmer's view (pawlow or twining position).	Allows lateral visualization of lower cervical and upper thoracic vertebrae between the shadows of the upper chest and shoulders especially in patients with wide shoulders and short necks.
Dynamic Assessment*	
Flexion-extension lateral views	Rotation about the X axis evaluated (flexion = +theta × rotation; extension = −theta × rotation). Normal glide/tilt, spinous fanning, and approximation and hence functional stability are assessed.
Lateral flexion Open mouth Lower cervical spine	Rotation about the Y axis evaluated (RLF* = +theta z rotation; LLF = −theta z rotation). Synkinetic or coupled motions and functional stability assessed).
Before positioning for these views, it should be determined that severe injury is not present.	
Rotational views AP open mouth with body rotation Lower cervical rotation	Rotation about the Y axis evaluated. Coupled motion assessed to determine joint fixation or hypermobile states where there is musculoligamentous loosening.

Table 2.1 *continued*
Radiographic Projections of the Cervical Spine

Projection	Purpose/Area Visualized/Points of Interest
Flexion or extension Oblique views (Boylston views)	Functional integrity of the facets and foraminal bony elements assessed. This method makes it possible to better examine the ligamentous structures under stress, one side at a time.
Tomography	Either hypocycloidal or linear tomography eliminates overlap of vertebral structures yielding thin "slices" of areas of interest. This is an indispensable tool in evaluating the nature and extent of obscure lesions or fractures.
Fluoroscopy	An extremely valuable tool in evaluating the cervical spine. Joint dynamics and structural integrity can be easily detected by the trained observer.

*RLF, right lateral flexion; LLF, left lateral flexion.

is important. While there is no precise definition of structural and functional normality, reasonable limits based on the literature available must guide the clinician's judgment.

Motion segment behavior of one cervical vertebra relative to the subadjacent segment can be described using the right-handed, three-dimensional coordinate system(15–19). About the three axes of the coordinate system, six forces along and six moments or torques are possible. Pure or isolated movements are nearly impossible(15) due to the modifying factors of the intervertebral disc, ligaments, capsules, articulating surfaces, and the muscles guiding individual intersegmental movements. The interplay of these complex movements contributes to a more generalized influence upon the contiguous vital tissues of the nervous and circulatory systems.

The traditional physiologic patterns of

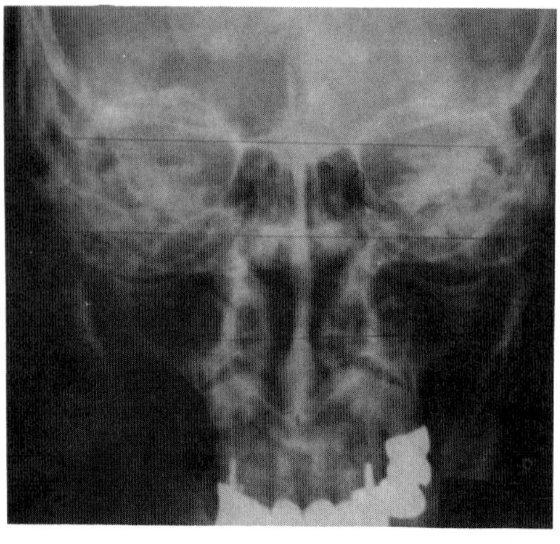

Figure 2.1. AP open-mouth view of the upper cervical spine, typically used by upper cervical practitioners.

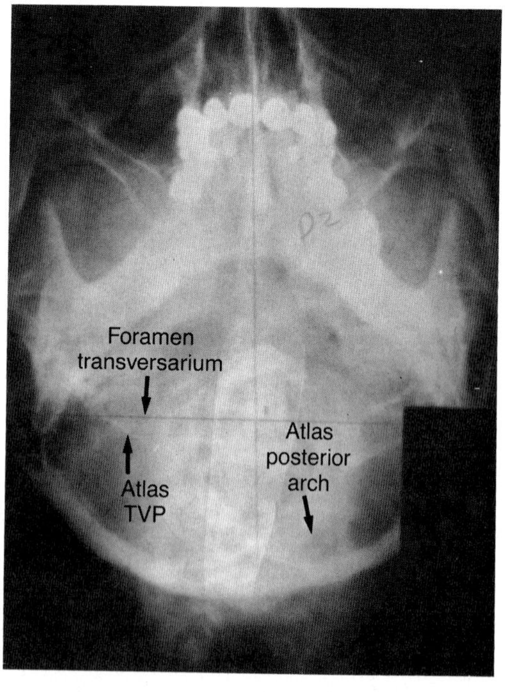

Figure 2.2. Basioposterior view of atlas, typically used by upper cervical practitioners.

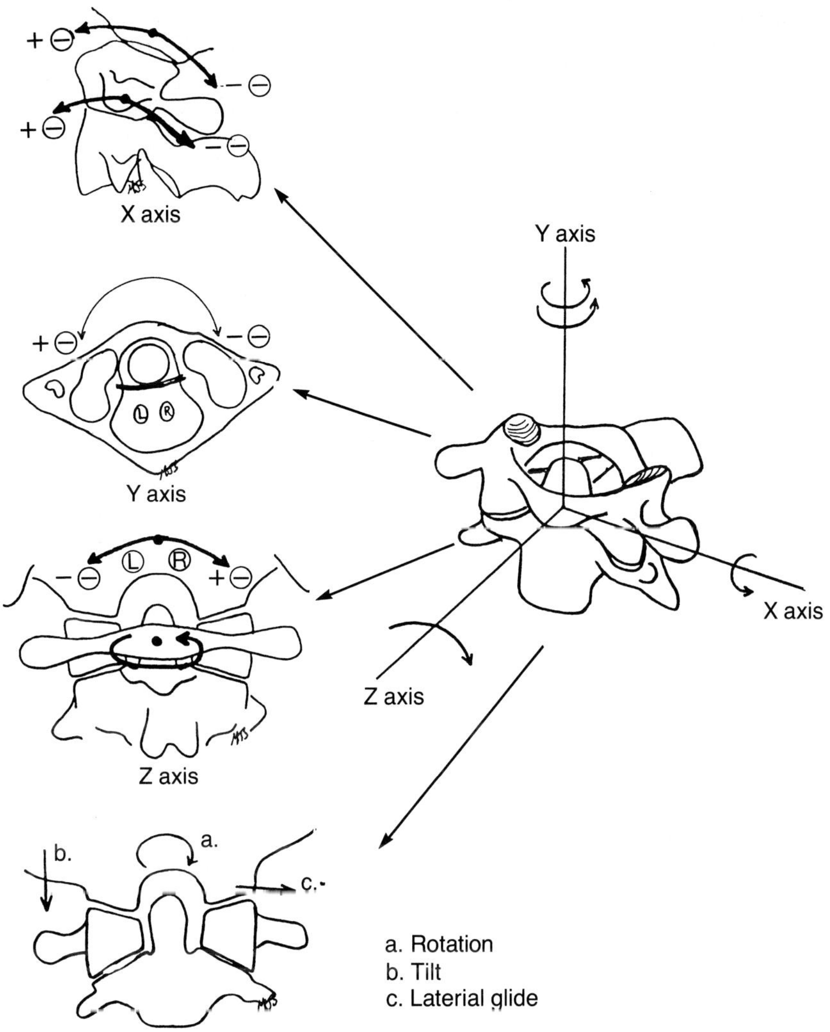

Figure 2.3. Orthogonal axes of motion in the upper cervical spine.

motion about the three axes are (see Fig. 2.3):

a) Rotation about the X axis
   i) flexion = +0 X rotation
   ii) extension = −0 X rotation
b) Rotation about the Y axis
   i) right rotation = −0 Y rotation
   ii) left rotation = +0 Y rotation
c) Rotation about the Z axis
   i) right lateral bending = +0 Z rotation
   ii) left lateral bending = −0 Z rotation

Translatory or gliding movements occur such that all parts of the vertebra at a given instant have the same direction of motion relative to a fixed point. These movements are

a) Translation along the X axis
   i) left lateral translation = +X axis
   ii) right lateral translation = −X axis
b) Translation along the Z axis
   i) anterior translation = +Z axis
   ii) posterior translation = −Z axis

One remaining movement is possible along the longitudinal axis of the spine and is described as

c) Translation along the Y axis
 i) distraction movement = +Y axis
 ii) compression movement = −Y axis

These rotational and translatory movements about and along the three axes comprise the six degrees of freedom of movement of one vertebra relative to another in all possible directions. A precise center of rotation for any given movement becomes difficult to plot especially when one realizes that coupled or synkinetic movements are more the rule than the exception(15, 16). Therefore, at any instant in time during the motion this center of movement is termed the instantaneous axis of rotation. The helical axis of motion is a three-dimensional description that superimposes rotation and translation about and along the same axis.

Radiographic functional analysis corroborates the findings of motion palpation of the vertebral motion segments. Various methods of examination of major sites of articular dysfunction can be determined(20–32). Recently, Henderson and Dormon(33) have assessed motion segment behavior of the cervical spine and a grading system was then assigned accordingly. The following charts demonstrate their findings (see Fig. 2.4 and Tables 2.2 and 2.3). The understanding of these mechanical concepts is essential in evaluating radiographs.

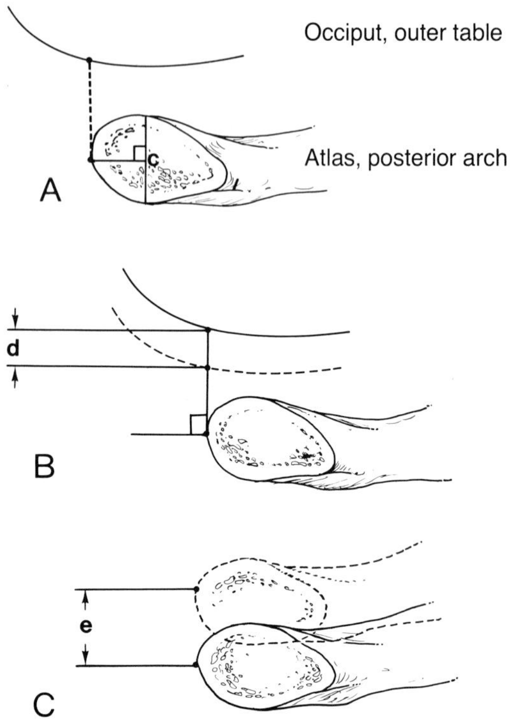

Figure 2.4. Roentgenometric analysis of occiput-C1 and C1-2 motion. (Reprinted with permission from Henderson and Dormon, J Manipulative Physiol Ther, 1985:8(4);219–227.) **A.** Determination of reference points. For atlas a point is chosen at the intersection of the cortex and a perpendicular bisector of the greatest vertial dimension of the posterior tubercle(c). **B.** Motion for occiput-C1 is expresed as absolute displacement of the reference point demonstrated in **A.** This motion value is not related to a vertebral dimension and is thus subject to magnification. **C.** Motion for C1–C2 is expressed as absolute displacement of the reference point demonstrated in **A.** This value is also subject to magnification.

TABLE 2.2
Mean and Standard Deviation Values for Intersegmental Motion from C2–3 through C6–7

	Proportion Sagittal Body Diameter Translation: Total Excursion*			
	Males		Females	
	Mean	S.D.	Mean	S.D.
C2	.33	.18	.47	.08
C3	.44	.12	.50	.11
C4	.49	.09	.55	.13
C5	.44	.13	.50	.11
C6	.31	.12	.34	.11

*Total excursion is indicated and expressed in percentage of sagittal body diameter.

Table 2.3
Mean and Standard Deviation Values for Occiput-C1 and C1–2 for Total Sagittal Plane Excursion

	Average Total Intersegment Motion—C0–C1*			
	Males		Females	
	Mean	S.D.	Mean	S.D.
C0	8.16	3.53	9.11	2.44
C1	7.97	2.75	8.93	2.68

*Values are expressed in millimeters.

Sagittal Measurement*

	Average up to Age 15		Adults	
At Level	Average	Range	Average	Range
C1	21.9 mm	18–27 mm	21.4 mm	16–30 mm
C2	20.9 mm	18–25 mm	19.2 mm	16–28 mm
C3	17.4 mm	14–21 mm	19.1 mm	14–25 mm

*FFD = 150 cm measured without enlargement factor.

ROENTGENOMETRICS

The value of roentgenometric evaluation cannot be overemphasized. Subtleties may be missed if the practitioner fails to apply basic principles. The following is a descriptive list of the most applicable and commonly used techniques of mensuration and evaluation.

Spinal Canal Diameter(34)

The sagittal diameter of the spinal canal is represented by the narrowest gap between the posterior edge of the vertebral body and the anterior edge of the vertebral arch (see Fig. 2.5).

Relative cord compression at the atlantoaxial level occurs between 15 and 17 mm in the adult. Absolute compression should be considered when distances are less than 14 mm. A general rule of thumb proposed by Steele(36) in 1968 (Fig. 2.6) considers the atlantal canal distance to be equally divided into thirds; each third is occupied by the dens, spinal cord, and free space, respectively. A proportionate loss of space equal to the diameter of the dens risks cord compression. This may occur in fracture or dislocation involving the atlas or axis. The transverse interpediculate diameter(35) is measured as: foramen magnum, 25–35 mm; C2, 25–30 mm; and C3, 20–25 mm.

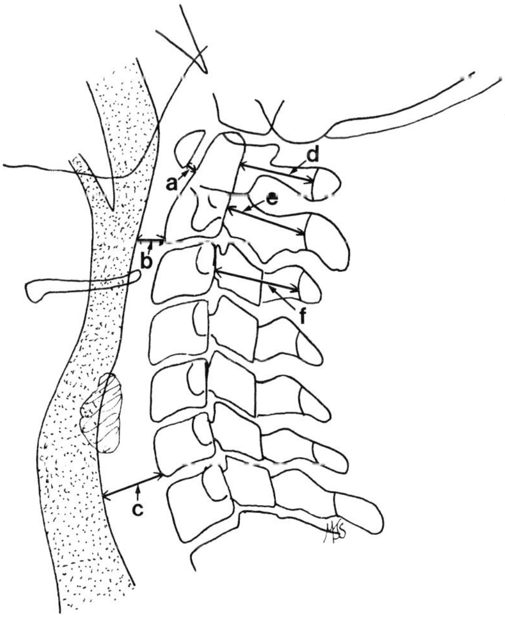

Figure 2.5. *a*, atlantodental interspace; *b*, retropharyngeal interspace; *c*, retrotracheal interspace, sagittal canal diameter; *d*, atlas; *e*, axis; *f*, C3–C7.

Condylar Angle(37)

These lines as seen on an anterior-posterior (AP) open mouth view are drawn along the axes of the atlantal condylar joints. In practice, a mean angle of 125°±10° is accepted as normal although angles greater

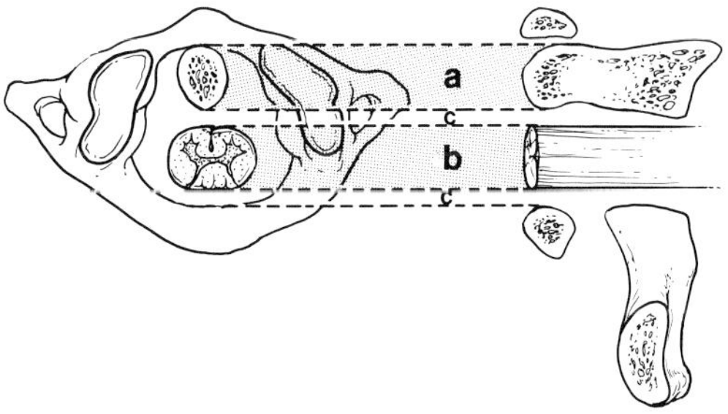

Figure 2.6. Steele's law of thirds. *a*, dens; *b*, spinal cord; *c*, space. (Adapted from Dvorak J, Dvorak V. Manual Medicine: Diagnostics. New York: Thieme-Stratton Inc, 1984:5.

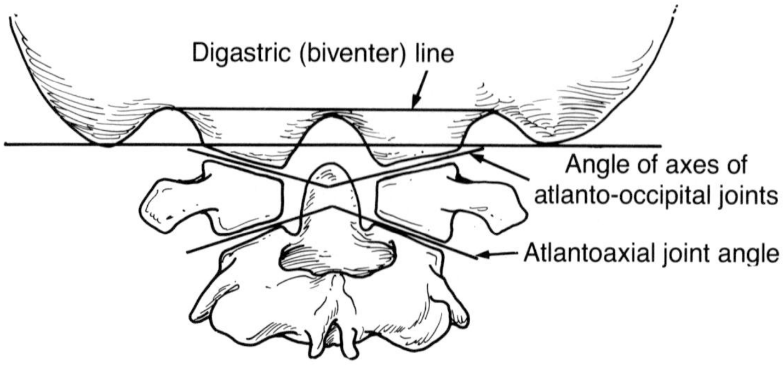

Figure 2.7. Roentgenometrics of the upper cervical spine (AP view).

than 137° represent condyle hypoplasia as described by von Torklus(38) (see Fig. 2.7).

Atlantoaxial Joint Angle (Fig. 2.7)

The planes of this joint are very nearly parallel to the contralateral condylar joint plane.

Usually the condylar angle is projected beneath the atlantoaxial angle, thus outlining a rhombus that appears to correspond to the anterior articular facet of the odontoid process (atlantodental joint).

Basilar Line(39) (Fig. 2.8)

A line drawn and extended downward along the plane of the clivus is termed the basilar line. The clivus is best depicted on tomograms. Under normal circumstances, the basilar line lies at an angle to the posterior aspect of the odontoid tip. This tangential relationship is physiological. Indeed the posterior aspect of the odontoid tip may be flattened in the direction of the basilar line(40). This tangential segment of the posterior aspect of the odontoid tip is often marked by cortical thickening, a sign of mechanical wear and tear. Significant differences of greater than 1 mm in the position of the odontoid and the basilar line viewed on extension and flexion films signify atlantodental joint hypermobility.

Basion-Odontoid Index(34) (Fig. 2.8)

On a neutral position lateral radiograph or median sagittal plane tomograph, the distance between the basion and the tip of the odontoid process is termed the Basion-Odontoid Index. Its value is about 5 mm in adults and may reach up to 10 mm in children(40). Normal values for this space are 3–6 mm. Upon flexion this value very nearly doubles during the forward sliding movement. Upon extension the value may increase but not much greater than the distance measured in a neutral position. Ligamentous damage of the occipitodental holding elements are revealed using this index.

The Atlantodental Interspace (Fig. 2.5)

The articular spacing between the posterior aspect of the anterior arch of atlas and the anterior margin of the dens is of immense clinical importance. The normal atlantodental interval distance at a 72-inch focus-to-film distance (FFD) should not exceed 2.5 mm in the adult(38, 41–43). One to 2 mm is the normal joint gap measurement depending on the articular cartilage thickness. In children larger distances are physiological. The distance is commonly 2–3 mm wide and should not exceed 5 mm as an extreme upper limit(41). In children, values above 4 mm should raise concern. (There are no statistical differences between the sexes.) The upper limit of measurement can best be seen on sagittal stress radiographs in flexion with narrowing observed on the extension film.

Widening of this interspace may be due to various arthritides(8, 44), infection, or trauma and has been recorded in up to 20% of Down's syndrome patients(45–47). Pathological rupture of the stabilizing transverse ligament encircling the posterior border of the odontoid accounts for the atlantoaxial joint dislocation seen on the neutral

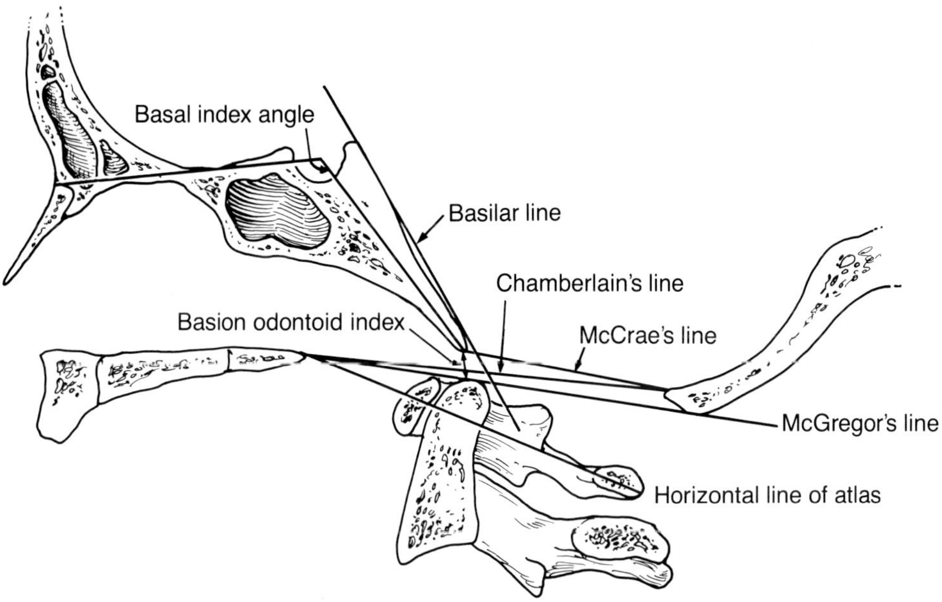

Figure 2.8. Roentgenometrics of the upper cervical spine (lateral view).

or stressed flexion radiographs. Any significant increase in the atlantodental interval will mean a reduction in the sagittal dimension of the spinal canal due to subluxation(44).

Chamberlain's Line (Fig. 2.8)

This line is drawn on a lateral skull radiograph, as an extension of the hard palate to a point represented by the opisthion (posterior margin of foramen magnum). The odontoid tip should not project more than 3.3 mm above the line(48, 49). If the odontoid protrudes further cephalad, this may indicate basilar impression.

McGregor's Line (Fig. 2.8)

This is a line drawn as an extension of the hard palate to the inferior aspect of the occipital squama. The tip of the dens should not exceed more than 4.5 mm above this line(48, 49). If the tip projects further, one should be suspicious of basilar impression or invagination.

McRae's Line (Fig. 2.8)

This line joins the anterior margin of the foramen magnum, the basion, to the posterior border of the foramen magnum. This is also called the basion-opisthion line. This is taken to represent the effective foramen magnum distance and should measure at least 19 mm at a FFD of 72 inches on the lateral cervical radiograph(38, 40). A value greater than this may indicate a possible congenital malformation such as the Arnold-Chiari malformation.

Atlantopalatine Angle (Method of Bull, 1955) (Fig. 2.8)

This angle is measured between Chamberlain's line and the horizontal line of atlas. Historically reported, the angle was not to exceed more than 13°. If the angle were greater than 13°, it would suggest an abnormal position of atlas relative to the skull. The angle was originally measured in patients in the prone position(49). More recently, Wackenheim(40) has determined normal values up to 30°. Angles greater than 30° are said to represent pathology.

Biventer Line (Bidigastric) (Fig. 2.7)

This is a line drawn on a 40-inch FFD AP upper cervical film joining the two digastric grooves (inscisura mastoidea) that lie just medial to the bases of the mastoid processes. The perpendicular measurement to the midpoint of the atlantooccipital joint from the digastric line should be within 3.8–20.5 mm (11.6 mm mean). Measured to the apex of the dens, a normal distance of between 1 and 20.4 mm is considered normal (10.7 mm mean)(40). Measurements are decreased in basilar impression.

Martin's Basilar Angle

On a true lateral skull film a line drawn from the nasion to the center of the sella turcica intersects a line from the basion to the center of the sella producing an angle of less than 140°. Angles exceeding 150° suggest the presence of basilar impression and angles less than 132° indicate basilar kyphosis(35).

Basilar Invagination

The foregoing lines and angles of Chamberlain, McGregor, and Martin are helpful in determining whether there has been vertical translocation of the upper cervical complex, or cranial settling, as found in basilar invagination and other bone-softening diseases.

In 1984 Redlund-Johnell and Pettersson(49) used a modified method to detect whether vertical dislocation of C1 and C2 was present. Since arthritic erosion, dyspastic changes and overprojection may obscure the apex of the dens and other osseous landmarks, this new method of measurement was introduced. The Redlund-Johnell (Fig 2.8) method uses a line extended cephalad to McGregor's line from end plate of C2. A distance between the lower end plate of C2 and McGregor's line of less than 34 mm in men and 29 mm in women has been proposed to define vertical dislocation of the upper cervical complex.

Atlantooccipital Hypermobility

Wiesel et al (1979)(50, 51) determined the normal odontoid-basion distance as 4–5 mm. Wackenheim(40) described a normal distance of 3–6 mm. Changes in this determined anatomic relationship are significant. Since atlantooccipital motion is essentially confined to flexion and extension, any horizontal translation of more than 1 mm in the relative positions of either flexion or extension compared to the neutral denotes hypermobility or instability. In the lateral cervical radiographs of flexion and extension, three landmarks are drawn:

1. The central and most dorsal aspect of the posterior arch of atlas;
2. The center of the anterior arch of C1; joining these two lines yields the horizontal line of atlas. The perpendicular line is then raised superiorly at the posterior edge of the anterior arch of atlas.
3. Point three represents the caudal tip of the clivus, the basion, which is found by following the clivus from the sella turcia to the base of the skull.

The shortest distance from the perpendicular tip of the basion (point 3) to the perpendicular line raised from the horizontal line of atlas is measured in flexion and extension. The normal range of horizontal translation at the occipital-atlantal articulation in flexion and extension is no more than 1 mm(50). Movement greater than 1 mm is clinically significant and suggests radiographic instability. Excessive motion may cause mechanical irritation to the brainstem or upper cord. This has been demonstrated in patients with high cervical segment fusion or congenital block fusion as in the Klippel-Feil syndrome. This method of detection for occipital-atlantal hypermobility can be effectively applied in cases of trauma or congenital or acquired fixation leading to mechanical instability.

Retropharyngeal Space

This represents the width of the prevertebral soft tissue shadow. This is measured from the lower edge of the anterior border of axis to the posterior edge of the pharyngeal gas shadow. In both children and adults the average distance is 3.5 mm with a range of 1–7 mm(35). This distance should not exceed 7 mm or roughly one-third of the midsagittal distance of the C2 body (Fig. 5). Widening of this space may be found in oropharyngeal infections (Grisel's syndrome), tuberculous cold abscess, osteomyelitis, tumors, traumatic hematoma, or edema.

Retrotracheal Space

The space may be widened as part of a linear fascial spread resulting from edematous or hemorrhagic extension. This distance is measured from the anterior aspect of C6 to the posterior margin of the tracheal gas shadow. The average measurement is 7–9 mm in children (range, 5–14 mm) and 14 mm in the adult (range, 9–22 mm)(35) (Fig. 2.5). This spacing, therefore, should not exceed 14 mm or 22 mm in the child or adult, respectively; i.e., the spacing should not appreciably exceed the midsagittal diameter or the C6 vertebra.

Once these lines, angles, and methods are understood and practiced, imaginary construction should suffice. Actual line drawings are necessary if abnormalities are suspected.

Congenital Abnormalities of the Upper Cervical Spine

Os Odontoideum (Fig. 2.9). Historically, the os odontoideum was first described in 1886 by Giacomeni(52, 53). Greenfield in 1953(54) recorded two such cases in which quadriplegia occurred following flexion of the head. In 1969 Michaels(55) noted this anomaly as a congenital failure of fusion between ossification centers. Recently Fielding et al(56) and Freiberger et al(57) have suggested a traumatic origin, after reviewing serial radiographs in patients who had normal atlantoaxial structures at the time of injury and later demonstrated evidence of os odontoideum. The latter authors concluded that nonunion at the fracture site was initially unrecognized and that a compromised blood supply prevented revascularization of the odontoid process. Schiff and Parke(58) described the consequent bone resorption that occurs and considered this sequela as an acquired os odontoideum.

Another contemporary theory proposes the etiology of an os odontoideum to be persistence of a transverse plane of mesenchymal tissue at the base of the odontoid that fails to undergo chondrification(52). Persistent biomechanical forces acting upon this mesenchymal persistency may result in separation of the dens from the body of axis. The radiological features of the os odontoideum are(59, 60)

i) persistence of a small round corticated ossicle of variable size separated from the base of the dens by a lucent cleft of varying width.
ii) The os may be orthotopic (undisplaced) or dystopic lying near the basion; at this site it may be separated or fused to the basion.
iii) The lucent gap of mesenchymal tissue between the portions of the odontoid lie above the plane of the superior articular processes of axis.
iv) The base of the odontoid may project upward with a peg-like appearance (cupola-shaped, cranial bulge); this represents a hypoplastic dens.
v) There is likely to be overdevelopment or compensatory cortical hypertrophy of the anterior arch of atlas with attenuation of the posterior arch of atlas (there may be nonunion). This constitutes evidence of an associated congenital bone anomaly and not recent trauma.
vi) Atlantoaxial dislocation seen on functional lateral stress radiographs; the os remains fixed to the anterior arch of atlas by the transverse ligament allowing translatory movement. Articular stability can be determined using tomography and/or functional studies in the sagittal plane. The forward slippage of C1 on C2 often seen on a flexion radiograph is presumptive evidence of spinal cord entrapment. Instability, especially associated with progressive neurological symptoms, requires immediate prophylactic surgical consideration.

Os Terminale (Bergmann) (Fig. 2.10). A much less common anomaly is the fusion failure of the apical secondary center of the dens (proatlas). Normally, prior to the 12th year the ossiculum terminale fuses with the body of the dens(38). Clinical symptoms arising from instability are infrequent.

Dysplasia of the Dens (Fig. 2.11). Disorders of segmentation and ossification can

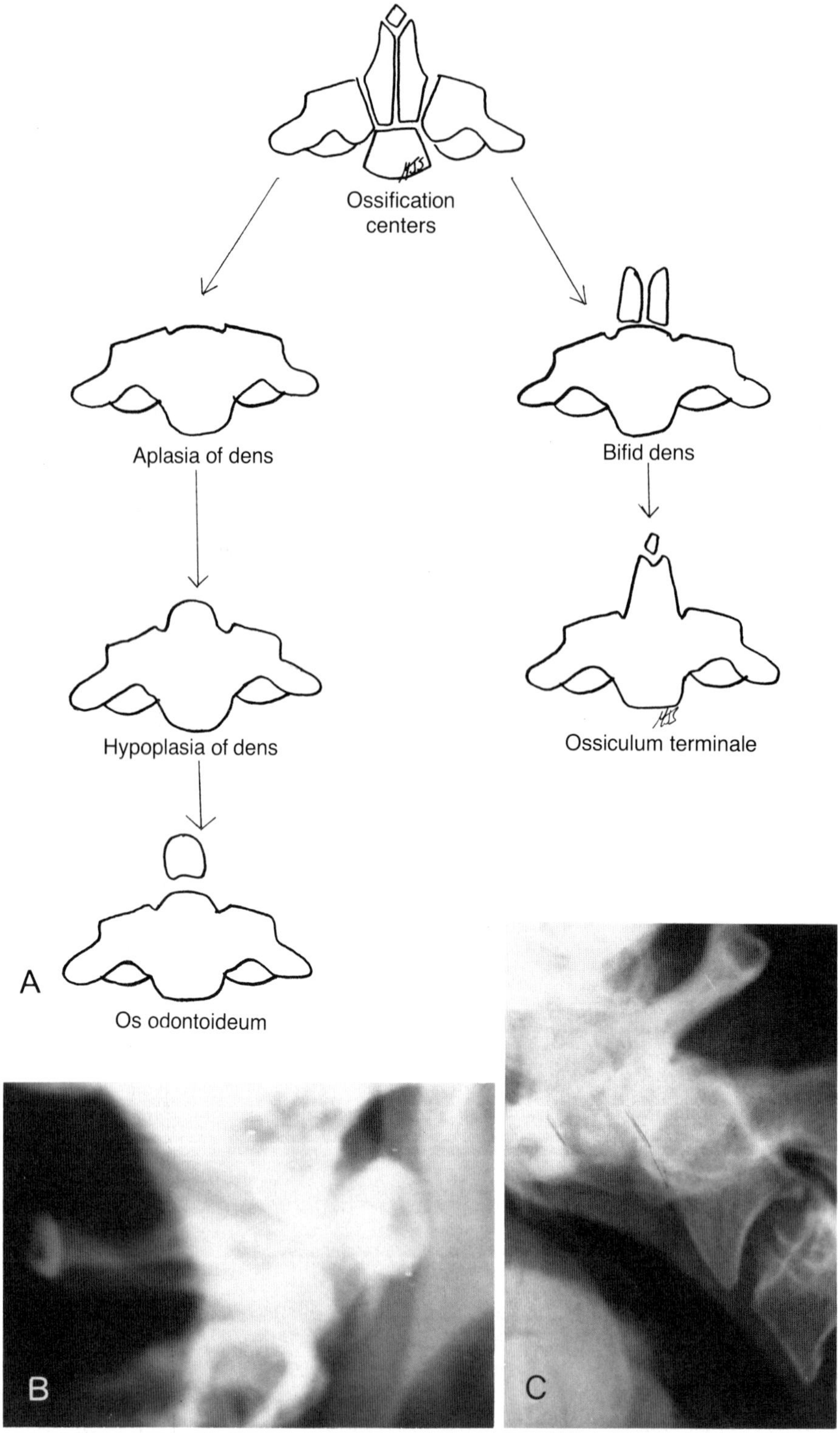

Figure 2.9. A. Development of axis and possible consequent anomalies. **B.** Os odontoideum. **C.** Increased atlantodental interval demonstrating instability.

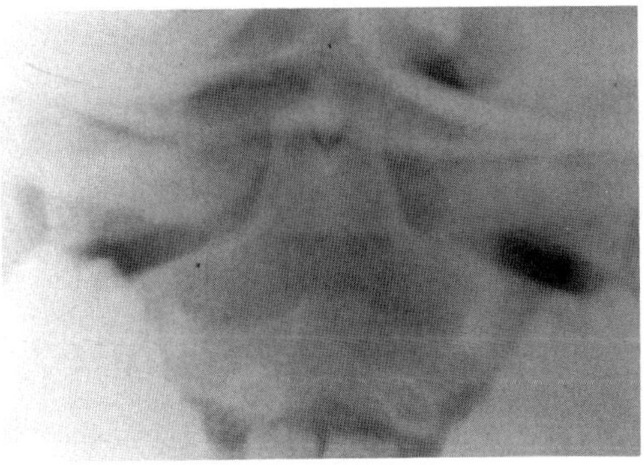

Figure 2.10. Ossiculum terminale.

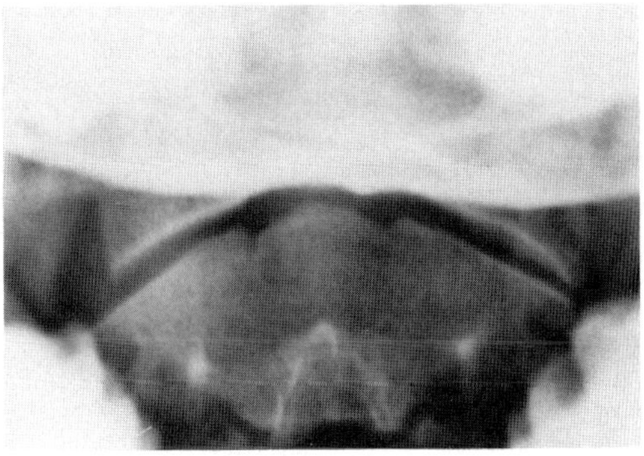

Figure 2.11. Aplastic dens.

lead to varied anomalies. For example, a bipartite (double tipped) dens termed dens bicornis may result from a fusion failure(38). This appearance may be simulated by the projection of the upper incisors over the dens (Mach effect).

Malformation or hypoplasia of the dens may demonstrate various subtle configurations. If this is combined with primary defects in the holding elements, instability may result.

Posterior and Lateral Ponticle of Atlas (Fig. 2.12). The ponticulus posticus, also called pons posticus, refers to a bony bridge of the posterior atlantooccipital membrane overlying the atlantosulcus for the vertebral artery. Arising from the lateral masses it forms a bony conduit, the foramen arcuale, allowing passage for the vertebral artery, the posterior recurrent autonomic chain, the suboccipital nerve, and venus plexus. Also called Kimmerle's variant, it is seen in about 10–12% of the roentgen examinations(61), either as a complete or incomplete bony ring. It represents an incidental finding of little clinical significance.

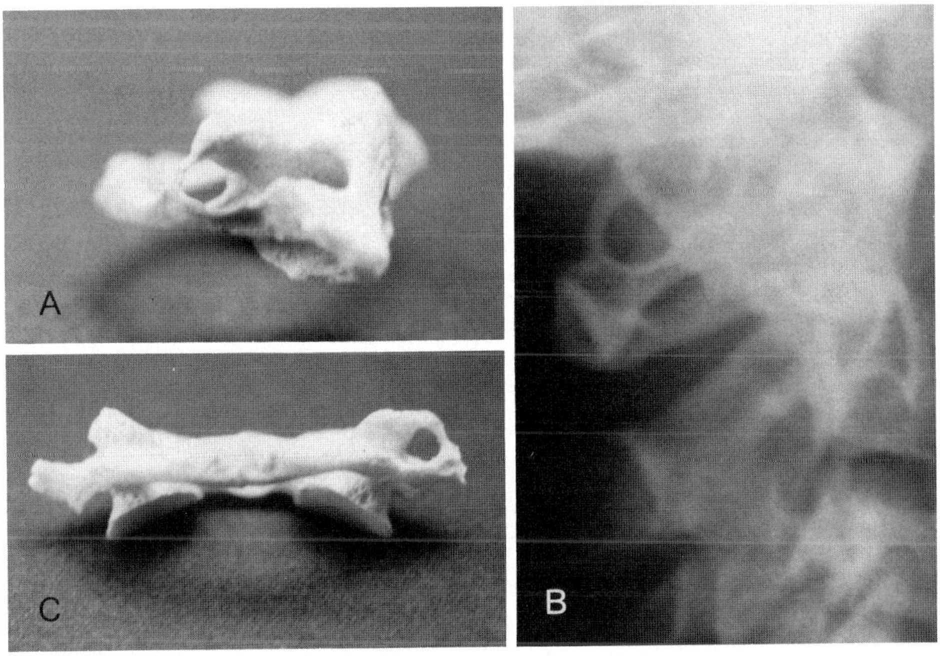

Figure 2.12. **A.** Posterior ponticle of atlas (dry specimen). **B.** Posterior ponticle of atlas (radiograph). **C.** Lateral ponticle of atlas (dry specimen).

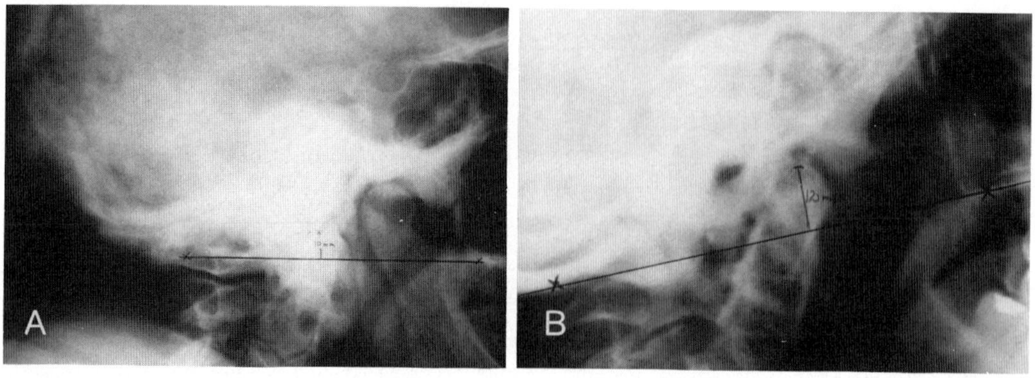

Figure 2.13. **A.** Basilar impression (Paget's disease). (Photo courtesy of Dr. James Grilliot.) **B.** Basilar invagination.

The lateral ponticle or pons lateralis may be seen with lesser frequency, about 3% of cases(38), forming a bony bridge between the lateral mass and transverse process of atlas. Running obliquely, it is not well seen and rarely represents a complete bony ring.

Basilar Impression (Fig. 2.13, a and b). A diversity of features best described as occipital-cervical dysplasia is generally termed basilar impression(40, 61). Clinically, basilar impression refers to the caudal indentation of the base of the skull due to primary congenital causes or secondarily acquired bone-softening diseases. Seen rarely, this occurs in Paget's disease, osteomalacia, achondroplasia, and osteoporosis. Similar changes may be seen in destructive bone diseases such as tuberculosis or rheumatic spondylitis. The term invagination has also been used to describe the inward projection of the upper cervical elements into the skull around the foramen magnum.

Platybasia refers to flattening of the base of the skull. This is considered anterior basilar invagination as a result of hypoplasia of the basiocciput(61). The clivus takes on a more horizontal slope with shortening and thinning of the basiocciput. This produces an elevation of the plane of the foramen magnum. The vasilar angle of Welcker or Martin is increased to greater than 150°.

Paramedian basilar impression is caused by a unilateral or bilateral median rise or thinning of the exoccipital bones(38). As a result there may be atlantooccipital fusion, flattening of the occiput, foramen magnum stenosis or distortion, and upward translocation of the odontoid process.

The clinical importance of these cervicobasilar changes is in their effect on the neurocranium and cervical cord. Signs and symptoms may simulate tumors of the posterior cranial fossa, demyelinating diseases, or syringomyelia. Pressure may be exerted upon the cerebellum causing herniation as may be seen in the Arnold-Chiari syndrome. If there is any suspicion of basilar impression, a neurologic evaluation is necessary in addition to further diagnostic imaging.

Radiographic diagnosis is based on the alternation of the craniometric relationships. These lines and angles of importance have been discussed under Roentgenometrics. Suspicion of basilar invagination should also be considered in those cases where osseous structures normally seen on the AP open-mouth view cannot be clearly demonstrated.

Condylar Hypoplasia. With flattening of the occipital condyles, a raised portion of the atlas and axis is present, which may or may not be associated with the paramedian type of basilar impression. The angle of the axes of the atlantooccipital joints' average is 125°. Angles greater than 137° are seen in condylar hypoplasia(38). The intersection of the joint axes commonly lies over the dens. In condylar assymetry this junctional intersection lies lateral to the dens. Clinically, there may be skeletal torticollis and atlantooccipital hypomobility. Medial prominence of the condyles may laterally narrow the foramen magnum.

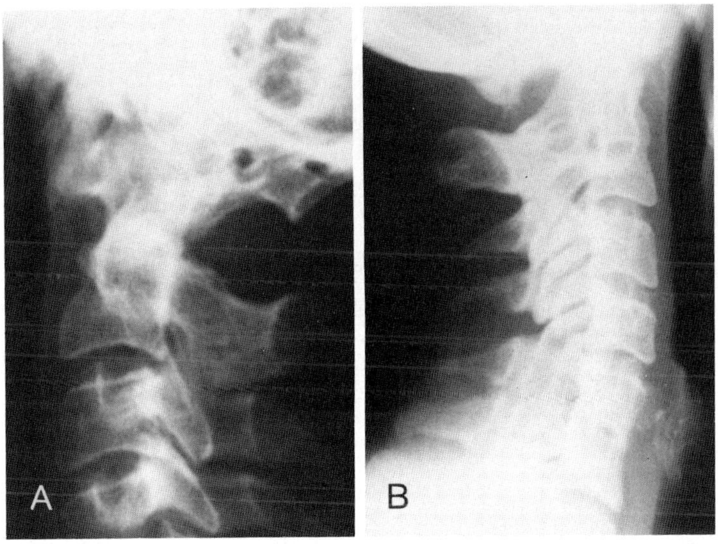

Figure 2.14. **A.** Occipitalization. **B.** Occipitalization with multiple block vertebrae.

Atlantal Assimilation (Occipitalization) (Fig. 2.14). Varying degrees of bony fusion between the atlas and occiput occur infrequently. In the majority of cases it is seen with other malformations such as basilar invagination, multiple block vertebrae, and spinal dysrhaphism(38, 52). The degree of assimilation cannot be accurately determined with the use of conventional radiography. Tomographic investigation is often necessary to determine the true extent of atlantal assimilation. With the loss of joint movement at the craniocervical joints, progressive stress may be placed upon the atlantodental joint leading to subluxation and instability(62).

Atlantal Arch Malformation (Fig. 2.15). A very rare occurence is aplasia(38) or complete absence of the posterior arch of atlas. An isolated paramedian remnant may be the only visible trace of bone in the area of the posterior tubercle. So long as the joint integrity remains, instability is not a feature.

Hemiaplasia, in which there is absence of one-half of the arch, is more common. Variation of hypoplasia of the arch may be associated with compensatory hypertrophy of the dens or os odontoideum.

Anterior arch developmental errors that include aplasia or hypoplasia are exceedingly rare. If discovered, considerable instability would result. Apparent hypoplasia may be associated with atlantodental or atlantoaxial synostosis. Hyperplasia of the anterior arch should lead to a suspicion of developmental anomalies in the area, or longstanding stress due to adjacent instability.

Posterior clefting of the arch is predominantly medial, with lateral clefting posterior to the lateral masses very uncommon. Geipel(63) finds that posterior clefting is present to some degree in 3% of the population. If the posterior tubercle is absent, the ends are bulbous and lack the spinolaminar demarcation as viewed on the lateral radiograph. Lateral clefting, if seen at all, may be visualized if the head is laterally tipped a few degrees bringing the posterior atlantal ring into better visual projection (Fig. 2.16).

Atlantal clefting may suggest dysrhaphism of the cord and meninges. As the atlas does not have a spinous process the term spina bifida is not used.

Atlantoaxial Fusion and Irregular Segmentation (Fig. 2.17). Except in complete fusion in cases of Klippel-Feil syndrome, atlantoaxial fusion is rare. Atlantodental fusion may be associated with hypoplasia of the anterior arch of atlas.

Segmentation irregularities may be associated with atlantal assimilation. Uneven joint displacements may be seen on the AP openmouth view in which the joints on one side are remarkably higher or lower than the other side(38). Odontal dysplasia may

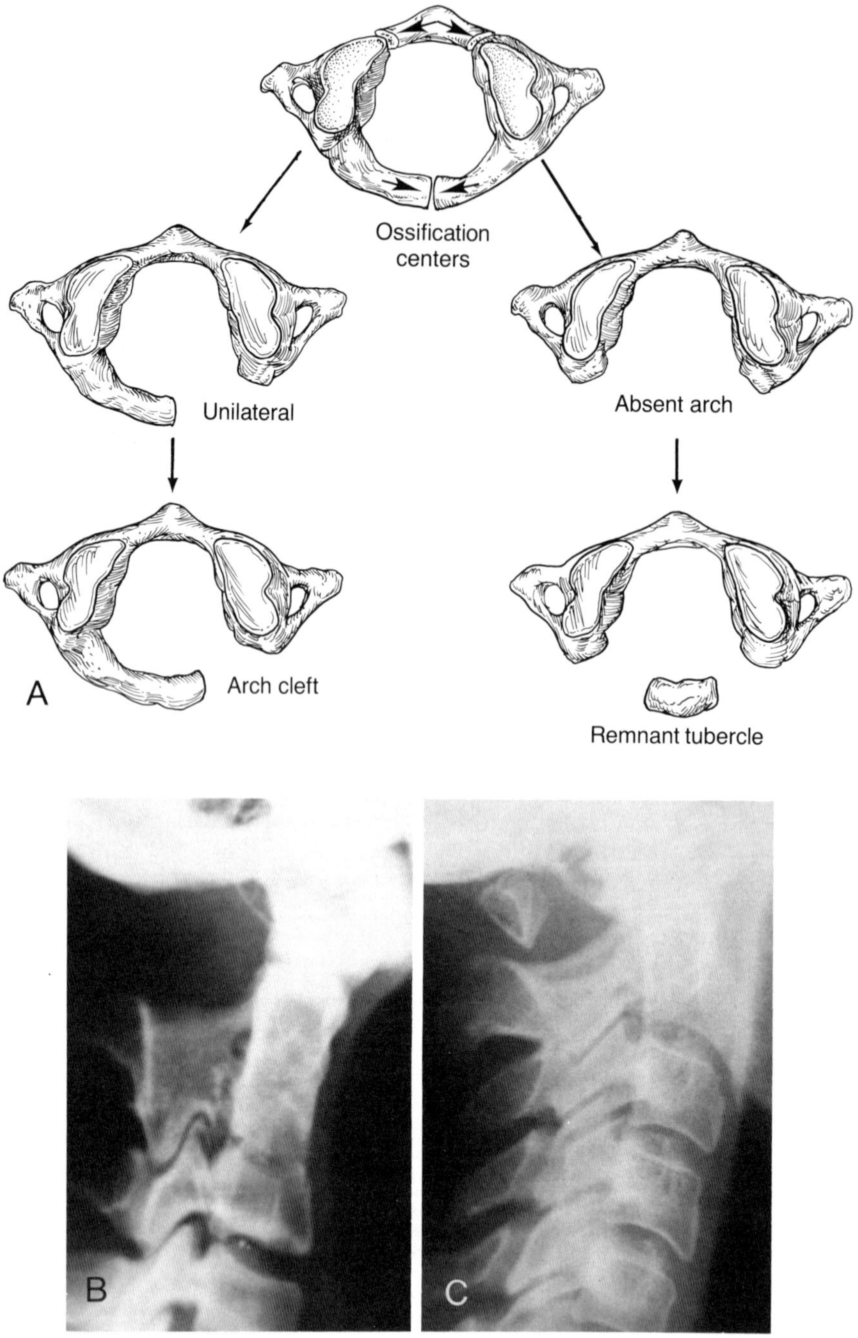

Figure 2.15. **A.** Atlas development and possible consequent anomalies. **B.** Aplasia of atlantal arch. **C.** Remnant tubercle of atlas arch. **D.** Incomplete arch of atlas (AP open-mouth view). **E.** Incomplete arch of atlas (lateral view). **F.** Nonunion of posterior arch of atlas.

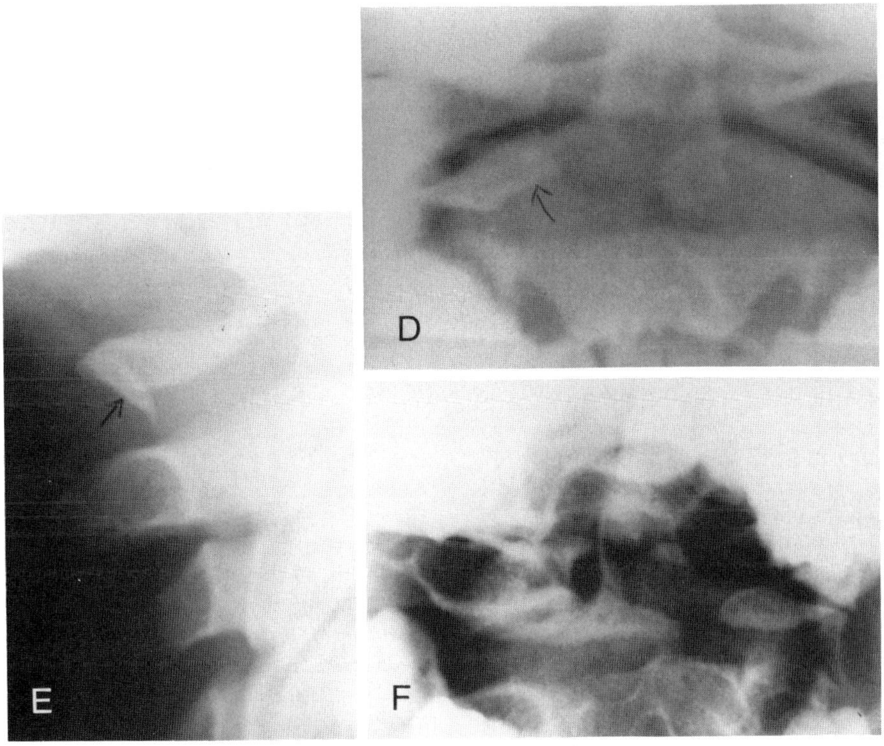

Figure 2.15. D–F

be seen in combination with irregular segmentation.

Spina Bifida of Axis. A split in the spinous process of axis is eight times less common than clefting of the atlas. A fibrous bridge covers the fissure and such anomalies do not impose any mechanical problems.

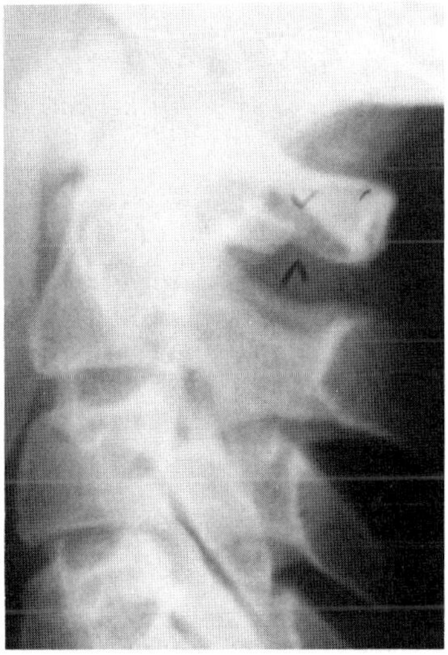

Figure 2.16. Lateral clefting, arch of atlas.

Congenital Block of C2–3 (Fig. 2.18). The most frequent site of congenital cervical fusion occurs at the C2–3 level(64). Due to early embryonic errors of somatic division, these segmental defects may involve the bodies, arches, posterior joints, and spinous processes. Typical of congenital fusion is the wasp-waist appearance in which there is constriction in the anterior and posterior diameter between the vertebrae. There is a smooth contour of the cortex on the anterior surface of the intersegmental rudimentary disc. Often the intervertebral foramina at the fusion site is smaller than normal(65). The Klippel-Feil syndrome usually is represented by complete intervertebral fusion of the C2–3 segment as part of its multiple block vertebrae appearance. Concern should be directed to the suprajacent hypermobility of the atlantodental joint. With advancing age, degenerative limitation of joint function elsewhere may further compromise the adjacent articulations.

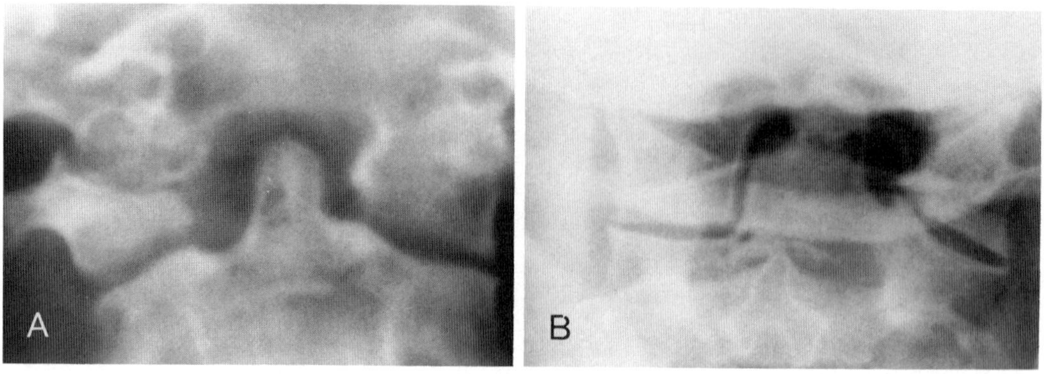

Figure 2.17. Segmentation defect or dysplasia.

Notochord Persistency Defects. Disturbance or regression of the chorda dorsalis (notochord) is visualized as dents in the inferior marginal endplates along its posterior half. These invaginated appearances are far more common elsewhere in the spine, particularly the lumbar area, but rarely occur at axis. They have little if any clinical significance.

Persistent Hypochordal Bow of Proatlas. Although extremely rare, signs of the persistency of the hypochordal bow of proatlas located extracranially are visualized at the anterior central margin of the foramen magnum(38). Various bony prominences may be seen anterior to the basion on lateral radiographs. This can vary from a basilar process, prebasioccipital arch, to a basilar accessory third condyle. This third condyle may form a pseudo joint with the dens, anterior arch of atlas or contribute to a joint interspace in dystopic os odontoideum. Occipital cervical joint restriction as well as positional anomalies of atlas are likely results. Tomography clarifies the suspected features of this anomaly.

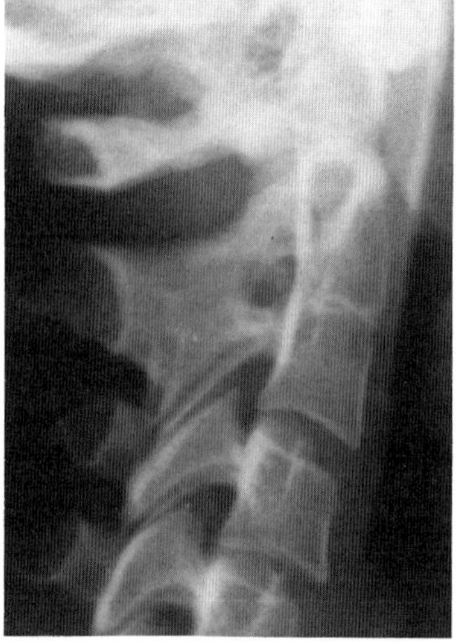

Figure 2.18. Block vertebrae C2–C3.

Paracondylitic and Epitransverse Processes (Fig. 2.19a). Between the lateral part of the occipital bone adjacent to the occipital condyle and the transverse process of atlas prominences or processes may be seen. The paracondylitic process is often plump and broad based, extending downward from the occiput in contrast to the more slender cephalic stalk or hook-like process arising from the atlantal transverse process. In some cases a true or false joint may be evident on the AP open-mouth view(38, 40). Unilateral fusion between the occiput and transverse process of atlas is also a possible variation. The result may be skeletal torticollis, modified joint function, and atlantal malalignment. Obliquity of atlas due to a tripod mechanism may result in scoliotic compensation of the cervico thoracic spine in an effort to level the head. These malformations should not be mistaken for a calcified styloid process seen to project anterior to the transverse process of atlas on the lateral view (Eagle syndrome) (Fig. 2.19b).

Dysostosis, Dysplasia Syndromes, and the Genetic Diseases

There are various diseases which affect the upper cervical complex. Only a few will be

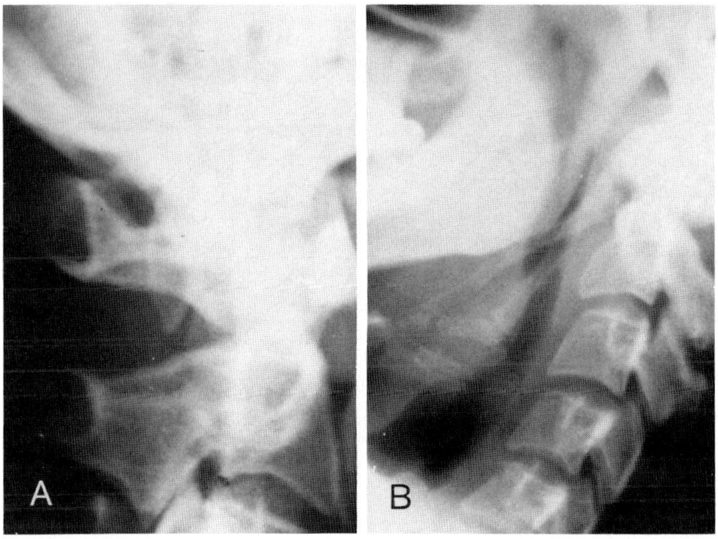

Figure 2.19. **A.** Paramastoid process. **B.** Calcified stylohoid ligaments (Eagle syndrome).

mentioned. Spondyloepiphyseal dysostosis (Morquio Brailsford) has been described in combination with odontal and posterior arch hypoplasia and basilar impression. Dislocation of atlas occurs in a significant percentage of Down's syndrome. The mucopolysaccharide disorders may also exhibit atlantoaxial instability and odontoid hypoplasia. The Arnold-Chiari malformation may demonstrate bony abnormalities of the occiput or cervical spine as well as osseous defects and myeloceles(66). Platybasia of the skull and neural arch defects of the spine may be seen in cleidocranial dysostosis.

Arthritides and Other Joint Disease

Rheumatoid arthritis is a generalized disease of the connective tissues (see Table 2.4). Spinal involvement is usually restricted to the sacroiliac joints and the cervical area. The basic pathological lesion is the same regardless of the site with the joint synovium being the target tissue of preference. Histological changes in the synovial joint can exist long before radiological evidence of joint erosion can be found. The dens and transverse ligament is surrounded by synovium and can therefore be a primary target of importance. With synovitis, juxtaarticular inflammation, distension, and stretching as well as erosion of the ligament and bone proceed leading to subluxation. The subluxation is the result of instability secondary to joint destruction and ligamentous laxity(67). Aside from mechanical reasons, the anterior atlantoaxial subluxation (AAS) characteristic of the

Table 2.4
Radiological Evidence Suggestive of Arthritic Involvement in the Upper Cervical Spine[a]

Atlantodental interspace widening with resultant canal stenosis in its sagittal width
Interruption of the posterior spinolaminar line
Increase in the retropharyngeal space
Flexion malposition of atlas upon axis greater than 10° and flexion instability upon flexion-extension views
Vertical translocation of atlas and odontoid of axis
Pseudo basilar invagination demonstrated by craniovertebral roentgenometrics
Erosive "whittling" or "frosting" of the odontoid process
Subchondral marginal sclerosis of joint surface and bony demineralization
Joint space narrowing with marginal articular irregularities
Apophyseal ankylosis (late)

[a]Adapted from Yochum TR, Rowe LJ. Arthritides of the upper cervical complex. In: Idczak RM. Aspects of Manipulative Therapy. Victoria. Lincoln Institute of Health Sciences. 1980:22–32.

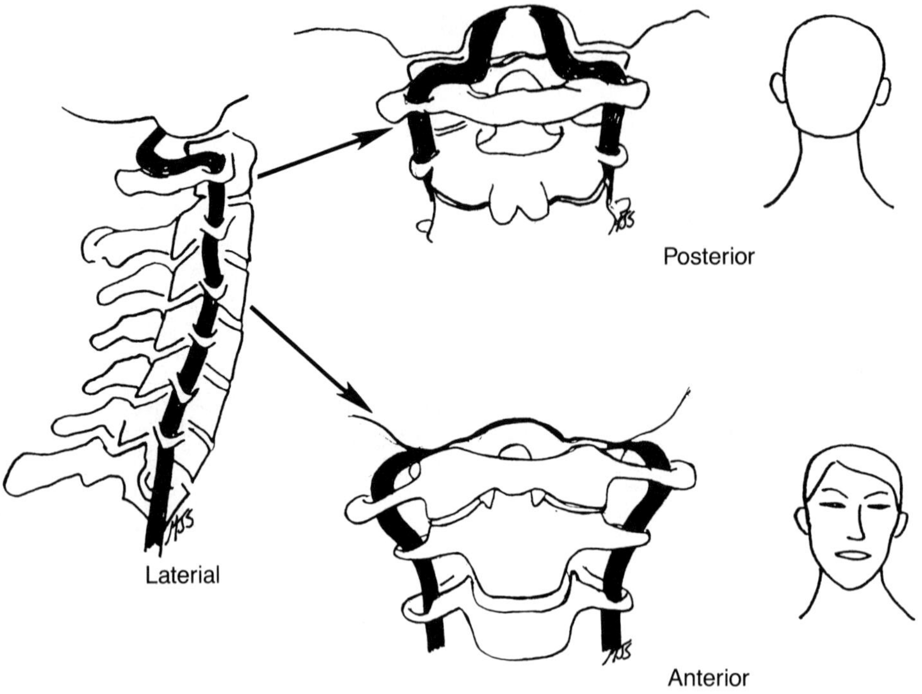

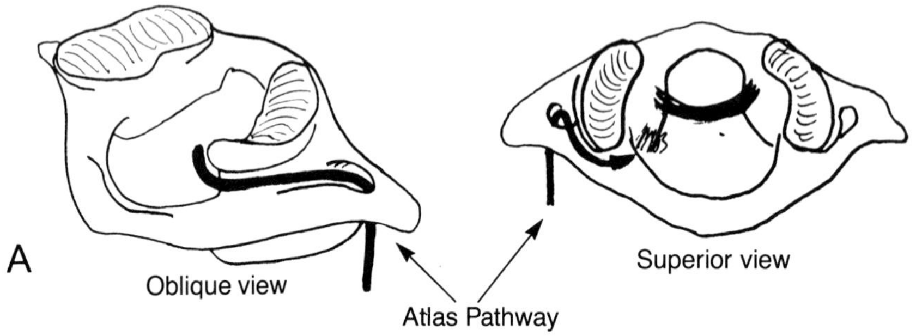

Figure 2.20. A. Orientation of the vertebral artery in the upper cervical spine. **B.** Effect of various head/neck positions on the vertebral artery (overleaf).

rheumatoid neck may be an adaptive change to increase the sagittal canal diameter as the pannus tissue accumulates. Cord lesions are secondary to ischemic compression by the resultant decrease in the canal diameter from rheumatic tissue or bony impingement. Emerging nerve roots may be involved in an entrapment neuropathy in the intervertebral tunnel, the compressive tissue being disc material (at the C2–3 level), dural, or perivascular adhesions. The clinical picture does not necessarily equate with the radiological changes.

Forward subluxation of the atlas upon the axis occurs following disease of the atlantoaxial joints. The transverse ligament may be destroyed and the dens may be eroded. An atlantodental interspace (ADI) measurement exceeding 3–4 mm is diagnostic of atlantoaxial subluxation(68–70). Commonly, AAS occurs in flexion and reduces in extension, however, the distance may persist due to granulation tissue within the ADI. With progressive atlantoaxial joint erosion, the odontoid may translocate vertically into the foramen magnum producing

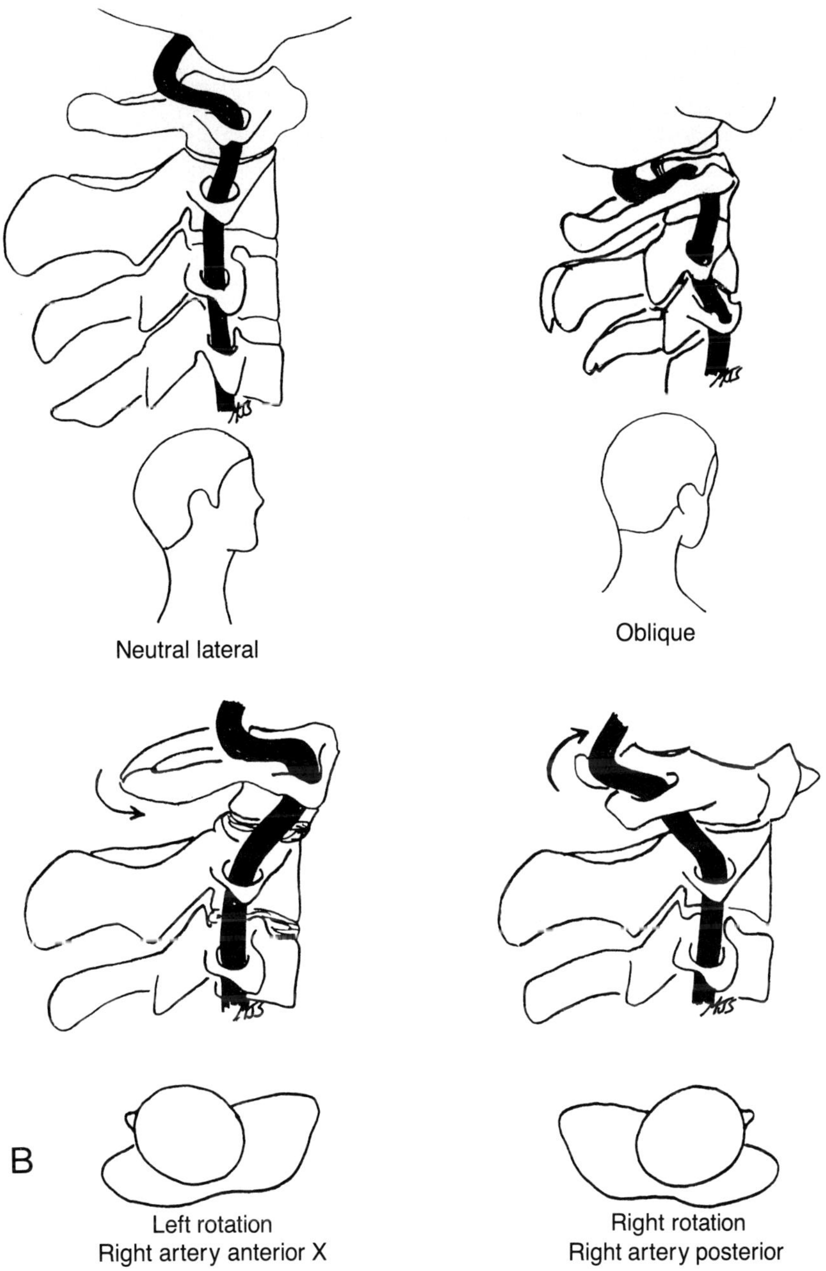

Figure 2.20B

pseudo basilar invagination. Roentgenometric lines denoting basilar invagination would be breached. Following odontal translocation, the atlas beds down between the body axis and the occiput as adjacent joints are narrowed and eroded by mechanical and inflammatory forces(48).

The anterior atlantoaxial subluxation can have potentially devastating consequences on not only the cord, but both vertebral and internal carotid arteries. The combination of the AAS with extension-rotation may result in serious vascular injuries. The vertebral artery in its complex sojourn in the upper cervical spine (Fig. 2.20, A and B) is subject to shearing forces at the intertransverse foramena at the C2 and C1 levels as well as the foramen magnum(71, 72). Vertical translocation of the dens can cause additional compromise. The internal carotid artery may be impinged upon by the lateral masses of atlas upon rotation of the head to the opposite side. Recognition of these developments is essential. Referral for surgical consideration may be life saving whereas manipulation may be disastrous.

Juvenile rheumatoid arthritis or Still's disease involving the upper cervical spine is similar to the adult form. The only subtle difference is the tendency to develop complete joint ankylosis as a late manifestation of the disease. Growth disturbances during the disease may cause a widening of the odontoid process and a hypoplastic appearance to the vertebral bodies(69).

Other arthritides that may produce changes similar to rheumatoid arthritis (RA) in the upper cervical spine include Reiter's disease, systemic lupus erythematosis, and lipoid dermoarthritis. Psoriatic involvement of the upper cervical complex, although rare, may follow a similar pattern to RA. Apophyseal joint ankylosis appears to be more likely. Radiographic appraisal of the sacroiliac joints is helpful in the diagnosis of rheumatoid-related diseases. A chronic inflammatory disease which characteristically involves the sacroiliac joints and ascends the spine in a skip-like fashion is ankylosing spondylitis. The incidence of upper cervical involvement varies between 2 and 15% depending on studies(69) and is not unlike the characteristic rheumatoid description. With intervertebral ankylosis, mechanical involvement may be direct or compensatory leading to stress at the atlantodental joint with subluxation. Trivial trauma may cause fractures at or near the fusion sites.

Remarkably, degenerative joint disease rarely involves the craniocervical area probably because of the relative persistence of mobility occurring in this region(73, 74). The absence of a disc at this level precludes the development of changes typical of spondylosis. Hypertrophic spondylotic changes in the lower cervical spine lead to progressive joint fixation. Compensatory hypermobility redistributed to more cephalic motion segments may result in relative increase in strain at the more mobile upper cervical joints. Additional trauma may further cause joint laxity and eventual increase in the atlantodental interspace. The usual uncomplicated course with aging produces narrowing of the ADI due to progressive thinning of the anterior cartilage. Marginal osteophytic formation at the atlantoaxial joints is proof of arthritic changes.

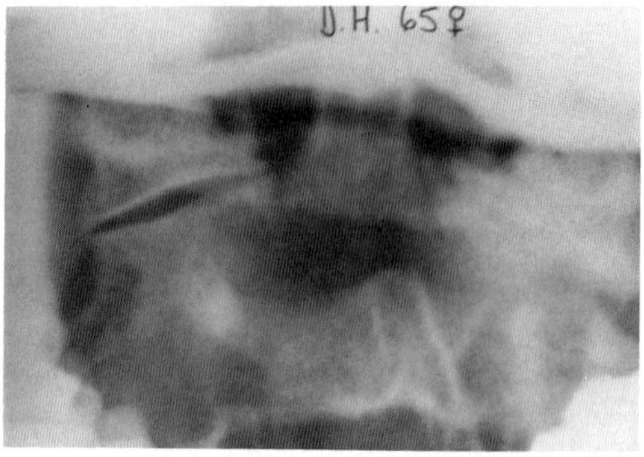

Figure 2.21. Unilateral atlantoaxial joint degenerative disease.

Arthrosis of the atlantodental joint is as common as in the lower intervertebral joints, while it is rarely seen at the atlantooccipital and lateral atlantoaxial joints (Fig. 2.21). The upper pole of the anterior arch of atlas is a common site for atlantodental arthrosis(38).

Spondylosis at the C2–3 level is rarely encountered in the absence of major degenerative changes lower in the cervical spine (Fig. 2.22). Spondylosis isolated to the C2–3 level suggests a traumatic origin or significant biomechanical fault. (The segmental occurrence and extent of posterior joint arthrosis differ from that of spondylosis.) Arthrosis is more common in the midcervical spine whereas spondylotic changes are more pronounced in the lower cervical spine(73).

Senile ankylosing hyperostosis of Forrestier, also called diffuse idiopathic skeletal hyperostosis (DISH), is a special atypical form of spondylosis. Exuberant calcification of the anterior longitudinal ligament is characteristic. Surprisingly for the degree of architectural change, disc spacing in these conditions is preserved longer than with degenerative spondylosis.

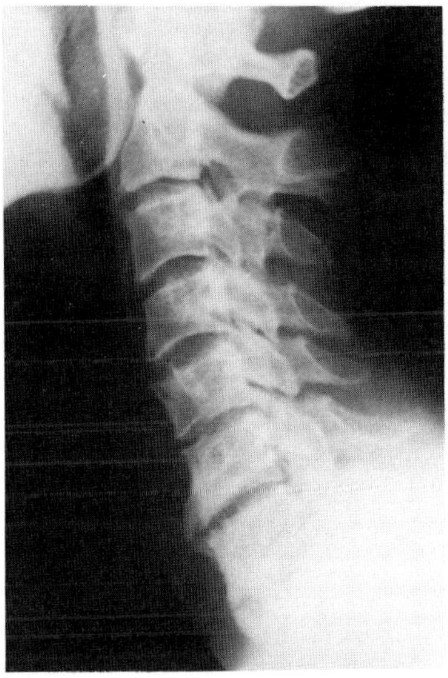

Figure 2.22. Spondylosis deformans.

Infection

Tuberculous spondylitis of the upper cervical spine is extremely rare and is hardly ever seen. Sometimes called malum suboccipitale it has been a reported cause of basilar impression(38).

Nasopharyngeal infection in children and adolescents causing wry neck was described by Grisel in 1930(75). Tonsillar infection spread via the lymphatic channels to invade the retropharyngeal space where prevertebral widening may be noted. Spinal involvement with atlantoaxial dislocation has been described with Grisel's syndrome.

Trauma

Diagnosis of fractures and dislocations is based on an interpretation of direct signs including fracture lines or fragments of bone as well as valuable indirect signs such as diastasis, malalignment, displacement, and soft tissue abnormalities. A single traumatic event or a series of successive traumata may be responsible for fracture development. This is best exemplified by the so-called "whiplash" injury in which a concentration of forces applied to points of lesser resistance results in certain typical fractures. Hyperextension injuries are generally considered more serious than hyperflexion injuries, however, this depends on many factors, the most notable being morphological variation(76–78).

A common fracture during hyperextension (lower body acceleration with inertial resistance of the head and neck) is the apical or superior odontal fracture. In the hyperflexion or declaration injury, the basal or inferior odontal fracture is frequently encountered (Fig. 2.23).

Fracture or dislocation sites not readily seen on neutral or standard radiographic views may be better visualized on functional examinations or other special projections. Extreme care should be exercised in the positioning of any view that is painful or otherwise awkward for the patient. A case in point was reported by De Rongemont in 1956(40) in which a congenitally luxated odontoid was complicated by vertebral artery thrombosis. Vertebral positioning is dependent on radiographic technique. Positional errors and normal variations in symmetry must always be considered. Muscular spasm and ligamentous injuries translated to the radiograph reveal malpositions often considered trivial and of no practical importance to the diagnostician.

Rotational subluxation at the level of the upper cervical spine due to vertical, oblique, or lateral forces is not an uncommon cause of acute torticollis. Spontaneous occurrence of upper cervical fixation or blocking is seen in the immature hypermobile cervical spine. This syndrome is unaccompanied by atlantodental interspace widening and anterior atlantal dislocation more often seen in cervical arthritis and fracture dislocation. In viewing the AP open-mouth film, in spite of rotation of the spinous process laterally, the head and atlas remain symmetrical(38). Helpful in the diagnosis are

a) congruence of the lower triangles of the lateral masses formed by the border of the posterior arch of atlas;
b) no malposition of the head; occiput remains level (biventer mastoid line);
c) lateral view shows separation of facet overlap. One articular surface projects anterior to the vertebral body.
d) a smaller interrupted posterior body contour line (George's line) with anterior shift of axis.

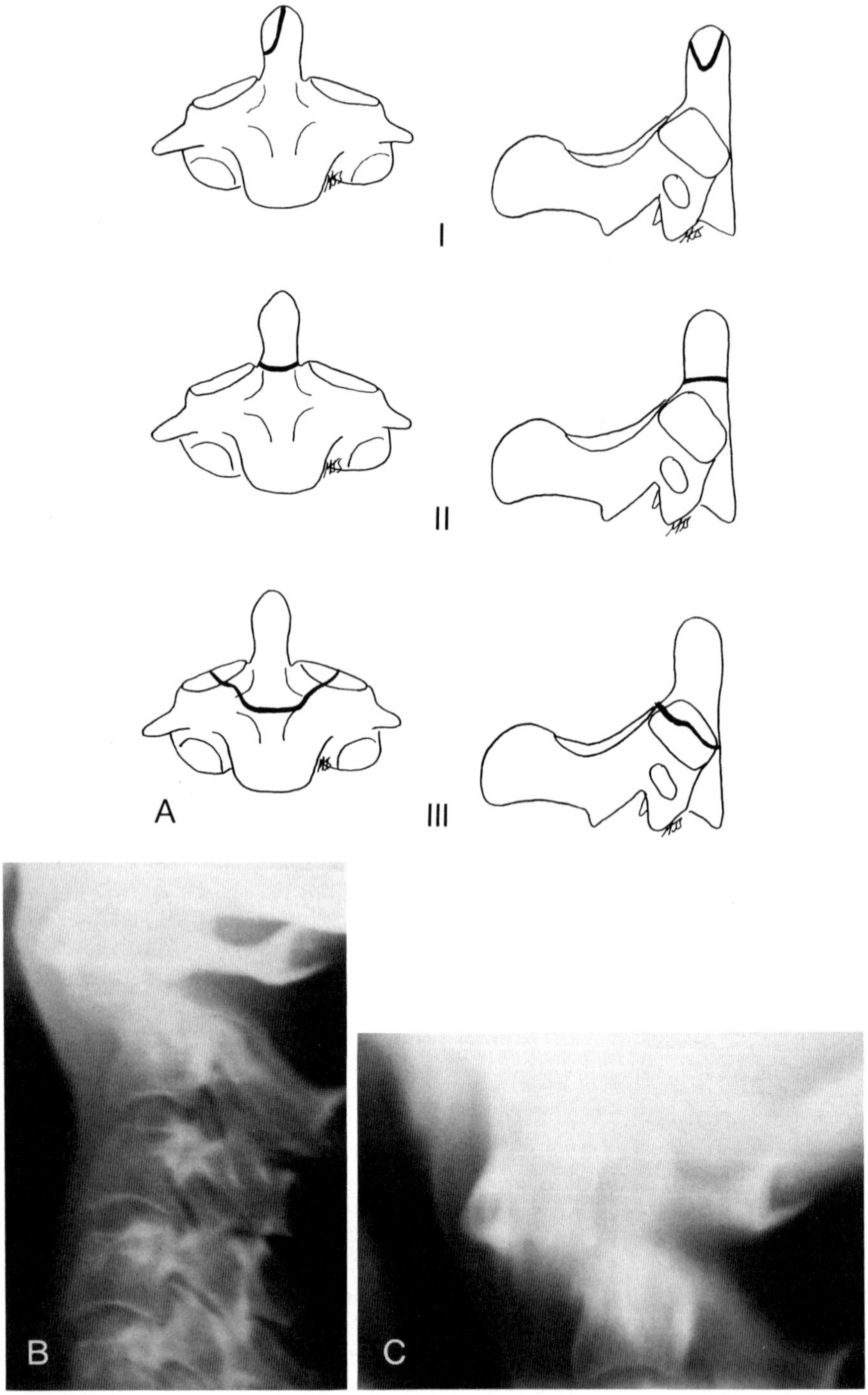

Figure 2.23. **A.** Odontoid fractures, types I–III. **B.** Odontoid fracture (lateral radiograph). **C.** Odontoid fracture (tomogram).

If rotational subluxation is seen at the atlantooccipital joints, the AP films show atlantal assymmetry in relation to the occiput. On the lateral view projectional separation of the lateral masses is seen despite good facet overlap in the caudal segments. Lateral mass overlap produces a pseudo narrowing of the anterior arch of atlas.

Clinical indicators govern the inclusion of these radiographic considerations before rotational subluxation is diagnosed. Anomalous assymetry must also be accounted for in the radiographic appraisal.

Finally, AP open-mouth views in lateral deviation of the spinous process of axis from the neutral position facilitate the diagnosis of articular fixation. Preexisting assymmetries taken into account, the spinous process of axis should normally deviate to the side away from lateral bending. Care and positioning for the lateral bending film is critical to the interpretation.

Pseudosubluxation

Apparent subluxation between C2–3 and C3–4 is a concern when flexion-extension films are taken in children up to the age of 16. A generous shifting or anterior step-off of 2–4 mm is found in healthy children due to the normal laxity of the joint capsules and ligament. This laxity gradually disappears after age 16(79, 80). The apparent hypermobility is due to the persistence of the relative horizontal intervertebral joint planes and the immature development of the uncovertebral joints. This tendency occurs in about 40% of children under the age of eight and about 20% of children up to age 16(61). The anterior laminar cortex of the C2 arch should not deviate more than 1 1/2–2 mm anterior of a spinolaminar junction line joining C1 to C3(79). If there is a greater deviation than this, a true unstable subluxation of C2 on C3 must be considered.

Observation of a subluxation should take into account postinjury signs and symptoms. There may be frank dislocation of the posterior joints in which the facets remain locked in a displaced position regardless of the motion plane and will not correct with normal reverse movement. If positional correction occurs and the clinical findings are unremarkable, pseudo subluxation is likely(68). Suffice to say that in all cases of persistent childhood torticollis, radiographic investigation is essential to rule out pathological subluxation and assess segmental hypermobility preparatory to manipulative intervention.

Subluxations and Ligamentous Lesions Classification

Anteroposterior Disclocation of the Atlas and Axis

Ligamentous injury to the cranial-vertebral transition may displace the atlas anteriorly and the axis posteriorly as a result of tearing or stretching of the transverse ligament of the atlas. Three signs favoring traumatic origin over congenital absence of the transverse ligament include(40):

i) the degree of atlantodental separation is often irreducible upon extension of the head.
ii) a radio-opacity is evident within the atlantodental interspace, representing a hematoma—a likely cause of the irreducibility;
iii) a breach of the basilar line overlapping the odontoid process very nearly equals the amount of separation at the atlantodental interval.

Transverse Dislocation Involving the Occiput, Atlas, and Axis

i) *Transverse atlantocondylar subluxation.* Viewed as a malalignment between the occiput and atlas, on frontal views, lateral displacement of the atlas is encountered as a subluxation.
ii) *Atlantocondylar diastasis.* A unilateral increase in the width of this interspace on the AP open-mouth view can be best identified on tomography.

Transverse Atlantoaxial Subluxation

Lateral displacement is demonstrated by overlap of the margin of atlas over the lateral margin of axis. This accounts for the corresponding differences in the periodontal spacing viewed on the AP open-mouth film.

Atlantoaxial Rotation and Subluxation

For discussion, see above.

Anteroposterior Dislocation of the Atlas and Axis on the Occiput

For discussion of this rare posttraumatic displacement see Roentgenometrics and Occipital Atlantal Hypermobility above.

Anterosuperior Tilting

Under normal circumstances McRae's foramen magnum line and the horizontal plane of atlas are almost parallel. Two malpositions may be seen:

i) *Anterosuperior tilting*
The anterior arch is raised and the posterior arch is lowered; this extended position of atlas may remain fixed relative to the axis during head flexion.
ii) *Anteroinferior tilting*
The atlantal inclination is flexed. This position is favored in traumatic damage to the transverse ligament.

Fracture Types

Jefferson's Burst Fracture (Fig. 2.24)

A sudden axial impact or blow upon the skull impacts upon a point of lesser resistance, the atlas, separating or bursting the atlas apart. With discal resorption of the forces, the unprotected atlas becomes a weak link in the vertebral chain. The AP open-mouth view shows a spreading of the lateral masses of atlas seen as bilateral overlap on the lateral margins of axis. This deformity is the result of fracture at the anterior and posterior arches of atlas(38).

Fractures of the Arches of Atlas

The sulcal groove for the vertebral artery is a point of lesser resistance to traumatic forces and fractures may readily be seen on the plain lateral film. Often seen is a Jefferson-type fracture in which there is articular offset as seen in the AP mouth view if the posterior and anterior atlantal ring is split(40, 76).

Fractures of Axis (Fig. 2.25)

Fractures involving the body of axis are usually the result of significant injury and, if present, are usually accompanied by fracture of the odontoid process. Fractures involving the posterior arch of axis, so-called "Hangman's" (better termed Hangee's) fractures, may be seen to best advantage on the lateral view. Fractures involving the body of axis are relatively rare.

Of special significance are fractures involving the odontoid process. Accounting for about 1–2% of all spinal fractures and 10% of cervical fractures, the most common causes include diving injuries and head injuries as a result of motor vehicle accidents(76). The position of the displacement of the dens relative to the axis body suggest the vector of mechanical forces sustained. Forward displacement of the dens is caused by a shearing break caused by transverse check ligament rupture during violent or sudden flexion of the head upon the neck (Fig. 2.23 *b*). Backward displacement is caused by sudden extension-type

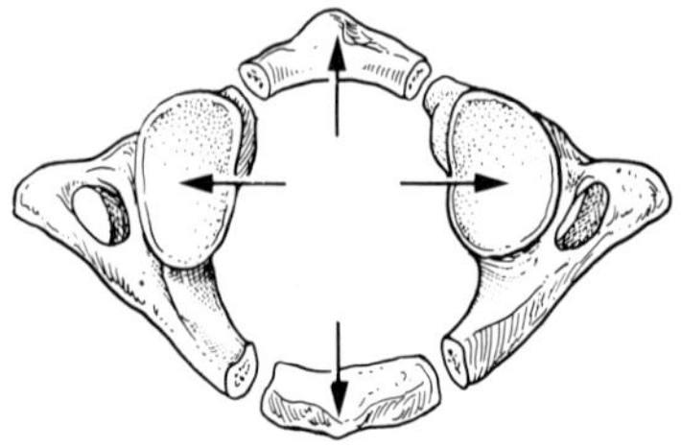

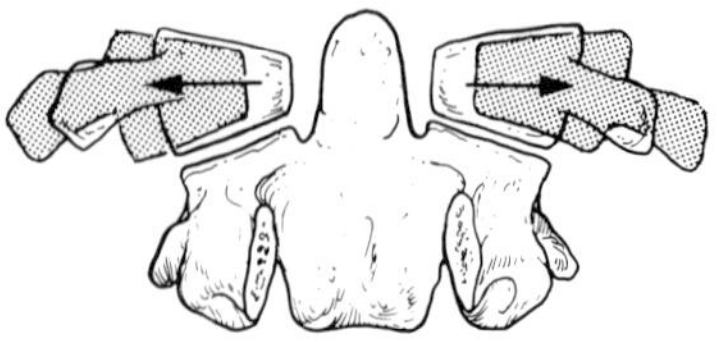

Figure 2.24. Jefferson's fracture of atlas.

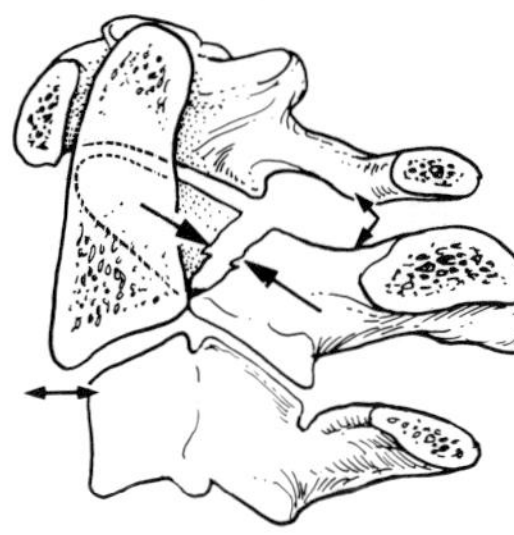

Figure 2.25. Hangman's fracture of axis.

forces imposed upon the dens by the anterior arch of atlas. The net result may be atlantoaxial fracture displacement as the transverse ligament secures the fractured odontoid in a position of deformity. Associated fractures may involve the skull, mandible, and atlas.

In children up to the age of eight years, separation of the epiphysis occurs at the cartilagenous anlage. Termed epiphysiolysis of the odontoid process, the odontoid may be displaced from its base or it may remain sufficiently positioned to ensure satisfactory healing.

Should complete separation of the epiphysis dentis occur, rarefaction may follow giving the false appearance of aplasia. Gone undiagnosed, the odontoid remnant may form a pseudo arthrosis. If union of the odontoid occurs following adequate immobilization over the course of about three months, deformity may be seen with the odontal segment placed slightly posterior to the inferior portion (Bayonette appearance) or anterior to it. The lower the fracture site the better the osseous healing(76, 81, 82). Functional studies identify instability.

Wackenheim described five radiological signs that help differentiate traumatic lesions from congenital or other variations in the upper cervical spine(40, 83):

1. Condyloatlantal diastasis—definite abnormality is diagnosed when one side is twice the width of the other side.
2. Increase in AP sagittal diameter of C2 over atlas. Normally atlas is 1–3 mm greater than axis. Reversal is abnormal.
3. Transverse dislocation of the cervicooccipital joint manifested by loss of symmetry of the atlantooccipital and atlantoaxial joints.
4. Functional blockage of the atlantooccipital or atlantoaxial joint such that there persists a constant relationship between segments during flexion, extension, and neutral positions of the neck.
5. Differentiation of an odontoid fracture from an os odontoideum, with the latter showing evidence of reduction with flexion and the former showing reduction usually with extension.

Fractures of the odontold have been known to go unnoticed and are found as serious incidental findings upon subsequent radiographic examination for hitherto unrelated symptomotology. The causes for misdiagnosis:

- unremarkable symptoms attributable to the upper cervical spine;
- obscuring effect of concommitant priority injurie of skull and brain;
- lack of obvious displacement of the odontoid;
- presence of a cervical collar or immobilization device during emergency radiography compromising film quality; and
- other radiographic positioning or technical difficulties.

Because of these reasons, the practitioner of manipulation should assume that these subtletics exist and radiographically reevaluate the posttraumatized patient. To do less may well lead to disastrous results if manipulative maneuvers are administered for palpably found dysfunction.

Tumor and Tumor-like Conditions of the Upper Cervical Spine

Tumors and tumor-like conditions of the cervical spine, both primary (benign and malignant) and secondary, are not common(84–89). However, the potential for morbidity or mortality is significant and thus important to review. Table 2.5 summarizes those tumors or tumor-like conditions described in the literature.

Tumors of the cervical spine impair static protection as well as postural and kinetic

Table 2.5
Cervical Tumors or Tumor-like Conditions

Primary Benign Tumors or Tumor-like Conditions	Primary Malignant	Secondary (Metastasis)	Intraspinal
Hemangioma Aneurysmal bone cyst Benign giant cell tumor Solitary plasmacytoma Solitary eosinophilic Granuloma Osteochondroma Osteoid osteoma Desmoid tumor Fibrous dysplasia (predominately occipital)	Multiple myeloma Aggressive solitary plasmacytoma Chordoma Chondrosarcoma Osteosarcoma Ewings Fibrosarcoma Lymphoma	Adult Breast (highest incidence) Lung (rare) Prostate Renal Colon Head and neck tumors Child Leukemia Neuroblastoma Retinoblastoma Ewings sarcoma	Tumors may be intramedullary or extramedullary (intradural and extradural); more likely to cause pedicle erosion or widening of interpedicular space. Primary tumors Neurofibromas Meningiomas Lipomas Gliomas Vascular tumors Hemanigiomas Desmoids Secondary tumors Carcinomas Melanomas Sarcomas Lymphomas

activities. This is due to the derangement of intrinsic spinal stability (Fig. 2.26). Because of the tumor locations, the vascular and neural structures may be affected. Signs of compression of the cord and its roots may result from displacement and instability or from direct compression due to the tumor outgrowth. One must also be aware of ischemia to the cord caused by the constriction of the feeding arterial system. Symptoms of local and radiating pain, tenderness, muscle spasm, and limited cervical range of motion are the most frequent presenting complaints. It has been reported that the earliest sign of tumor in the atlantoaxial region is the loss of rotary motion. The most common locations of tumors, however, are found at levels C2–C7.

Plain roentgenograms of the cervical spine are extremely valuable. One may visualize foraminal enlargement or body scalloping from neurofibromatosis. Changes in bone texture may be noted in multiple myeloma. Other radiographic signs of vertebral body or posterior element disruption, postural changes, and deformities may be seen. Radiographic features of instability may also be evident. Benign tumors will most likely be demonstrable on the plain film at the time of symptomology but this does not necessarily hold true for malignant tumors.

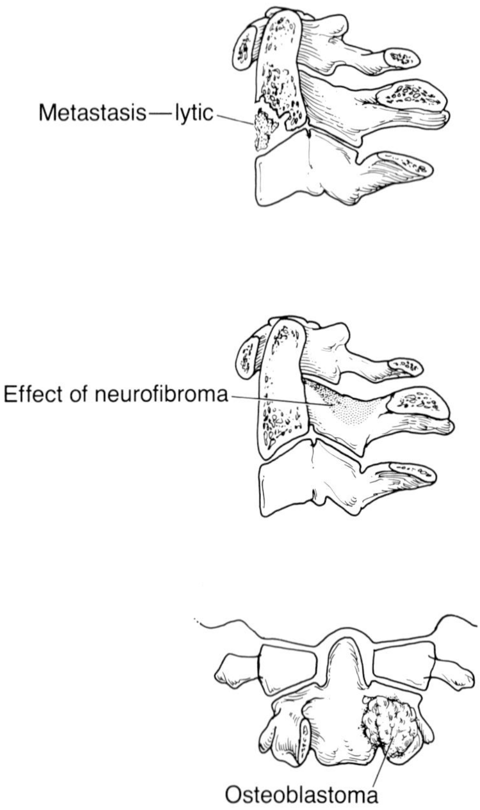

Figure 2.26. Tumors of the upper cervical spine. *Top,* metastasis. *Middle,* neurofibroma. *Bottom,* osteoblastoma.

Metastatic involvement of the cervical spine is by far more frequent than primary tumors, especially in the adult. With primary tumors, the incidence of benign tumors is greater than malignant ones in the child. The cervical spine overall is the least common location for spinal metastasis. According to Bailey, the most common cervical tumor in the adult spine is multiple myeloma.

Hemangiomas of the vertebral body are the most frequent benign tumors of the cervical spine in the adult and generally involve a single vertebra. The typical coarse vertical striations are its hallmark.

Aneurysmal bone cysts are relatively common in the cervical spine. This lytic, soap-bubble, expansile lesion may cause destruction of contiguous segments. The axis appears to have a higher predilection for this tumor than atlas.

Osteoblastoma is another expansile tumor of the posterior elements. One must be aware that there may be difficulty in differentiation of an aneurysmal bone cyst, giant cell tumor, and osteoblastoma as well as differentiating an osteogenic sarcoma that may appear as benign as the aforementioned tumors.

A giant cell tumor, like a hemangioma, involves the veretebral body. This tumor is considered quasimalignant. It may be well defined or appear to be quite invasive.

Osteochondromas can produce a well-delineated large mass with or without a calcified cartilaginous cap.

A chordoma is a rare malignant neoplasm arising from the vestigial remnants of the embryonic notochord especially in the cervical-occipital area and is seen as an expansible osteolytic lesion with progressive destruction.

Neurofibromatosis may demonstrate scalloping of vertebral bodies or show foraminal enlargement. Other radiographic changes include loss of the cervical lordosis, atlantal rotary subluxation, or a fixed anterolisthesis of C2 upon C3. The patient may or may not have symptomatic pain on motion or neural deficits on examination.

Other rare tumors, desmoid tumors, or fibromatosis, may be mono- or multifocal and are considered to be of two types involving the spine. There are extra abdominal desmoids that may originate in the vertebral ligaments themselves or the desmoidplastic fibromas that develop inside the bone from the endosteum.

In differentiating tumors from infection, it must be noted that the infection usually affects the disc space with apparent reactive sclerosis.

Once a lesion has been established or there is a high index of suspicion without radiographic confirmation, further diagnostic workup such as tomography, bone scanning, computed tomography, magnetic resonance imaging, anteriography, and myelography is necessary or manditory. Treatment often involves surgical stabilization, radiation, or chemotherapy.

CONCLUSION:

The use of radiography as both a clinical and investigative tool requires that we reflect on the wisdom of a quotation in Sir John Herschel's "On the Study of Natural Philosophy," 1830:

> A bone is a framework of the most curious carpentry; in which occurs not a single straight line nor any known geometrical curve, yet all evidently, systematic, and constructed by rules which defy our research.

And thus the primary health care practitioner must rely on knowledge and experience as well as consultation for those elusive cases.

References

1. Sherman RA. Chiropractic x-ray rationale. J Can Chirop Assoc 1986;30:33–35.
2. Stoddard A. Manual of osteopathic practice. New York: Harper & Row, Publishers, 1969:87, 284.
3. Stoddard A. Manual of osteopathic technique. 9th ed. London: Hutchison & Co. (Publishers) Ltd., 1977:36
4. Korbelas PA, Henderson DJ. Fracture-dislocation at the atlanto-axial junction: a case report to demonstrate the importance of radiographic examination in chiropractic practice. J Can Chirop Assoc 1980;24:157–160.
5. Brewerton DA. The doctor's role in diagnosis and prescribing manipulation. In: Maitland GD. Vertebral Manipulation. London: Butterworth & Co, LTD, 1973:1–8.
6. Bourdillon JF. Spinal manipulation. 2nd ed. New York: Appleton-Century-Crofts, 1973:58–59.

7. Phillips RB. The use of x-rays in spinal manipulative therapy. In: Haldeman S. Modern Developments in the principles and practice of chiropractic. New York: Appleton-Century-Crofts, 1980: 189–208.
8. Yochum TR, Rowe LJ. Essentials of skeletal radiology. Baltimore: Williams & Wilkins, 1987:1–94.
9. Coelho LR. Spinal radiographic techniques, quality assurance, and radiation safety. In: Haleman S. Modern developments in the principles and practice of chiropractic. New York: Appleton-Century-Crofts, 1980:209–229.
10. Merrill V. Atlas of radiographic positions. 4th ed. St Louis, CV Mosby Co., 1975.
11. Hildebrandt RW. Chiropractic spinography. Des Plaines, IL: Hilmark, 1977:59–78.
12. Meschan I. Radiographic positioning and related anatomy. 2nd ed. Philadelphia: WB Saunders, 1978.
13. Buehler M, Pugh J, Sandman T. Physics and technology in routine radiography. Lombard, IL: National College of Chiropractic. 1979:7–170.
14. Bolyston BF. Oblique roentgenographic views of the cervical spine in flexion and extension: an aid in the diagnosis of cervical subluxations and obscure dislocations. J Bone Jt Surg 1957;39:1302–8.
15. White AA, Panjabi MM. Clinical biomechanics of the spine. Toronto: JB Lippincott Co, 1978:35–42, 61–74.
16. White AA, Panjabi MM. Kinematics. The research status of spinal manipulative therapy. National Institute of Neurological & Communicative Disorders and Strike Monograph 1975;18:93–102.
17. Shafer RC. Clinical biomechanics, musculo-skeletal actions and reactions. Baltimore: Williams & Wilkins, 1983:264–272.
18. White AA, Panjabi MM. The clinical biomechanics of the occipito atlanto axial complex. Symposium on the upper cervical spine. Ortho Clin North Am 1978:9;4:867–878.
19. Worth DR. Kinematics of the cranio-vertebral joints. In: Idczak RM. Aspects of manipulative therapy. Victoria Lincoln Institute of Health Sciences. 1980:39–44.
20. Carrick FR. Cervical radiculopathy: the diagnosis and treatment of pathomechanics in the cervical spine. J Manipulative Physiol Ther 1983; 6:129–137.
21. Jirout J. The dynamic dependence of the lower cervical vertebrae on the atlanto-occipital joints. Neuroradiology 1974;7:249–252.
22. Wackenheim A. Functional atlanto-occipital block. Neuroradiology, 1971;3:80–81.
23. Watkins RJ. Upper cervical mechanics. J Clin Chiro.
24. Conley RN. Stress evaluation of cervical mechanics. J Clin Chirop 1974;1:3.
25. Grice AS. Preliminary evaluation of 50 agittal cervical motion radiographic examinations. J Can Chirop Assoc 1977;21:33–4.
26. Hviid H. Functional radiography of the cervical spine. Ann Swiss Chirop Assoc 1963;3:37–65.
27. Prantl K. X-ray examination and functional analysis of the cervical spine. Man Med 1985;2:5–15.
28. Jirout J. Comments regarding the diagnosis and treatment of dysfunctions in the C2-3 segment. Man Med 1985;2:16–17.
29. Arlen A. Biometrishe rontgenfunktionsdiagnostik der halswirbelsaule. Fischer, Heidelbert (Schriftenreihe Manuelle Medizin, Bd 5). 1979.
30. Lane GR. Cervical spine: its movement and symptomatology. J Clin Chirop Arch. 1st ed. Spring 1971.
31. Lysell E. The pattern of motion in the cervical spine. In: Hirsch C, Zotterman Y. Cervical pain. Toronto: Pergamon Press, 1972:53–58.
32. Penning L. Functional pathology of the cervical spine. Baltimore: Williams & Wilkins, 1968.
33. Henderson DJ, Dormon TM. Functional roentgenometric evaluation of the cervical spine in the sagittal plane. J Manipulative Physiol Ther 1985;8:219–227.
34. Wholey MH, Brewer HL, Baker HL. The lateral roentgenogram of the neck. Radiology 1958; 71:350.
35. Meschan I. Synopsis of analysis of roentgen signs in general radiology. Toronto: WB Saunders Co. 1976:214–222.
36. Dvorak J, Dvorak V. Manual medicine: diagnostics. New York: Thieme-Stratton Inc. 1984: 5.
37. Schmidt H, Fischer E. Die okzipitale dysplasie. Thieme, Stuttgart. 1960.
38. von Torklus D, Gehle W. The upper cervical spine. New York: Grune & Stratton. 1972.
39. Thiebaut F, Wackenheim A, Vrousos C. Un nouveau repère pour de la dent de l'axis dans les traumatismes et les malformations de la charniere cervico-occipitale. Rev Oto-neuro-ophthal.
40. Wackenheim A. Roentgen diagnosis of the craniovertebral region. New York: Springer-Verlag, 1974;82–96.
41. Hinck VC, Hopkins CE. Measurement of the atlanto-dental interval in the adult. Am J Roent 1960;84(5):945–951.
42. Locke GR, Gardner JI, van Epps EF. Atlas-dens interval (ADI) in children. Am J Roent 1966;97:135.
43. Jackson H. Diagnosis of minimal atlanto-axial subluxation. Br J Radiol 1950;23:672.
44. Buehler MT, Sandman TD. Anterior atlanto-axial subluxation: clinical and radiographic depiction. J Manipulative Physiol Ther 1978;(14):223–227.
45. Tishler J, Martel W. Dislocation of the atlas in mongolism. Radiology 1965;84:904.
46. Kobori M, Takahashi H, Mikawa Y. Atlanto-axial dislocation in Down's syndrome spine. Spine 1986;11:195–200.
47. Poznanski AK. Congenital anomalies of the cervical spine. In: Bailey RW. The cervical spine. Philadelphia; Lea & Febiger, 1974:47–90.
48. Redlund-Johnell I, Pettersson H. Vertical dislocation of C1 and C2 vertebral in rheumatoid arthritis. Acta Radiol Diagn 1984;25:133–141.
49. Redlund-Johnell I, Pettersson H. Radiographic measurements of the craniovertebral region. Acta Radiol Diagn 1984;25:23–28.
50. Wiesel SW, Rothman RH. Occipito-atlantal hypermobility. Spine 1979;4(3):187–191.
51. Wiesel SW, Kraus D, Rothman RH. Atlanto-occipital hypermobility. In: Sherk HH, Fielding JW. Symposium on the upper cervical spine. Orthop Clin North Am 1978;9(4):969–972.

52. Truex RC, Johnson CH. Congenital anomalies of the upper cervical spine. In: Sherk HH, Fielding JW. Symposium on the upper cervical spine. Orthop Clin North Am 1978;9(4):891–900.
53. Giacomeni C. Sull' esitenza dell "os odontoideum" nell. Uomo, Gior: Accad. Med. Torino 1886;49:24.
54. Greenfield J. Malformations et dégénerscence des disques intervertebraux de la région cervicale. Rev Med Suisse Rom, 1953;73:229.
55. Michaels L, Prevost M, Crang D. Pathologic cases in a case of os odontoideum. J Bone J Surg 1969;51(A):965.
56. Fielding JW, Hawkins R, Thompson W. Os odontoideum: congenital or acquired? J Bone J Surg 1976;58(A):413.
57. Freiberger R, Wilson P, Nichols J. Acquired absence of the odontoid process. J Bone J Surg 1965;47(A):1231.
58. Schiff D, Parke W. The arterial supply of the odontoid process. J Bone J Surg 1973;55(A):1450.
59. Grilliot JR. Os odontoideum. ACA J. Chirop. 1985;19:67–69.
60. Guebert GM, Thompson JR. Os odontoideum. ACA J Chirop 1986;20:69–71.
61. Schmorl G, Junghanns H. The human spine in health and disease. 2nd ed. New York: Grune & Stratton 1971:409–413.
62. Brocher JEW. Die wirbelsaulenleiden und ihre differential—diagnose. Stuttgart: Aufl Thieme, 1966:4.
63. Geipel P. Doppelte spaltbildung des atlas. Med Klin 1936;2:1302.
64. Fried K. Der wirbelblock. Radiol Diagn 1963;4:165.
65. Hadley LA. Anatomico-roentgenographic studies of the spine. Springfield IL: Charles C Thomas, 1973.
66. Schut L, Bruce DA. The Arnold-Chiari malformation. In: Sherk HH, Fielding JW. Symposium on the upper cervical spine. Orthop Clin North Am 1978;9(4):913–922.
67. Jeffreys E. Disorders of the cervical spine. London: Butterworths, 1980;106–118.
68. Sandman TD, Sandman KB. Rheumatoid arthritis of the cervical spine: examination prior to chiropractic manipulative therapy. J Manip Physiol Ther 1981;4(1):19–20.
69. Yochum TR, Rowe LJ. Arthritides of the upper cervical complex. In: Idczak RM. Aspects of manipulative therapy. Victoria: Lincoln Institute of Health Sciences, 1980; 22–32.
70. Redlund-Johnell I. Atlanto-occipital dislocation in rheumatoid arthritis. Acta Radiol Diagn 1984;25:165–168.
71. Lyness SS, Simeone FA. Vascular complications of upper cervical spine injuries. In: Sherk HH, Fielding JW. Symposium on the Upper Cervical Spine. Orthop Clin North Am 1978;9(4):1029–1038.
72. Henderson DJ. Significance of vertebral dyskinesia in relation to the cervical syndrome. J Manipulative Physiol Therap 1979;2(1):3–15.
73. Hirsch C. Some morphological changes in the cervical spine during aging. In: Hirsch C, Zoltermann Y. Cervical pain. Toronto: Pergamon Press, 1972;21–31.
74. Sager P. An osteoarchaeological study of spondylosis cervicalis. In: Hirsch C., Zolterman Y. Cervical pain. Toronto: Pergamon Press. 1972;33–42.
75. Grisel P. Enucléation de l'atlas et torticollis nasophargyngien. Presse Méd 1930;38:50.
76. Braakman R, Penning L. Injuries of the cervical spine. Exerpta Med Int Congr Ser, 1971.
77. Harris JH. The radiology of acute cervical trauma. Baltimore: Williams & Wilkins, 1978.
78. Shapiro R, Youngbert AS, Rothman SLG. The differential diagnosis of traumatic lesions of the occipito atlanto-axial segment. Radiol Clin North Am 1973;11(3):505–526.
79. Pope TL, Riddervold HO. Pitfalls in interpreting cervical films. Diagnosis 1980;(Dec)23–31.
80. Fechtel SG. Pseudosubluxation of the cervical spine in adolescents: a case report. J Manipulative Physiol Ther 1983;6(2):81–84.
81. Amyes EW, Anderson FM. Fracture of the odontoid process: report of 63 cases. Arch Surg 1956:72;377.
82. Alexander EH, Forsyth F, David CH, Nashold BS. Dislocation of the atlas on the axis—the value of early fusion of C1, C2 and C3. J Neurosurg 1958;15:353.
83. Henrys P, Lyne ED, Lifton C, Salciccioli G. Clinical review of cervical spine injuries in children. Clin Orthop Relat Res 1977;129:172–176.
84. Bailey RW, ed. The Cervical Spine Research Society. Philadelphia; JB Lippincott Co, 1983.
85. Bailey RW, ed. The cervical spine. Philadelphia: Lea & Febiger, 1974.
86. Boklman H, et al. Neoplasms of the cervical spine. J Bone Jt Surg 1986;86(4).
87. Hirsch C, Zotteman Y, eds. International Symposium Series. Cervical pain. Vol. 19, January. Toronto, Peragamon Press, 1971.
88. Huvos AG, ed. Bone tumors: diagnosis, treatment and prognosis. Philadelphia: WB Saunders Co., 1979.
89. Jeanmart L, ed. Tumors—radiology of the spine. Springer-Heidelberg:Springer-Verlag, 1986.

3 Neuroanatomy and Neurophysiology of the Upper Cervical Spine

Don E. Fitz-Ritson, B.A., D.C.

Since the inception of chiropractic it has been propounded that spinal adjustments or manipulations exert an effect on the human nervous system. This theory justifies our anecdotal experience with a wide array of clinical symptomatology whose relief appears to be due to effects far more complex and profound than those that might arise from mechanical changes induced by spinal manipulation. While numerous authors as summarized by Gitelman (1) invoke systematic theories of the neurological effects of spinal manipulation, much remains unknown. I would like to review some basic principles of neurological thought before applying them to the upper cervical spine.

DEVELOPMENT

In the embryonic development of man and higher vertebrates, two major systems begin developing and functioning in the first 3 weeks of life. The cardiovascular system is first, followed very closely in time by the development of the primitive nervous system. The cardiovascular system matures rapidly unlike the nervous system which takes up to 2 decades, or longer, before it reaches full functional and emotional maturity. Initially, the neural tube begins closing at cervical levels of the spinal cord. With additional maturation, tubal closure continues cephalically at a slightly faster rate than caudally. From this basic developmental pattern the cephalocaudal law of development was established. However, if one correlates phylogenetic developmental patterns with embryonic development along with onset of function, the cephalocaudal law, per se, needs to be modified. Instead, the law should be restated as the cervicocephalocaudal law of development.

Placing emphasis upon the cervical levels in regard to growth, development, balance, coordination, and function establishes the importance of this area of the nervous system and the body, especially in relation to (re)habilitation. It is interesting to note that just as the nervous system begins developing here, the mature nervous system also expresses, both structurally and functionally, the importance of this area. For example, the majority of ascending or descending pathways begin or end here. Granted, a large component of these fibers, destined for cervical levels, are necessary for upper limb functions. But many are for afferent and efferent regulation of neurons that fine-tune the neck musculature.

Similarly, many of the critical reflex responses of the body originate at cervical levels before spreading up, down, and across the system to affect the rest of the organism. The tonic neck reflexes and labyrinthine (vestibular) reflexes (also known as the postural and righting reflexes) may act initially at cervical levels. Visual reflexes to peripheral stimuli and auditory reflexes to sound are mediated via specific tracts to cervical levels. The chain reflexes or body-on-body reflexes as well as most of the primitive avoidance reflexes all manifest themselves in movement, initially at cervical levels. Suffice it to say that the cervical levels of the neuraxis are critical and must be considered as a primary area for restoration of function following nervous system insult.

Lack of stability at cervical levels results in decreased stability in the rest of the trunk as well as the shoulder and hip girdles. Instability in these areas is radiated into the appendages, including the head, and especially into the distal parts of the limb. Instability in the appendages, along with lack of head control, sets up a multitude of aberrant feedback signals, especially from the visual vestibular and other proprioceptive systems that coordinate head-neck and body movements (1a).

The essence of movement is mediated by the central nervous system (CNS). How does the CNS control movement, especially in the upper cervical region? We know that the architecture of the joints determines the direction and range of specific segmental and regional movements, but the information from joints, muscles, and capsules is used by the CNS to monitor and thus determine the extent of character and complexities of these movements.

What is the purpose for these movements at the upper cervical area? And why is it that Bach-y-Rita (1a), the foremost authority in rehabilitative medicine, can make a statement as follows: "It is almost impossible for all other systems of the nervous system to function normally when there is a lack of stability, coordination, and purposeful movement patterns including normal feedback information at the cervical level of the body. This area is the key point for controlling the head, and the rest of the body in relation to the head." What are some of the tissues and their pathways into the CNS that provide this information that is so vital for maintaining posture or initiating movements?

MUSCLE MECHANISMS

For excellent reviews see Fitz-Ritson(2); Kendal E, and Schwartz,(3); and Mountcastle VB(4). There are, however, certain features of the cervical paraspinal muscles that require special mention. These features of paraspinal muscles with reference to the cervical muscles are taken from papers of Bakker et al., Richmond et al., and Richmond and Abrahams(5–9). First, spinal nerves do not fuse, as in peripheral nerves. Thus, spinal nerves innervate different parts of a muscle.

The peripheral muscles are supplied usually by branches of a number of spinal nerves. However, spinal muscles receive separate nerves to specific parts, thus exercising more direct control of the portion of the muscle.

Second, paraspinal muscles contain more spindles than any equivalent muscle mass in the body. Muscle spindles are exceptionally dense by location in intervertebral muscles, i.e., interspinous, intertransverse, and spinal rotators.

The majority of muscle spindles occur as members of elaborate spindle arrays consisting of 2–12 muscle spindles linked together in complexes such as paired, parallel, and tandem configurations.

Myelinated 1A afferent from paraspinal muscles have conduction velocities in the range of 90 m/sec, whereas peripheral afferents have conduction velocities of 120 m/sec.

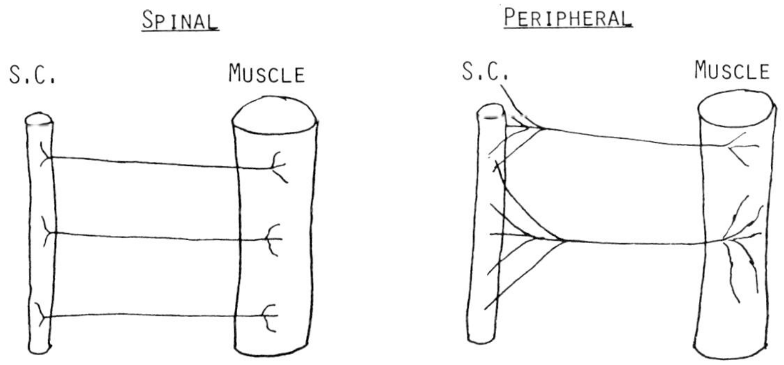

Figure 3.1. Innervation of spinal and peripheral muscles.

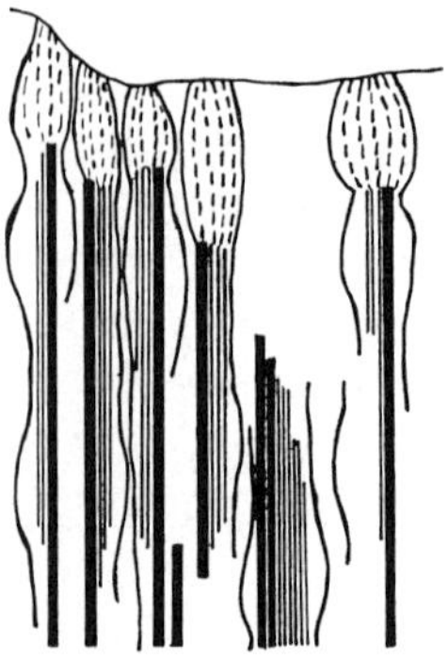

Figure 3.2. Diagram of spindle complex located in the intertransverse muscle group of the C2–C3 joint region. Tendons are shown as strippled regions. Golgi tendon organs at the ends of spindles are shown as encapsulated regions containing broken lines. (Adapted from Bakker D, Richmond F. Muscle spindle complexes in muscles around upper cervical vertebrae in the cat. J. Neurophysiol 1982;48:62–74.)

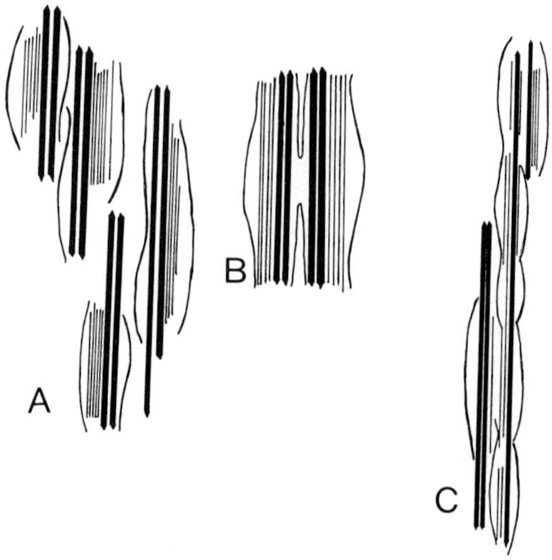

Figure 3.3. Diagrams of muscle spindles in various configurations. **A.** Four paired spindles. Note that no intrafusal fibers are shared. **B.** Parallel spindles. Note the capsule discontinuity at the equatorial regions of spindles. **C.** Spindle array in which five spindles exist in tandem sharing one common nuclear bag fiber. (Adapted form Richmond F, Abrahams V. Morphology and enzyme histochemistry of dorsal muscles of the cat neck. J Neurophysiol 1975;38:1312–1321.)

The gamma fiber content in hind limb muscle motor fibers is usually less than 55%, whereas in paraspinal muscle motor nerves, the gamma fiber content in individual nerve fibers ranges from 55% to 95%. This is because of the increased number of spindles.

The afferents from the Golgi tendon organs rarely fire spontaneously when neck muscles are passively stretched within their optimum length range, but they begin to fire regularly and with progressively increasing frequency as the muscle is passively stretched to very long muscle lengths.

Richmond(9) and colleagues have shown that the fiber architecture of the splenius muscle is different in its medial and lateral parts. In the medial splenius, muscle fascicles run uninterrupted from the muscle origin to its insertion, while in the lateral splenius, separate compartments of muscle fascicles are linked in series by two tendinous inscriptions.

Experiments using glycogen depletion showed that nerves from different spinal segments innervate different muscle regions. Nerves from C1 supply muscle fibers in a small rostromedial zone. Nerves from C2–C4 have motor domains that extend from the medial to the lateral muscle edge and are arranged in series. In the lateral splenius, the motor domains are separated by tendinous inscriptions.

Compared with other compartmentalized muscles, splenius stands out because its division into motor subvolumes has a complex pattern that does not follow any simple rule. Rostromedially, the motor domain of the C1 nerve is arranged parallel to the rest of the muscle, whereas more laterally, motor domains supplied by C2, C3, and C4 are organized in series. Further, the serial arrangements between motor domains are different in lateral and medial muscle regions. In lateral muscle regions, all motor units supplied by a segmental nerve were found to attach onto a single tendinous inscription. During contraction, the motor units must exert their forces jointly onto this inscription and thus presumably provide an evenly distributed pull on all of the muscle fibers inserting on the opposite side. However, in the medial splenius, no tendinous inscriptions were present. Fibers of one segmentally innervated domain inserted within a fascicle by

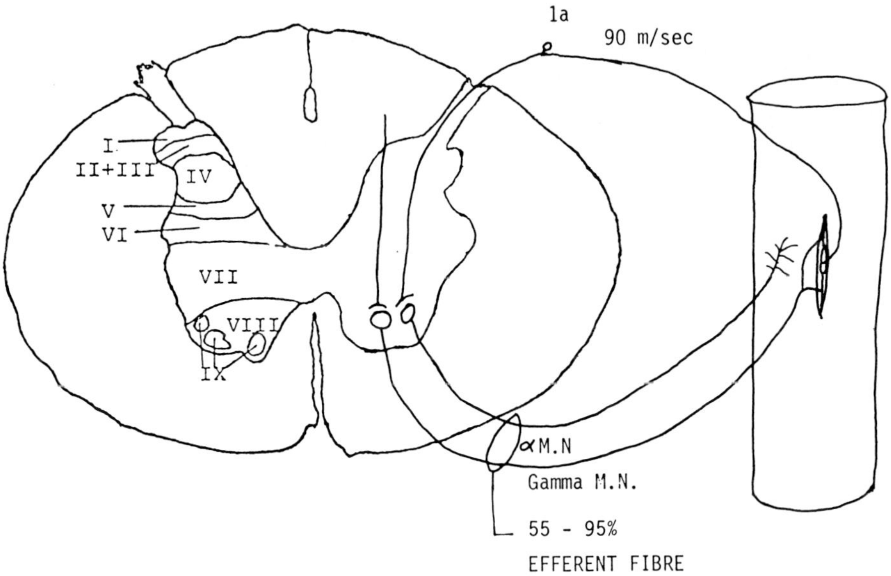

Figure 3.4. Cross section of spinal cord showing relationships of 1, α m.n., and gamma m.n.

interdigitating alongside fibers in the same fascicle that were supplied from a different spinal segment.

This form of interface has not been well characterized. It may allow the tension generated by individual fibers to be transferred more selectively to a few fibers of serially linked motor units. Alternatively, it might allow forces to be dispensed more evenly throughout a volume of fibers rather than concentrating them into a single collagenous structure.

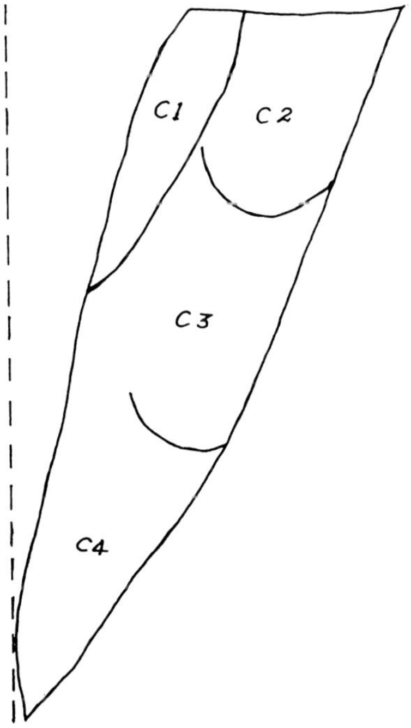

Figure 3.5. Compartmentalization of splenius capitis muscle and segmental innervation.

The mechanical and functional consequences of serial linkages between extrafusal fibers have seldom been modeled or examined experimentally, yet this information may be important for understanding the physiological operation of many long muscles. Richmond et al(9) summed up these concerns: "If a muscle gave only a local contraction at one end during a fractional response, it would do so with a loss of effectiveness to the muscle as a whole, . . . a wasteful stretch of the fibres at the other end must result." How does the central nervous system control a highly compartmentalized muscle such as splenius? Clearly, in-series compartmentalization may place constraints on the recruitment of motor units, especially during the first turning movements for which splenius is mechanically suited. The nervous system has mechanisms that coordinate the actions of different motor domains. In the alert cat, highly synchronous electromyographic (EMG) activity patterns are recorded in different parts of splenius during visually directed or optokinetically driven head movements. This evidence suggests that commands governing the activity of splenius must be distributed to motoneurons supplying different in-series compartments of the muscle.

However, underlying mechanisms for this coordination are not well understood. Both the elaborate motor-unit distribution and the specialized spinal organization of splenius suggest that this muscle is a more sophisticated motor machine than most muscles on which our concepts of muscle physiology are based. It is not yet clear what benefits occur to this muscle as a result of its compartmentalized organization. However, it is clear that the considerations of a central motor control must take into account the peripheral specialties of splenius and must explain the manner in which motor performance is monitored and balanced in diffrent muscle regions.

Brink et al (10) showed that afferents make monosynaptic connections with motoneurons of their own in rostral areas (i.e., C1 and C2) and disynaptic connections with motoneurons in more caudal areas (i.e., C3 and C4).

MECHANORECEPTORS

For excellent reviews se Wyke(11), Haldeman(12), Newton(13), and Wyke(14). However, the pertinent features of the mechanoreceptors are outlined herein.

Joint mechanoreceptors are classified as types I–III (diagrams modified from Newton R. Joint receptor contributions to reflexive and kinesthetic response. Physiother Can 1982;62:22–29).

TYPE I

These are located in the stratum fibrosum of the capsule and ligaments. They are higher in density in proximal joints and are active at rest and during movement. They are slow adapting, and they signal joint angle through normal ranges, therefore making an important contribution to position sense.

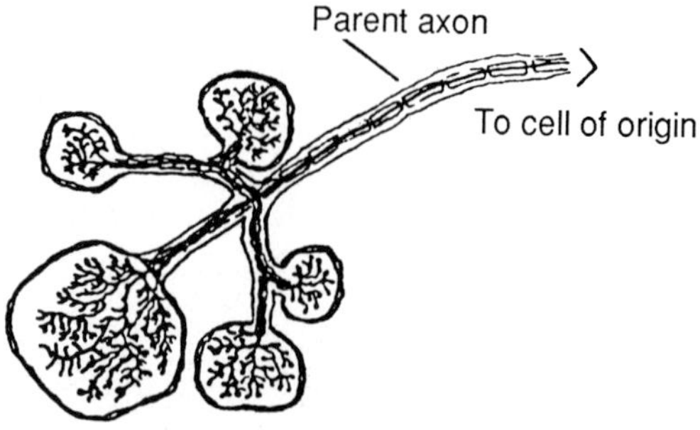

TYPE I SENSORY UNIT

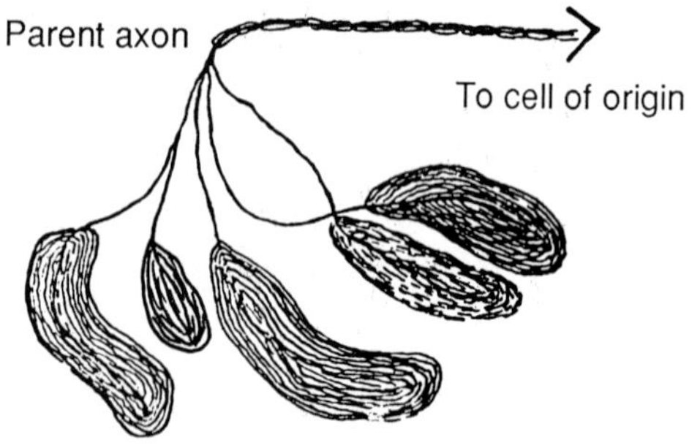

TYPE II SENSORY UNIT

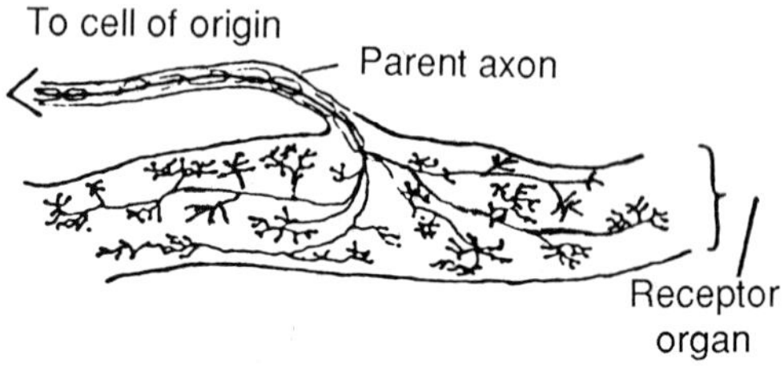

TYPE III SENSORY UNIT

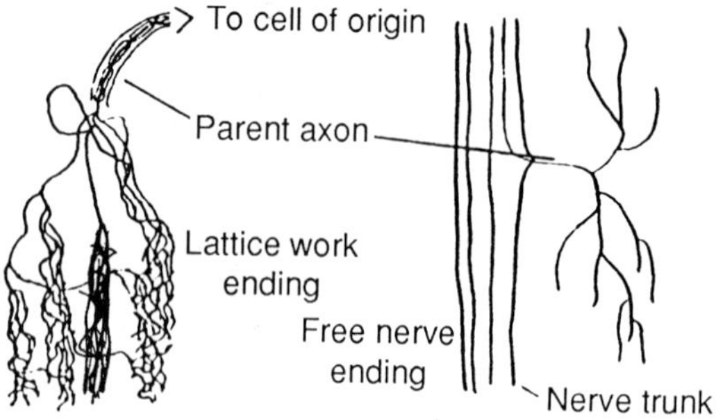

TYPE IV SENSORY UNIT

TYPE II

These are located at the junction of synovial and fibrosum of the capsule. They are also found in intraarticular and extraarticular fat-pads. They are higher in density in distal joints and are active at onset and termination of movement. They are rapidly adapting.

TYPE III

These are located in collateral ligaments and are not found in the intraspinous ligaments of the cervical region. They are active at the end of joint range and are slowly adapting.

These mechanoreceptors are 5–20 cm in diameter and enter the spinal cord synapsing in the apical spinal nucleus (laminae II and III).

Within the apical spinal nucleus, the mechanoreceptor afferents project 3–5 segments cephalad and caudal and interact with second order neurons at these segments. The second order neurons from the apical spinal nucleus project to the basal spinal nucleus (lamina V).

TYPE IV

The type IV mechanoreceptor (Wykes(3) classification) also is a free nerve ending and it responds to pain stimulus. These are located in ligaments, capsule, and articular fat-pads. They are absent in synovial tissue. They are active only to extreme mechanical or chemical irritation and are slow adapting.

The parent axon for these free nerve endings are called unencapsulated nociceptive afferents and they are less than 5 mm in diameter. These nociceptive affer-

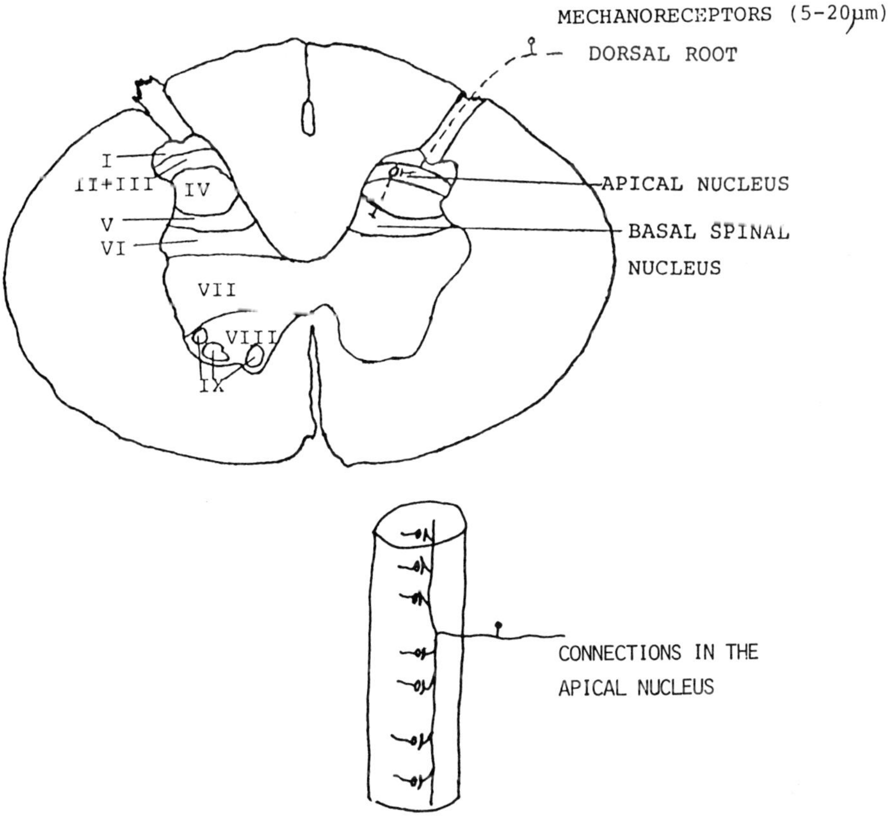

Figure 3.6. Cross section of spinal cord showing interaction of mechanoreceptors.

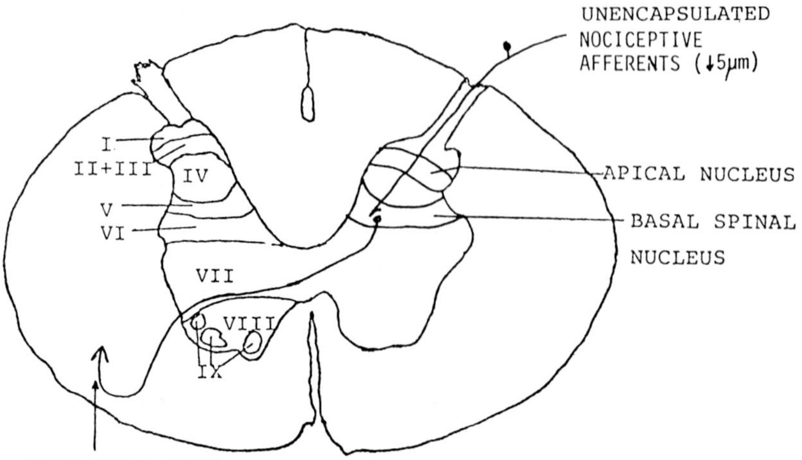

Figure 3.7. Cross section of spinal cord showing interaction of the nociceptive afferents.

ents enter the spinal cord and synapse in the basal spinal nucleus (lamina V). The second order neuron crosses the midline of the spinal cord forming the anterolateral tract, which projects to the thalamus.

If we observe the interaction of the unencapsulated nociceptive afferents and the mechanoreceptors in the spinal cord, we will see that the nociceptors have a direct input to the basal spinal nucleus, whereas the mechanoreceptors via their second order neurons in the apical spinal nucleus have an indirect effect.

JOINT AND PAIN MECHANISMS

It was mentioned above that the interaction of the unencapsulated nociceptive afferents and the mechanoreceptors is in the baal spinal nucleus (lamina V).

If we look at the details of the connections in the basal spinal nucleus, we will see that the second order mechanoreceptors from the apical spinal nucleus (laminae II and III) make axoaxonic synapses on the unencapsulated nociceptive afferents.

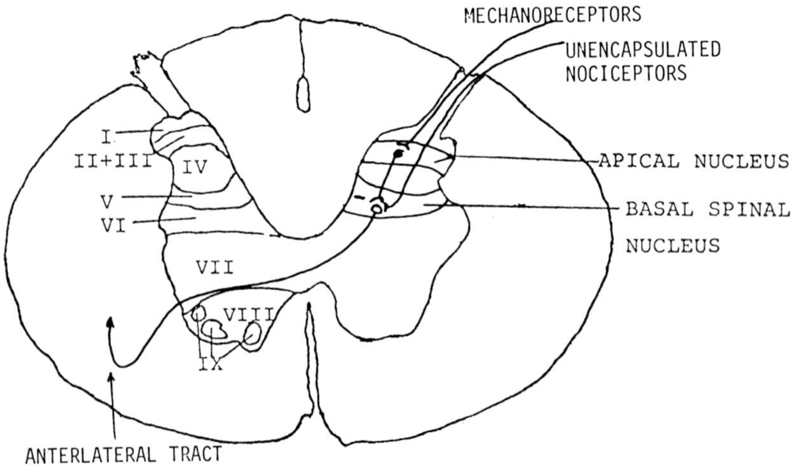

Figure 3.8. Cross section of spinal cord showing interaction of the mechanoreceptors and nociceptors.

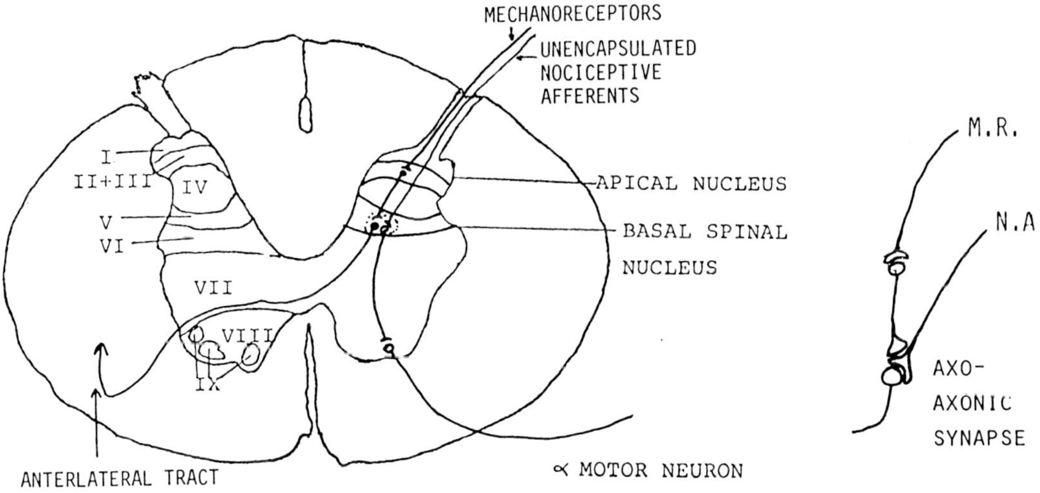

Figure 3.9. Cross section of spinal cord showing detailed interaction of the apical and basal spinal nucleus.

These unencapsulated nociceptive afferents synapse directly on the second order neuron, which crosses and forms the anterolateral tract, and also on interneurons that project to alpha motor neurons.

If we address a few studies that show the interaction in the spinal cord from different tissues, we will begin to appreciate the complex nature of the nervous system as it controls and integrates our response to the environemnt.

Schomburg and Steffens(15) showed that afferents from low threshold mechanoreceptors (hair follicles, pacinian corpuscle) and from nociceptors of the skin converge onto common interneurons in reflex pathways to facilitate alpha motoneuron response. They concluded that this would allow a functionally useful cooperation of these two types of afferents in spinal motor control.

Dvorak and Dvorak(16) and Terrett and Vernon(17) have shown that with a chiropractic adjustment, one obtains a decrease in pain and muscular tone because the mechanoreceptor activity resulting from a manipulation is inhibitory. Also, Fitz-Ritson (unpublished data) showed that with a chiropractic adjustment to a flexed ilium in 15 subjects, there was a statistically significant decrease in muscle tone of the hamstring of the ipsilateral side, which lasted for a minimum of 10 minutes.

Siegel and Tomaszewski(18) showed that somatosensory information derived from muscle and joint receptors elicits a profound reticular formation response during postural adjustments and movements. They concluded that the CNS recalibrates proproceptive signals from the axial musculature and vertebral joints. This demonstrates that, because of the widespread connections of the reticular formation, any changes that are made within the vertebral motion segments (i.e., spinal manipulation) will affect pain and muscle tone and will have an effect on the CNS.

NECK PROPRIOCEPTORS

Recently, much attention has been paid to the role of nuchal proprioceptors not only in the direct control of neck muscles(19, 20) but also in more general perceptual and postural processes. Proprioceptors in the neck are thought to provide signals that permit a subject to recognize rotations of the trunk with respect to the head(21). They initiate reflexes that alter the excitability of limb motoneurons(22), and they interact with reflexes derived from the visual and vestibular systems to produce postural changes that stabilize the head and the visual field(23). It is interesting in light of these multiple functions to find that the main projections from suboccipital proprioceptors are found in precerebellar nuclei.

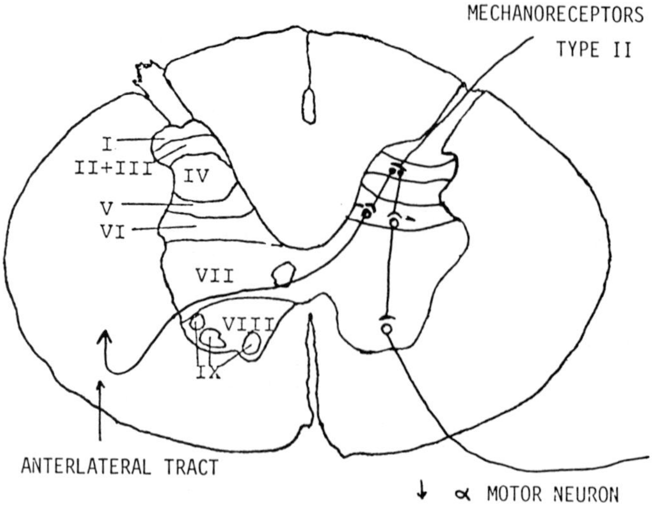

Figure 3.10. Cross section of spinal cord showing interaction of type II mechanoreceptors with α-motor neuron.

Most obvious are the strongly labeled terminations in the central cervical nucleus (CCN) and the external cuneatus nucleus (ECN)(24,25), two regions already known to supply nuchal information via mossy fiber projections to the anterior lobe of the cerebellum(26). However, there are three other populations of cells in the intermediate laminae of C1–C3 that may also transmit nuchal information to the cerebellum by separate ascending pathways, namely, the spinoreticular and two separate spino-olivary pathways(24). The special nature of information from suboccipital muscles that might be transmitted by different precerebellar pathways has not yet been explored in detail. However, nuchal projections have been described in several regions of the cat cerebellum(26–28). These observations have led to the suggestion that the cerebellum has a major role in a variety of postural adjustments that rely on nuchal afferent input for their appropriate execution(28). However, more work is still needed to understand the particular involvement of different precerebellar pathways from the neck in the control of eye-head-neck movements and posture.

In order to appreciate the pathway of the upper afferents from the upper cervical spine, Fitz-Ritson(25) found that while a number of studies had addressed this area, no study had specifically assessed the direct connections of any of the nerve roots into the spinal cord and brain stem nuclei. The relationship between these projections and neck-head-eye movements, eye-head-neck control, and coordinated movements has also not been explored. To begin to answer these queries, literature will first be reviewed, after which new research data will be presented to provide a basis for undertsanding the neural connections and interactions of eye-head-neck afferentation-efferentation.

LITERATURE REVIEW

There have been many studies of the central projections of spinal dorsal root fibers. However, the majority of these investigations have utilized the Marchi method(29–37), which stains only the degenerating fragments of myelin. The major drawback of this method is that by definition it cannot show the terminals of fibers, which are generally unmyelinated, nor can it demonstrate degenerating unmyelinated fibers.

More recent studies of dorsal root fibers(38–43) using silver staining methods have provided new data concerning (1) the distribution of these fibers in the spinal gray, and (2) their mode and patterns of termination in medullary nuclei. Most investigations utilizing the Nauta staining method can be used for unmyelinated as well as myelinated fibers. The method shows degeneration as far as the preterminal axon and perhaps as far as the synaptic bouton. Studies have been done on the cat and have been based upon sections of a limited number of dorsal roots in restricted regions of the spinal cord. A notable exception is Liu's(44) study of the dorsal root afferents to the dorsal and accessory cuneate nuclei in the cat. In addition to the spinal afferents mentioned above, there are a few dorsal root fibers of the upper cervical roots that appear to terminate in the vestibular nuclei (nucleus X) of different animal species such as cat, rabbit, and monkey(33–35, 37). The number of these fibers appears to be scanty as shown by the fact that they have been missed in the Nauta study applied on squirrel monkeys(45).

Other studies have looked at projections into the spinal gray and lesions of the spinal gray itself in an attempt to understand the anatomy of the upper cervical area(46–51).

More recently, Bakker et al(52) examined the central projections of suboccipital muscle nerves following four hours of exposure of cut peripheral nerves to the tracer horseradish peroxidase (HRP). Labeled fibers entered the C1 and C2 dorsal roots and ramified extensively throughout medial parts of the intermediate laminae, in and around the central cervical nucleus. Labeled fibers also projected toward the ventral horn. In cats subjected to ventral root section at the time of peripheral nerve exposure, a modest distribution of reaction product was observed deep in the ventral horn. In cats that did not undergo ventral root section, anterograde projections in the ventral horn were obscured by the simultaneous retrograde filling of motoneurons both in the ventromedial nucleus and on the medial and lateral borders of the gray matter. Labeled axons also coursed rostrally into the medulla where they formed a circumscribed bundle between the main cuneate nucleus and the spinal nucleus of V. Three consistent regions of HRP deposition could be identified at medullary levels. Dense accumulations of reaction product were present in circumscribed regions of the external cuneate nucleus throughout its rostrocaudal extent. A second zone of dense labeling occurred in the intermediate nucleus of Cajal, where it appeared to form a continuing column rostral to the central cervical nucleus in C1–C3. Sparse labeling was restricted to a third zone in the ventrolateral part of the main cuneate nucleus. Because of the short time of exposure, the labeling of the spinal and medullary nuclei is limited.

It is easy to see the lack of a precise assessment in the upper cervical ara. Some studies have assessed lesions to the cervical nerves, others have used the Nauta method and horseradish peroxidase.

The purpose of my research(25) of the spinal dorsal root of C2 in the monkey was to determine (1) the direct connections of the peripheral fibers within the spinal cord and (2) the projection and patterns of termination of ascending fibers in the medullary relay nuclei.

MATERIALS AND METHODS

Anterograde Tracer Methods

Experiments were performed on 3 adult Macaca Irus monkeys that were anesthetized with sodium pentobarbital and nembutal (30 mg/kg i.p.). All surgical procedures were carried out in a stereotactic apparatus using aseptic precautions. The right dorsal ganglion of C2 was exposed, and all injections were made using a glass micropipette with a tip diameter of 30–70 μm, which was attached to a microsyringe (10 μl) via polyethylene tubing. This micropipette was driven by a Sage syringe pump No. 341. The micropipette contained a solution of [^{3}H]leucine at a concentration of 37.5 μci/μl and a volume of μ1. Using a dissecting microscope, the end of the micropipette was broken off with forceps and the tip was introduced into the ganglion. The μ1 was injected over a period of 30 minutes.

The wound was then closed in layers and an antibiotic coverage (125 mg Ampicillin) was administered. The animal was permitted to survive for 45 hours, and following induction of euthanasia with sodium pentobarbital, the monkeys were perfused with an initial washing solution of 6% dextran followed by 10% buffered formaldehyde solution. Brains and spinal cords were removed, and the spinal cord was sectioned into respective segments from C3–L7 and C2. The brainstem and portions of the cerebellum were left as a unit and all were postfixed in 10% buffered formaldehyde solution. The brainstem and spinal segments of each animal were blocked in paraffin and transversely sectioned at 10 μm. Every third section was histologically processed according to the autoradiographic technique of Cowan et al(53), with modifications (methodology of Dr. D. Schwarz's lab). Silver grain distribution was examined in light- and darkfield and mapped onto enlarged cross-sectional drawings.

RESULTS

The cytoarchitectonic atlas of Rexed(54) and his nomenclature for cell groups of the spinal cord have been used in describing the anterograde tracer results from C2 dorsal root ganglion. While it is realized that these studies are based on the cat, there appears to be a fairly close general correspondence for the monkey. The use of Rexed's terminology also provides a basis for more precise description. The diagrams of the medullary area comprised a composite taken from these studies(55–59).

From Fig. 3.11, which shows the extent of the labeling in the spinal cord, the following major locations will be discussed:

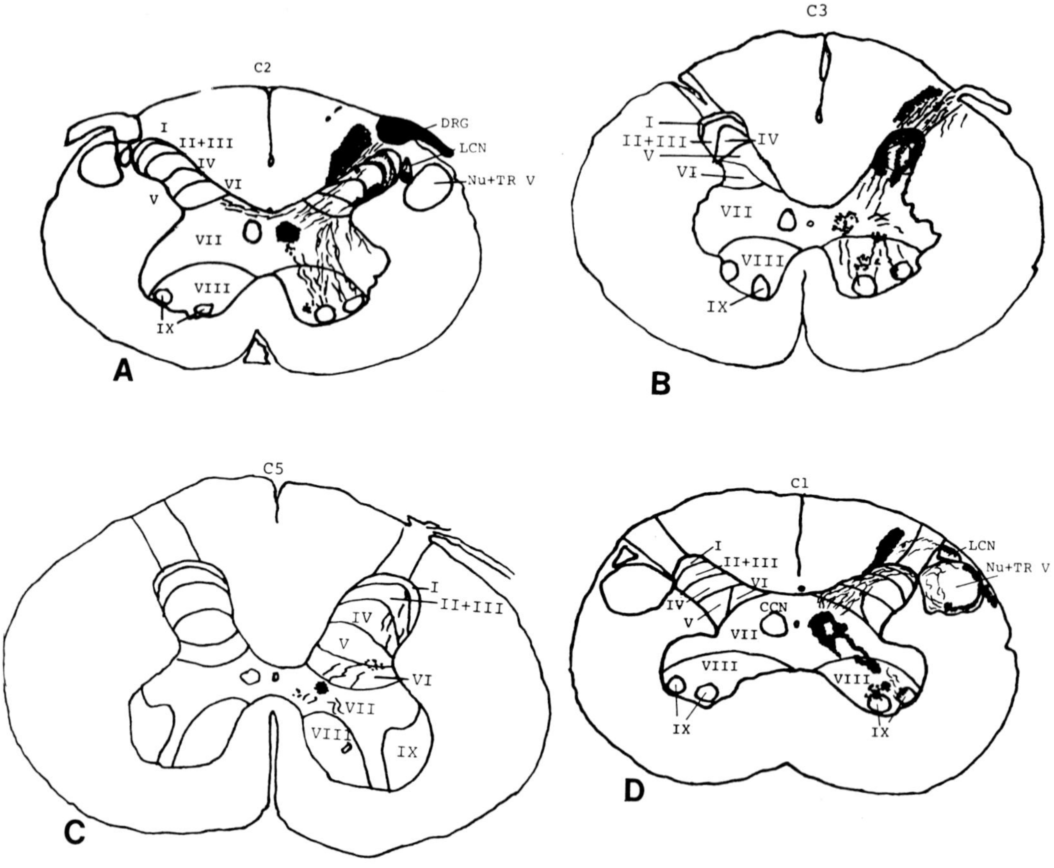

Figure 3.11. **A.** C2 injection level. **B.** Fibers from C2 into C3. **C.** Fibers from C2 into C5. **D.** Fibers from C2 into C1. (Adapted from Fitz-Ritson D. The direct connections of the C2 dorsal root ganglia in the Macaca Irus monkey: relevance to chiropractic therapautics. J Manipulative Physiol Ther 1985;8(3):147–156.

3.11A—C2 injection level

Labeling is seen in the

1. lateral cervical nucleus
2. fasciculus cuneatus
3. laminae II, IV
4. central cervical nucleus in lamina VII

Moving first caudally, labeling is seen in

3.11B—C3

1. fasciculus cuneatus
2. laminae I, II, III, and V
3. central cervical nucleus, lamina VII

3.11C—C5

1. lamina V
2. central cervical nucleus, lamina VIII

Then, moving cephalad, labeling is seen in

3.11D—C1

1. lateral cervical nucleus
2. fasciculus cuneatus
3. lateral aspect of the nucleus and tract of (Cn V) trigeminal
4. central cervical nucleus, lamina VII

C1—Medulla Junction (Fig. 3.12)

1. fasciculus cuneatus
2. anterior portion of the cuneatus nucleus
3. lateral portion of the nucleus traction solitarius

Caudal Medulla (Fig. 3.13)

1. anterior pole of the lateral cuneatus nucleus
2. interior cerebellar peduncle
3. anterior and lateral portions of the cuneatus nucleus
4. nucleus and tract of trigeminal (CnV)
5. anterior portion of the nucleus tractus solitarius
6. a fiber bundle dorsal to CnXII.

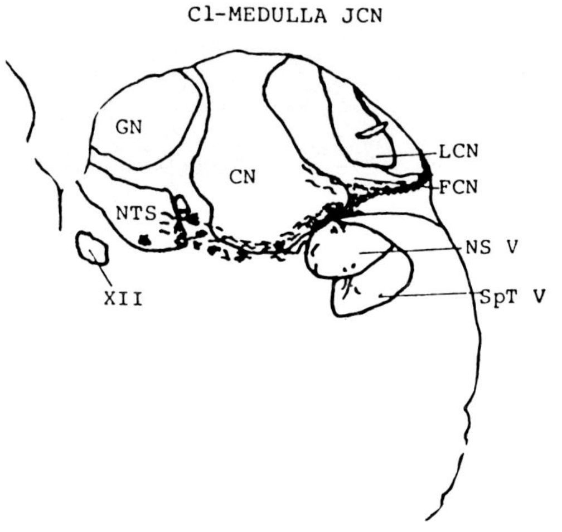

Figure 3.12. Section at C1-medullary junction. Adapted from Fitz-Ritson D. The direct connections of the C2 dorsal root ganglia in the Macaca Irus monkey: relevance to chiropractic therapeutics. J Maniuplative Phsyiol Ther 1985;8(3):147–156.

Medulla (Fig. 3.14)

1. anterior lateral portions of the lateral cuneatus nucleus
2. anterior portions of the nucleus cuneatus
3. nucleus intercalatus

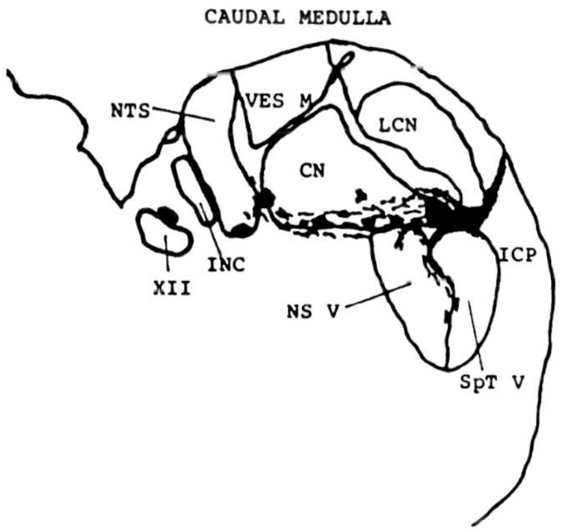

Figure 3.13. Section at the caudal medulla. Adapted from Fitz-Ritson D. The direct connections of the C2 dorsal root ganglia in the Macaca Irus monkey: relevance to chiropractic therapeutics. J Manipulative Physiol Ther 1985;8(3):147–156.

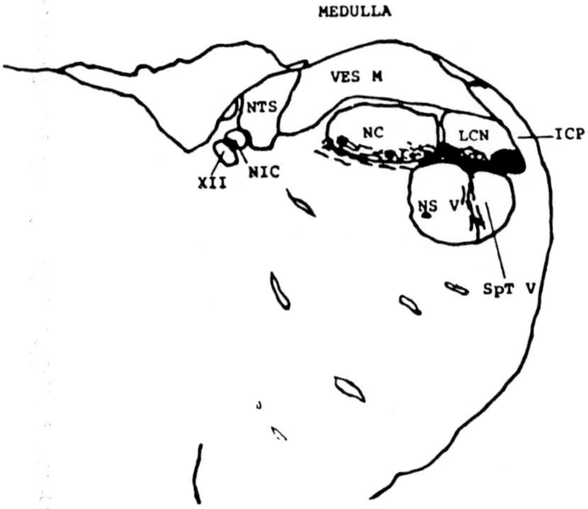

Figure 3.14. Medullary section showing nucleus cuneatus, and lateral cuneatus nucleus. Adapted from Fitz-Ritson D. The direct connections of the C2 dorsal root ganglia in the Macaca Irus monkey: relevance to chiropractic therapeutics. J Manipulative Physiol Ther 1985;8(3):147–156.

Medulla (Fig. 3.15)

1. anterior pole of the lateral cervical nucleus
2. nucleus and tract of trigeminal (CnV)
3. dorsal and lateral portions of the cuneatus nucleus
4. anterior portions of the medial vestibular nucleus

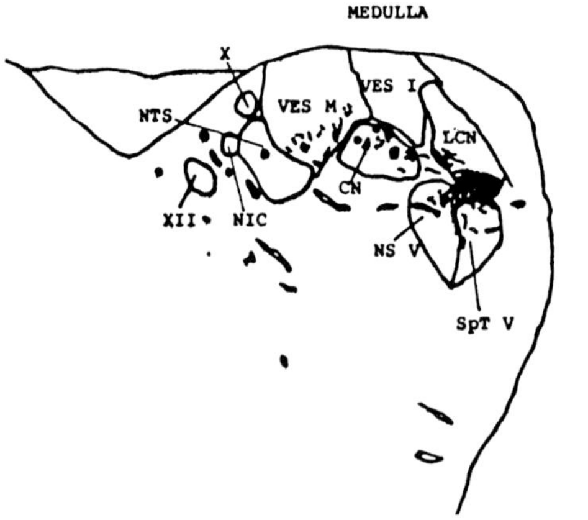

Figure 3.15. Medullary section showing medial vestibular nucleus. Adapted from Fitz-Ritson D. The direct connections of the C2 dorsal root ganglia in the Macaca Irus monkey: relevance to chiropractic therapeutics. J Manipulative Physiol Ther 1985;8(3):147–156.

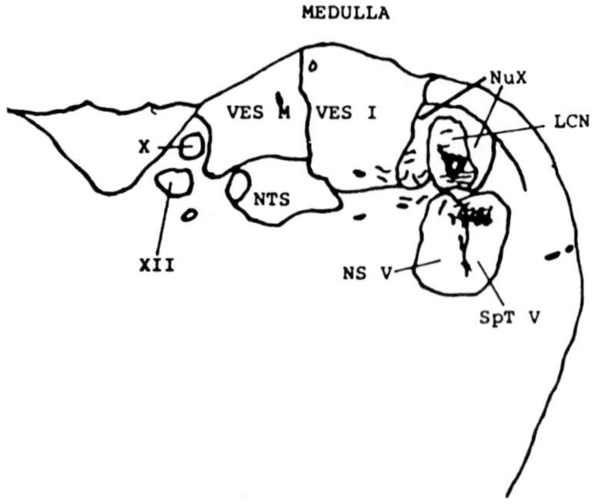

Figure 3.16. Medullary sections showing lateral cuneatus nucleus. Adapted from Fitz-Ritson D. The direct connections of the C2 dorsal root ganglia in the Macaca Irus monkey: relevance to chiropractic therapeutics. J Manipulative Physiol Ther 1985;8(3):147–156.

Medulla (Fig. 3.16)

1. lateral cuneatus nucleus
2. nucleus and tract of trigeminal (CnV)

Rostral Medulla (Fig. 3.17)

1. nucleus X of the vestibular system.

At the level of injection, labeling was seen in the lateral part of the fasciculus

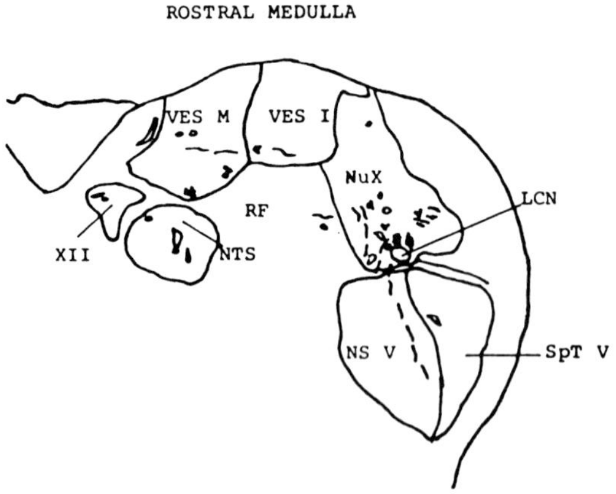

Figure 3.17. Section of rostral medulla. Adapted from Fitz-Ritson D. The direct connections of the C2 dorsal root ganglia in the Macaca Irus monkey: relevance to chiropractic therapeutics. J Maniuplative Physiol Ther 1985;8(3):147–156.

cuneatus from which site part of the fibers traversed lamina II and terminated primarily in the lateral regions of lamina IV (Fig. 3.11*A*). A bundle of fibers traversed central parts of laminae V and VI to arborize profusely about large cells of the central cervical nucleus, which projected caudally to C5 (Fig. 3.11*C*). Descending C2 root fibers in the lateral part of the fasciculus cuneatus could be found at C3 but not more caudal segments. Root fibers arborized extensively about cores of the central cervical nucleus at C3, C4, and C5 levels.

In the C1 segments (Fig. 3.11*D*), the distribution and amount of ascending C2 root fibers were less in the fasciculus cuneatus and not present in lamina IV, but more extensive arborization was seen in the central cervical nucleus. Ascending fiber tracts passed to the lateral cuneatus nucleus, cuneatus nucleus, nucleus tractus solitarius (Fig. 3.13), nucleus and tract of trigeminal, nucleus intercalatus (Fig. 3.14), and nucleus X of the vestibular system (Fig. 3.17).

Figure 3.18 shows a comprehensive diagram of the direct connections of the C2 dorsal root ganglion.

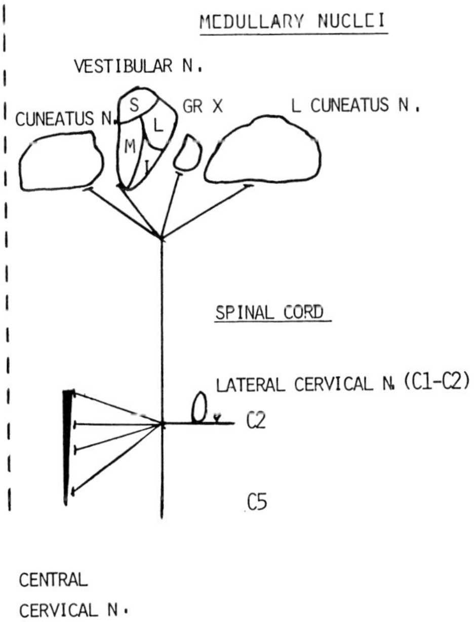

Figure 3.18. Direct connections of C2 dorsal root ganglion.

DISCUSSION

This study provides data for the Macaca Irus monkey concerning the distribution and termination of fibers from the C2 dorsal root ganglion. With the injection into the ganglion, we may be assessing only peripheral input into the spinal cord and brainstem nuclei.

Spinal Projections

Fiber projections to the spinal gray: The local distribution of labeling fibers from the C2 dorsal root ganglion appear similar to that described in the cat following the section of selected individual dorsal roots(43). At the level of injection, fibers occupy the root entry zone and most of the part of the posterior funiculus (Fig. 3.11*A*). From this site, dorsal root fibers enter the posterior horn by traversing the medial portions of, or by coursing medially around, laminae II to IV (i.e., nucleus proprius(43, 60).

A small number of labeled fibers in the lateral portions of laminae V and VI is notable both in the cat and monkey. From portions of laminae VI and VII, fibers pass ventrally to lamina VIII to reach cell groups in lamina IX(58).

The posterior horn in the upper cervical region (i.e., C1 to C2) merits special consideration because portions of it contain the nucleus caudalis of the spinal trigeminal nucleus. According to Olszewski(61) and Torvik(38), the nucleus caudalis has the same fundamental cellular arrangement as the head of the posterior horn—substantia gelatinosa (lamina I). Torvik(38) found that the C2 and C3 dorsal roots projected fibers into the substantia gelatinosa and the nucleus proprius at these levels, but none entered the posterior horn at C1. This study showed labeled cells in the nucleus and tract of trigeminal at C1 but not at C2, the level of injection. Lamina VII contains the central cervical nucleus. Afferent fibers to this nucleus are derived chiefly from the upper five cervical dorsal roots, and the extent of the nucleus was verified as C1 to C5 (Fig. 3.11, *A–D*).

Lamina IX

In the present study, the C2 dorsal root projected fibers to the motor neurons of the anterior horn at the level of root entry, and in adjacent spinal segments, these findings are similar to those reported(35, 41, 44, 62). In all animals, the amount of labeled fibers in lamina IX was greater in the C2 injection segment.

These findings disagree with those of Ranson et al(31) and Corbin and Hinsey(33), indicating that fibers from the upper three cervical dorsal roots do not descend more than two segments, but agree with those of Corbin et al(34), Yee and Corbin(35), and Liu(44), who reported that fibers of C1 and C2 dorsal roots extend caudally for three segments and those of C3 for three to four segments.

Lateral Cervical Nucleus

Rexed(63) was the first author to describe and name this nuleus. The nucleus is located at C1–C2 levels, ventrolateral to the dorsal horn. It receives afferents from lower levels of the spinal cord and sends its fibers to the cerebellum. Brodal and Rexed(64), in a detailed study, showed that spinal afferents from all levels of the cord terminate within the nucleus and all belong to the gray matter. The nucleus projects fibers to the cerebellum. Other authors(65–67) have shown the nucleus but at a more rostral level forming a band medial to the C1 fibers.

The above results have been verified additionally(68–70), and the following features of the lateral cervical nucleus (LCN) have been defined: (1) It receives afferents from ipsilateral Clarke's nucleus. (2) It receives afferents from the ventral spinocerebellar tact. (3) The limbs are more prominently represented. (4) Cats, dogs, and racoons are anatomically and physiologically similar. More recent studies in monkeys and humans have shown that 90% of the LCN cells project to the thalamus, while up to 45% send axons to the tectum(71).

Boivie(68), using monkeys, investigated the projection of the LCN using lesions. The cervicothalamic fibers cross the midline and ascent to the thalamus via the medial lemniscus tract to the posterior nuclear group (PNG) and ventral posterior lateral (VPL) nuclei of the thalamus. The lateral cervical nucleus (LCN) receives its ascending afferent input via the spinocervical tract (SCT), and the predominant source of activation for spinocervical tract neurons as well as for LCN cells are low threshold cutaneous mechanoreceptors. The present study showed the location of the LCN C3–C1 spinal levels (Fig. 3.11, *A–D*) with terminal labeling.

Central Cervical Nucleus

Several previous anatomical and physiological studies have shown that the central cervical nucleus (CCN) is a major source of spinocerebellar afferents(72–76). It has also been shown that the CCN receives primary afferent fibers of the cervical spinal nerves(77, 78) and from the trigeminal nerve(52,79). Recent studies also have demonstrated lower spinal cord and vestibular projections to the CCN(78, 80). More recently, it has been shown that the cervical primary afferents terminate heavily in the region of the CCN cerebellar projection neurons. Electron miroscopic findings demonstrate that primary afferent fibers of cervical dorsal roots synapse mainly with distal dendrites of CCN neurons projecting to the cerebellum(81).

Afferent fibers from superficial and deep (suboccipital) muscles project to the central cervical nucleus. However, electrophysiological evidence suggests that the projections from deep and superficial muscles may be organized differently in the CCN. Hirai and colleagues(82) have shown that potent short-latency excitation is evoked in spinocerebellar cells of the CCN when electrical stimuli are applied to upper cervical dorsal roots or soft tissues (capsules)(83) close to the vertebrae, but few short latency responses can be demonstrated by the stimulation of dorsal nerve rami supplying superficial neck muscles.

Medullary Projections

Lateral Cuneatus Nucleus

This nucleus is considered to be the medullary equivalent of the dorsal nucleus of

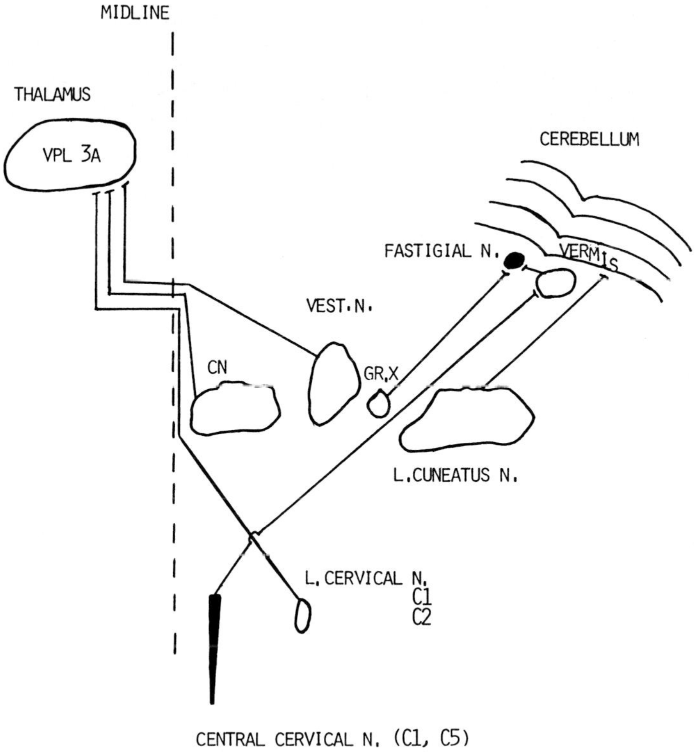

Figure 3.19. Spinal and medullary nuclei connections.

Clarke(32). Dorsal roots C1 through T7 project fibers to the lateral cuneate nucleus, also shown from C2 of the present study (Figs. 3.13–3.16). Clasically, the cuneocerebellar tract is considered to be related primarily to the upper extremity and neck, while the posterior spinocerebellar tract is considered to be related primarily to the lower extremity and trunk(84).

Shriver et al(58) showed that C5–C7 dorsal roots project to both the lateral cuneate and basal nuclei, while C1–C4 dorsal roots supply only the lateral cuneate nucleus.

According to Torvik(38) who used rats, fibers from the upper three cervical dorsal roots terminate in the most ventral and lateral parts of the lateral cuneate nucleus. In addition, Shriver et al(58) noted that the number of fibers projected to this nucleus is related to the level of the dorsal root.

Nucleus Cuneatus

All three dorsal roots of C2 studied in this series projected fibers to specific parts of the cuneate nucleus (Figs. 3.12–3.15). Carpenter(85) showed that dorsal roots T8 and L1 project a small number of fibers to this nucleus. Cervical root projections to the cuneate nucleus have been reported from levels as low as T8 in the rhesus monkey(86).

The most detailed analysis of dorsal root projections to the cuneate nucleus was made by Kuypers and Tuerk(87). Using the Nauta technique in the cat, dorsal rhizotomies of C2–C3, C7–C8, and T12 were analyzed. These authors found that degeneration from C2–C3 dorsal roots in caudal parts of the nucleus cuneatus was dense ventrolaterally and diffuse in the base of the nucleus.

Shriver et al(58) showed that fibers from C1 dorsal root are located most ventrolaterally in the rostral two-thirds of the nucleus. Fibers of the C2 dorsal root occupy the ventrolateral border of the caudal third of the nucleus.

Thoracic dorsal roots terminate in an orderly sequence in both exclusive and overlapping zones. Also fibers from T2–T7 are less numerous and exhibit more overlap.

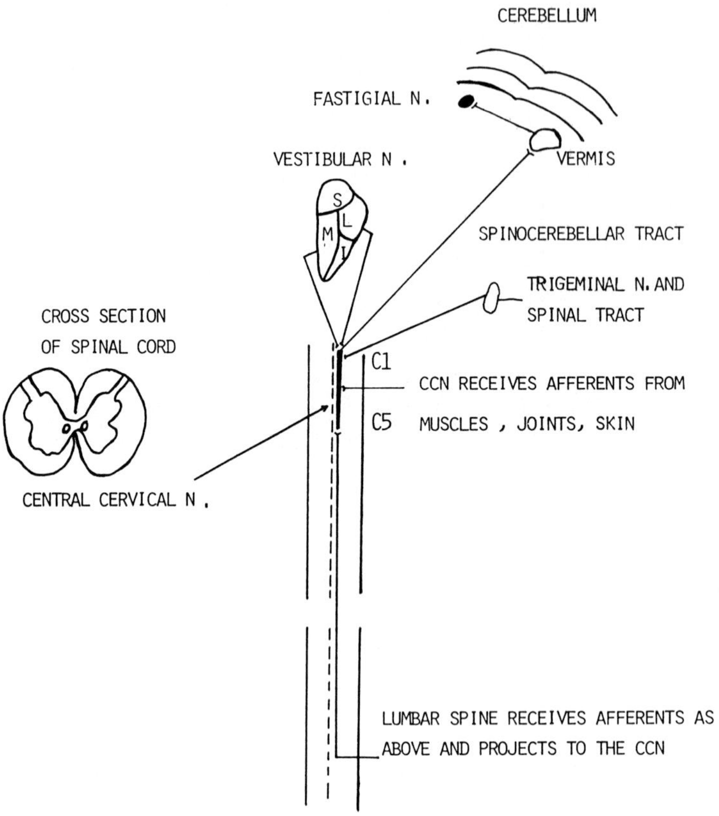

Figure 3.20. Connections with the central cervical nuculus (CCN).

Other Medullary Nuclei

Several authors have reported that ascending fibers from upper cervical dorsal roots project to the nucleus and tractus solitarius(31, 33, 35, 38, 44). This was shown as a weak projection in this study (Figs. 3.12 and 3.13). The nucleus intercalatus(38) was also shown in this study (Fig. 3.14). It is possible that the projection via this route is affected either by the small number of fibers or by a slower uptake of the isotope by the fibers. There is a distinct tract (Fig. 3.13) which projects to the caudal pole of the nucleus intercalatus (Fig. 3.12), but it is not evident in Figure 3.15.

Vestibular Nucleus

Group X Nucleus

Labeled terminals were also seen in the group X nucleus. Brodal(88) described the nucleus as a small aggregation of cells lateral to the caudal part of the inferior vestibular nucleus and rostral to the accessory cuneate nucleus. This cell group (nucleus) has been considered by some as part of the inferior vestibular nucleus(89). Spinovestibular afferents to this nucleus course with fibers of the posterior spinocerebellar tract. In the present study, nucleus X was drawn using cell size differences of the inferior vestibular and lateral cuneate nuclei. Figure 3.17 shows the labeling in the ventral region above the rostral tip of the lateral cuneate nucleus. This suggests that there is a direct pathway from the periphery via the C2 dorsal root to group (nucleus) X.

Anatomical studies have demonstrated a spinal dorsolateral fascicle input to X. High spinal lesions cause massive terminal degeneration(90, 91). Fibers from the levels of L4 or caudal to it again project both to the dorsolateral part of X(90) and to its dorsocaudal portion(91).

Hand(42) described a massive degeneration in X following transection of dorsal roots L6–S1 but did not specify its distribution within the nucleus. Johansson and Silfvenius(92) suggest that neurons in the rostral main cuneate nucleus (MCN) and in the region of the descending vestibular nucleus and the nucleus (DV-X) receive and relay information from ipsilateral hind limb group I muscle afferents and from cutaneous fibers of low electrical threshold. Such an organization is perhaps unexpected but may be homologous with the organization in the forelimb bulbar nuclei in the cat, where the MCN, the external lateral cuneate nucleus ECN, and neurons in the cervical cord are monosynaptically activated by spinal forelimb group I muscle afferents.

On the basis of anatomically defined connections, Brodal(88), suggested that nucleus X, which does not receive primary vestibular fibers, is a spinocerebellar relay nucleus that relays information both to the cerebellum (bilateral to the fastigial nuclei and ipsilateral to the flocculus and to the contralateral medial longitudinal fasciculus). The fastigial nuclei project fibers directly to the vestibular system, thus, there is a circuit: cervical spine-nucleus X,-fastigial nuclei of cerebellum-vestibular nuclei.

Johansson and Silfvenius(92) suggest that the DV-X could function as a correlator of precise motor acts in the ipsilateral hind limb and neck muscles, as there is anatomical evidence for a massive input to nucleus X from high spinal levels and physiological evidence for a neck input both to the anterior cerebellar lobe, from which antidromic activation was obtained in some DV-X cells, and to the flocculus onto which the nucleus X projects(88). Converging information from those afferents could be relayed to the vestibular part of the cerebellum, which could utilize it for descending control of posture, limb position, and cephalad for eye movement control. Fitz-Ritson(93) has reviewed all of the major descending tracts to and the major ascending tracts from the cervical spine. This helps one to appreciate the importance of the cervical area.

SUMMARY

The following is a review with special attention paid to the pathways and the information that initiates the coordinated movement of eye-head-neck mechanism.

Figure 3.21 is a summary of the afferents into the CNS. The joint and the muscle afferents project directly into the central cervical nucleus CCN. This nucleus projects directly to the cerebellum as outlined previously, the joint and muscle afferents project to other brainstem nuclei such as the vestibular and cuneatus nuclei, while muscle afferents project to the lateral cuneatus nuclei and joint afferents project to the group X nucleus *(vestibular N.)*

Figure 3.22 shows the direct connections into the group X nucleus and from this nucleus, into the fastigial nucleus and flocculus of the cerebellum.

If we assess the joint afferent input to the CNS, it will give us some understanding of a possible route for the sensation of vertebrogenic vertigo from which the patient may be alleviated after the chiropratic adjustment.

Using cats and stimulating the C2 dorsal root and the atlantoxial joint, Wilson et al(94) found that neck activity arises, at least in part, in joint receptors and that the relay is located principally in the group X nucleus of the vestibular nuclei. The results provide further evidence that impulses in neck afferents reach the flocculus by a mossy fiber (MF) route in addition to the climbing fiber (CF) pathway described previously. The pathway from neck to flocculus via the group X nucleus is quite specific. Input from neck receptors is ipsilateral and there is no obvious interaction at the brainstem level between neck and either forelimb or labyrinthine impulses.

Neck-evoked activity may, however, interact less directly with other inputs at the level of group X. This group of cells receives fibers from both the vestibulocerebellum, at least from the nodulus and uvula, and from the fastigial nucleus.

Figure 3.23 shows efferents from the fastigial nucleus. The fastigiospinal fibers arise from cells in all parts of the fastigial nucleus of the cerebellum. They cross the midline and synapse on neurons in the upper cervical (C1–C4) levels. These projection fibers are activated by labyrinthine and somatic stimuli(95–98).

Figure 3.24 shows that the fastigial nucleus and the flocculus also send projection

AFFERENTS	SPINAL CORD	BRAIN STEM N.	OTHER AREA
PAIN (LOW GRADE CUTANEOUS MECHANORECEPTORS)	LATERAL CERVICAL N.		THALAMUS (VPL)
	LAMINAE I, IV, V	ANTEROLATERAL TRACT	THALAMUS (VPL)
JOINTS			
JOINTS	CENTRAL CERVICAL N. (VIA SPINOCEREBELLAR TRACT)		CEREBELLUM
		VESTIBULAR N.	THALAMUS
		CUNEATUS N.	THALAMUS
		GR. X N. (VEST.N.)	CEREBELLUM
MUSCLES (IA, IB)	CENTRAL CERVICAL N. (VIA SPINOCEREBELLAR TRACT)		CEREBELLUM
		LATERAL CUNEATUS N.	CEREBELLUM
		VESTIBULAR N.	THALAMUS (3A)
(MINOR)		CUNEATUS N.	THALAMUS

Figure 3.21. Summary of afferents into the CNS.

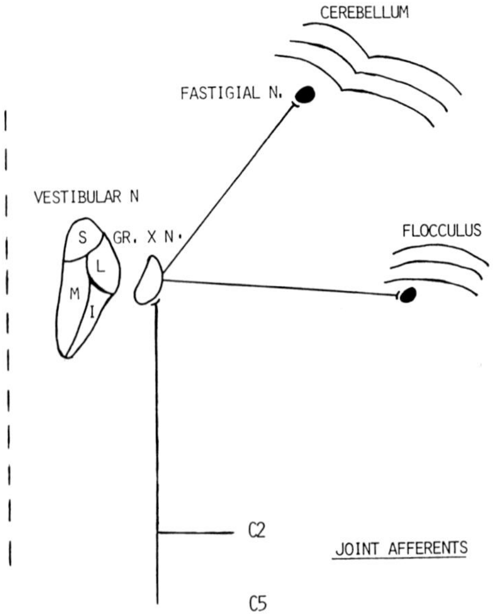

Figure 3.22. Joint afferents to cerebellum via group X nucleus.

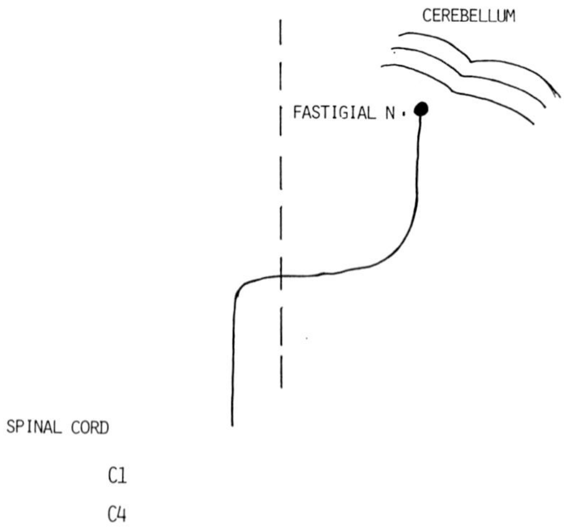

Figure 3.23. Cerebellar projections to the cervical spine.

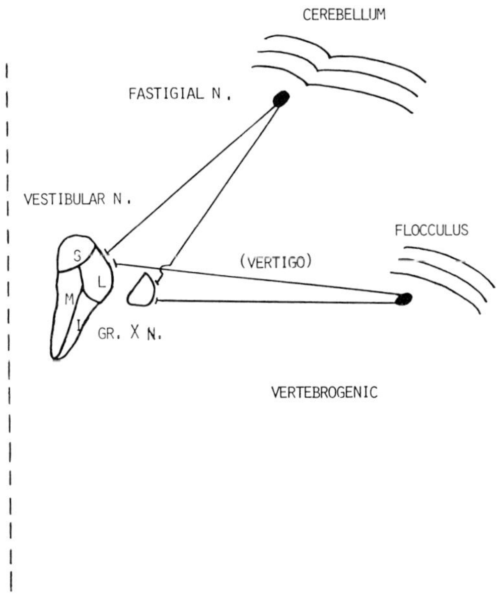

Figure 3.24. Cerebellum interactions with the vestibular and group X nuclei.

fibers to both the lateral vestibular and group X nuclei. It is via this pathway of group X nucleus to flocculus that, if there is a mismatch of normal afferentation from the joints, the sensation of vertigo is experienced. The cerebellum, because of its function to fine-tune movement, responds to this sensation. Via the fastigial nucleus and flocculus, it excites the lateral vestibular nucleus, which, being excitatory to extensor paraspinal muscles, increases the tone in the cervical spine (and the rest of the spine). This provides more stability in the area, thus helping to decrease the vertigo from the abnormal head-neck movements.

Second Order Connections: Eye Movements

The vestibular nuclei not only receive afferents from the cerebellum and respond by helping to control the cervical spine, but they also receive and send information to a number of brainstem nuclei as shown in

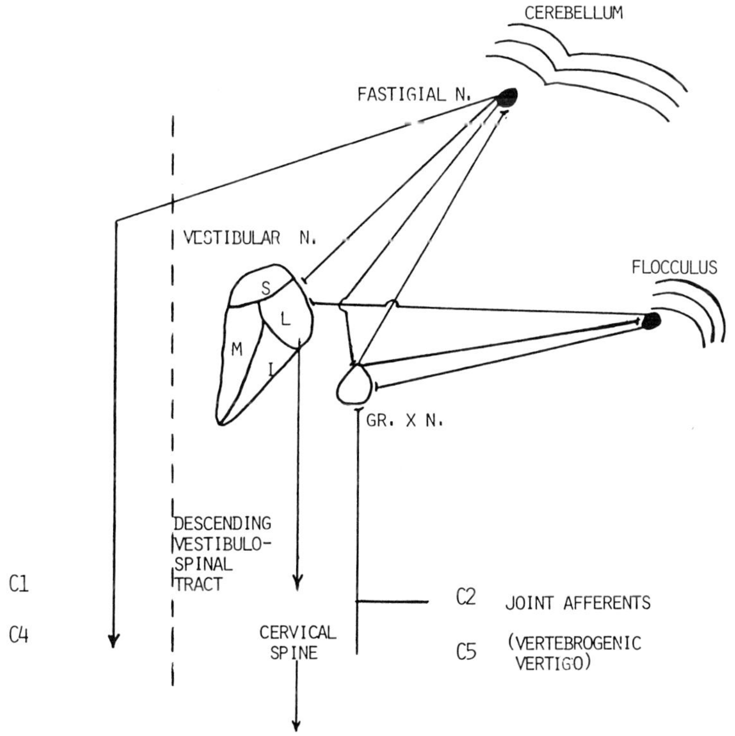

Figure 3.25. Cervical joints, group X nucleus, cerebellum, vestibular nucleus, and cervical area interactions.

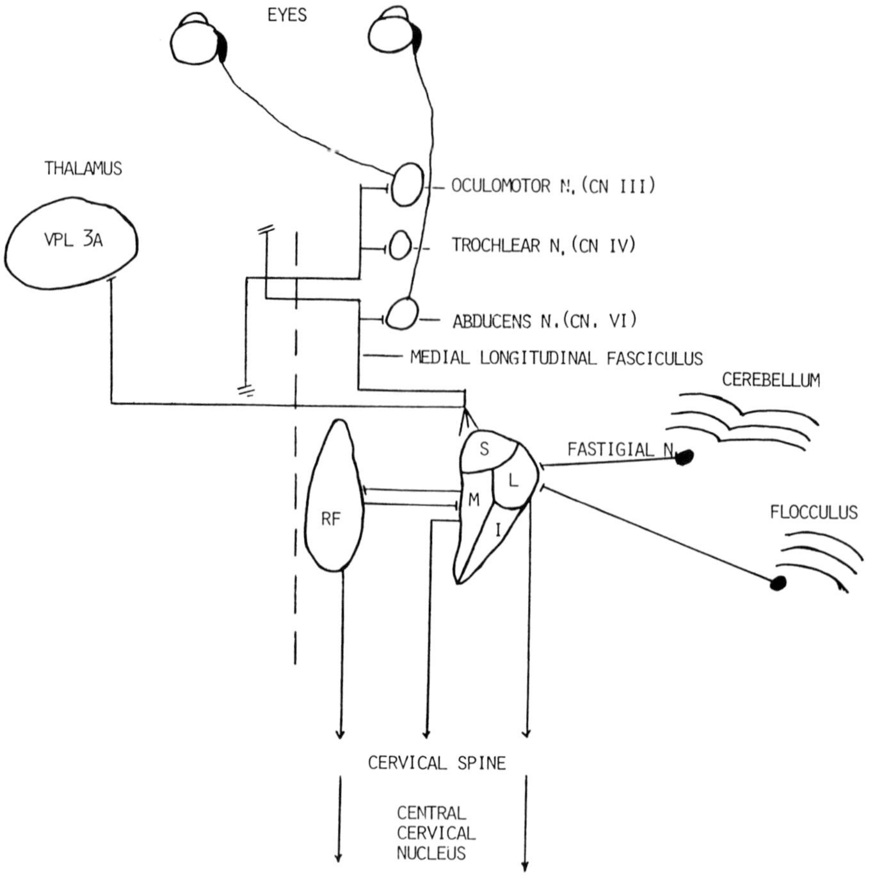

Figure 3.26. Vestibular nuclei connections.

Figures 3.26 and 3.27. Note that the vestibular nuclei via the cranial nuclei (Abducens VI, Trochlear IV, Oculomotor III) have a potent effect on the movement of the eyes.

Shaw and Baker,(99) have demonstrated monosynaptic projections to facial motoneurons from both vestibular and trigeminal nuclei. The trigeminal inputs exerted powerful excitory effects of facial motoneurons with fast rise time and large amplitude. The trigeminal input to the facial nucleus, being much stronger than the vestibular, is likely to be involved in facial reflexes, especially blinking and grimacing, which are known to be mediated via trigeminal input.

The influence of vestibular afferents on facial motoneurons activity is clearly much less than that of trigeminal afferents, as is found in abducens motoneurons that are also involved in the blink response. The vestibular activity affects dramatically the synaptic effect by providing a high background firing rate.

The secondary vestibular axons that project to both oculomotor and facial nuclei carry activity relating to head and eye movement. Inputs to neck muscles, probably from these same vestibular neurons, are also known to carry eye position-related activity(100). Thus, the most likely role for the vestibular projections to facial motoneurons is the coordination of facial movements with eye and head movements in an integrated orientation response. The vestibular nucleus is surely not the only structure involved in such coordination. The superior colliculus also projects to oculomotor, facial, and cervical nuclei. Cells in and around the oculomotor complex may also participate in such coordination, being also premotor to facial and oculomotor

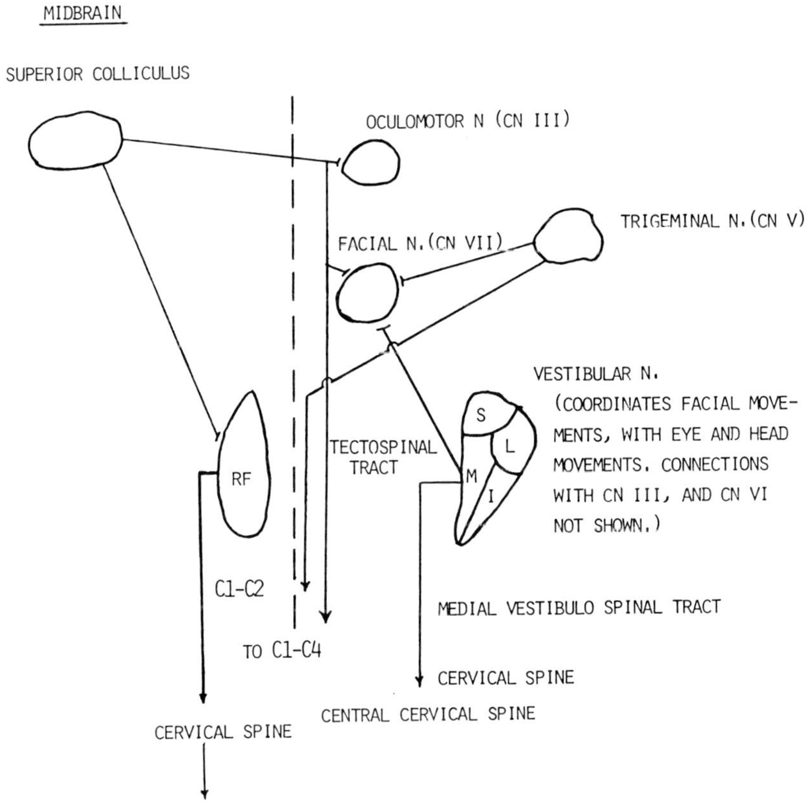

Figure 3.27. Connections of the superior colliculus.

nuclei and the cervical spinal cord(100). Also, the superior colliculus in the midbrain, via its projection to the oculomotor nuclei (CN III), has an effect on the movement of the eyes in relation to the cervical spine. Because the tectospinal tracts, (originated from the superior colliculus in the midbrain) cross at that level, they project only to the cervical spine, with the majority terminating in the upper four cervical spinal segments. The tracts mediate reflexes in postural movements in response to visual and auditory stimull.

Figure 3.28 shows an integrated schemata of the connections of the vestibular nuclei and other pertinent areas of the CNS in their relationship to the control of the eyes with that of the cervical spine.

I have covered some of the basic pathways and major nuclei and areas in the spinal cord, brainstem, and CNS that receive cervical afferents and have some affect on the control of the eyes. The central question is: Do the eyes and their control mechanism have any effect on the cervical spine? The following is a brief review of the eye-head-neck interactions.

Neural Mechanisms Involved in the Control of Eye-Head-Neck Movements

Head motion plays an important role in gaze and in the interaction between eye and head movements involving both their shared role in direction gaze and the compensatory vestibular ocular reflex. Coordinated gaze movements normally have an initial eye-in-orbit saccade onto the target followed by a synkinetic and much slower head movement. At the level of EMG signal latencies, these are synchronous; but because the viscoinertial dynamics of head and neck muscles are different from the viscoelastic dynamics of eye and extraocular muscles, the saccade is over before head position has changed. The vestibular oc-

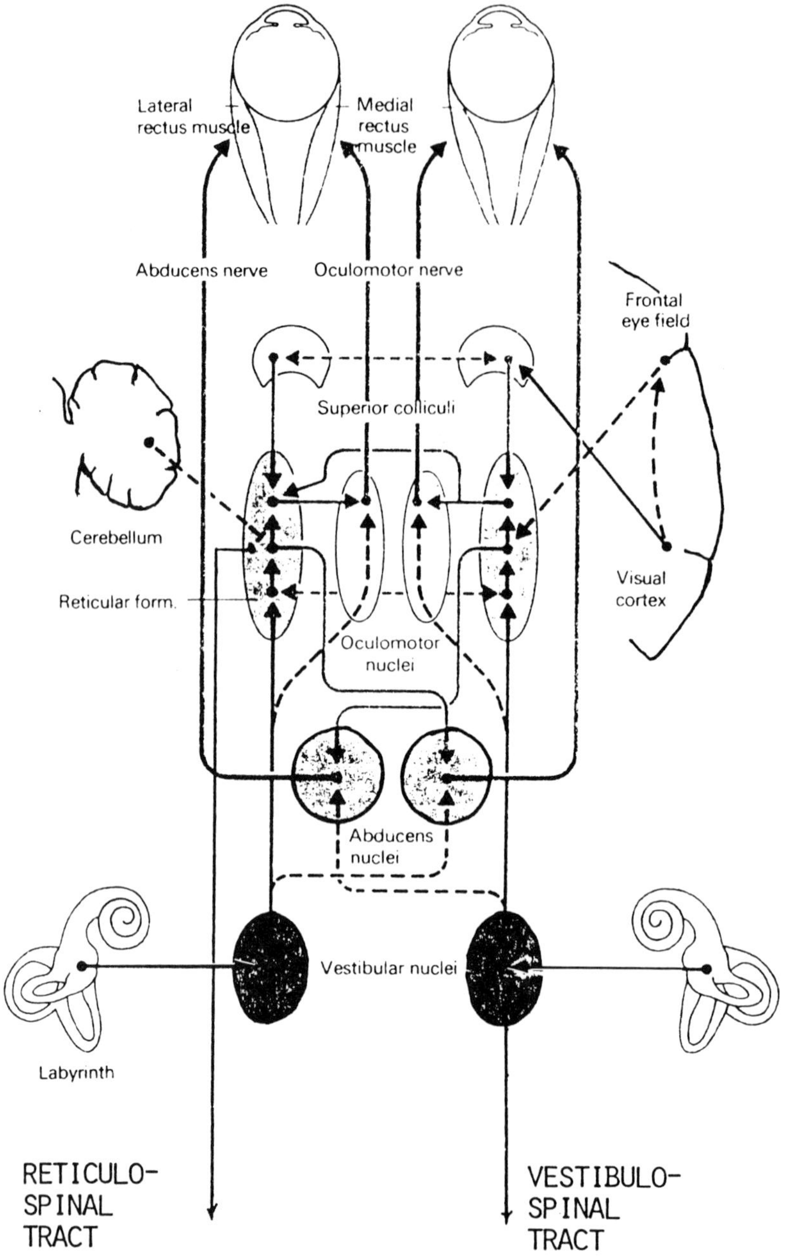

Figure 3.28. Nuclei involved in the coordination of eye movements and the cervical spine. Modified from Schmidt R. Ed. Fundamentals of sensory phsyiology. New York: Springer-Verlag, 1981, p. 174.

cular reflex (VOR) generated by head acceleration drives the compensatory eye movement (CEM), eye in orbit, in the opposite direction so that gaze, eye in space, remains on target. The CEM and its VOR component are influenced by visual input and other factors that modify gain: resultant overshoots or undershoots are corrected by later saccades(102). For more detail on what follows, see Reference 93.

Biguer et al(103) evaluated the time occurrence of eye, head, and arm movements directed at the same visual target in five human subjects. Although the overt movements are sequentially ordered (i.e., eye movement, then head, and finally arm), the EMG discharges are synchronous with respect to the eye movement onset. This is in agreement with the Zangemeister study and indicates a clustering of segmental motor programs for target-oriented actions.

Head movements are synkinetic with eye movements in gaze. Although similar to eye movements in overall properties, head movements show a contribution of stretch reflexes. There are also differences in detailed dynamic features. Electromyograms representing samples of neurological controller signals can be used to predict head rotations, which may be time optimal depending upon a subject's intent. A major property of neurological control signals is reciprocal innervation; both pairs of head-rotating muscles, the splenius capitis and sternocleidomastoideus muscles, demonstrate this. Reciprocally-innervated pairs of horizontal rotating muscles become cocontractors for vertical rotation. Cocontraction, the stretch reflex, fatigue, and supraspinal influences responding to complex stimuli contribute to variance in both EMG signals and head accelerations. Latency studies demonstrate the causal chain from target input to agonistic EMG (200 msec), to head acceleration (20 msec) and initial change in head position (45 msec), and to final head position (240 msec) for 20° head rotations. Antagonistic EMG, obeying reciprocal innervation, begins about 70 msec after agonistic EMG beings(102).

It can be asked whether the termination of movement and the subsequent maintenance of posture depend on a readout of proprioceptive afferent input generated during the movement itself or whether Instead it is centrally programmed. During head movements, the neck proprioceptive apparatus provides a wealth of afferent signals from which tension velocity of contraction, muscle length, and joint position can be extracted. Bizzi et al(104) address these problems by performing bilateral labyrinthectomy 3 months prior to the actual experiment even though Dichgans et al(105) showed that chronically vestibulectomized monkeys recover their ability to perform very effective visually triggered eye-hand movement.

Bizzi and coworkers(106) also utilized cervical rhizotomy (C1–T3) to study the effect of neck proprioceptors during head movements; thus all other sources of afferent input were eliminated. They showed that the final head position is an equilibrium point, dependent in part on centrally programmed patterns of neural activity, and that these patterns are not reset by the afferent proprioceptive impulses generated during the intended movement. However, in the intact animal, in parallel with this basic process, the proprioceptive system participates in the attainment of final position by increasing muscle stiffness when a load disturbance is applied. In fact, any stimulation of the proprioceptive apparatus, by virtue of its reflex connections, will modify the firing rate and the recruitment of alpha motoneurons and will therefore force the selection of a new length-tension curve(106).

The splenius muscle of the cat, a lateral flexor of the head, is subdivided into compartments that are innervated by different spinal nerves(9). This organization is reflected in the behavior of the different compartments during proprioceptive reflexes. The question arises as to how the different splenius compartments are activated by other stimuli. The splenius, in response to horizontal optokinetic stimulation, is known to evoke head movements.

Wilson(107, 108), using three cats, assessed this phenomenon. The results confirmed similar observations made by Vidal(109) that in response to optokinetic stimulation, as during saccades and vestibular nystagmus, the activity of the splenius muscle of the alert cat is closely related to eye position. He further suggested that the descending signals triggered by optokinetic stimuli do not influence the different compartments of splenius differentially, but activate or depress the muscle rather uniformly. The distribution of 1A afferents from the splenius muscle is asymmetric but related to its compartmentalization. Afferents make monosynaptic connections with motoneurons of their own in rostral rather than caudal segments(19). This suggests that there may be, in functional situations, selective reflex activation of rostral parts of the muscles. Recent experiments have in fact shown that cervicocollic reflexes evoked by sinusoidal lateral flexion in the yaw plane are distributed unevenly within the splenius, with its rostral part modulated more strongly and sometimes selectively(9).

Ezure(110) examined the cervicocollic reflex evoked by horizontal rotation of the head of decerebrated labyrinthectomized cats as it related to the splenius muscle. He found that when the cervicocollic reflex (CCR) is evoked by rotation of the head about a vertical axis, the modulation of EMG activity is higher in the rostral rather than the caudal compartments. In some cases, the rostral compartments can be modulated selectively, and if the axis of rotation is shifted caudally, the rostrocaudal gradient of modulation is absent.

In the muscles that had been completely detached from their origin and insertion, the pattern of activation of the CCR was similar to that observed in intact muscle, although the gain of the reflex fell by two-thirds. This strongly suggests that receptors in the splenius muscle make an important contribution to the CCR. Such localization or compartmentalization of activity is a feature of proprioceptive reflexes, but not necessarily of activation of the muscle by other means.

Under normal conditions, gaze is influenced by both eye position within the head and head position in space. When changes in head position are allowed to occur, three additional gaze-stabilizing reflexes must be considered; one of vestibular origin acting on neck muscles to move the head (the vestibulocollic reflex or VCR) and two originating from receptors in the neck and acting on extraocular and neck muscles (the cervicoocular reflex, or COR, and cervicocollic reflex, or CCR). In recent years, vestibular reflex experiments have been extended by investigation of the VCR so that the dynamic properties and neuronal substances of this reflex are now reasonably well understood(109–114). Considerable attention has also been directed to investigation of the COR, leading to the conclusion that this reflex plays a relatively minor role in gaze stability, except possibly at low rotational frequencies despite its relatively direct synaptic connectivity(115, 116).

The CCR has been less well studied. It is basically a neck stretch reflex in which information from neck proprioceptors act back on neck muscles in a negative-feedback fashion to minimize neck rotation. Appropriate anatomic substrates for such a reflex have been identified by Bakker et al(5), Richmond and Abrahams(7.8) and Bakker and Richmond(6).

Corresponding electrophysiological studies have described a monosynaptic reflex in the neck similar to (but weaker than) that in the limb muscles, as well as neck actions on brainstem neurons projecting back to the spinal cord.

Recent data(117) indicate that in the decerebrate cat, the VCR and CCR not only behave approximately linearly when evoked in isolation, but also combine by simple linear summation when evoked together. When the head is rotated on a stationary body, the two reflexes act in a synergistic fashion to oppose the rotation. Thus the pattern of VCR and CCR interaction described here appears to be a relatively inflexible characteristic of the neck motor system, which is probably preserved to prevent debilitating mechanical instability of the head.

Visual Afferents

Gentalucci et al(118) have shown that in the postarcuate cortex, visual information is coded in terms of head or body coordinates, considering that the premotor function of the area is cytoarchitecturally part of Brodmann's Area 6. This type of coding appears to be the most appropriate for the organization of visually guided movements directed to peripersonal space. It has been suggested that fixation neurons of the parietal lobe and the various types of intralaminal units compute the position of stimuli in space from information about the position of the eyes in the orbit and the part of the retina that is stimulated. Soma-related visual neurons very likely compare the position of the visual stimulus with the vision of a body part and/or with the knowledge of its position based on proprioceptive cues. Thus, the ability to know the position of an object in space appears to depend on at least two different mechanisms: one strictly related to oculomotion, and the other to the knowledge of the position of the body.

Mountcastle and Motter(119) showed that in response to a visual cue, responses were observed in Brodmann's Area 7 of the cortex. No movement of the eye is necessary for this response to occur and the stimuli can be outside of foveal vision. The greater response was seen with dynamic and directionally specific stimuli. Area 7 projects to the premotor cortex, supplementary motor cortex, and the periarcuate region.

Godschalk et al(120) also found cues responding in the periarcuate region when monkeys foveated and reached for food.

Kubota and Funahash(121) demonstrated that periarcuate prefrontal neurons responded in a visual tracking task. These neurons were activated prior to movement onset of the wrist. He suggested that the activity of periarcuate prefrontal neurons seems responsible in part for the quick movement onset via unknown facilitatory pathways to the motor cortex. It would seem from the above that the periacuate area is involved in the synthesis of visual cues to initiate serial ordering of movement parameters.

Berson and McIlwain(122) showed that the visual cortex in cats receives information from the retina and projects to and exerts a significant influence on cells of the deep superior colliculus. He concluded that one obvious function of the superior colliculus would be to transform spatial information received in what are probably several different formats into a common code appropriate to the organization of the target motor structures of the brainstem and spinal cord. This may mean that the inter-

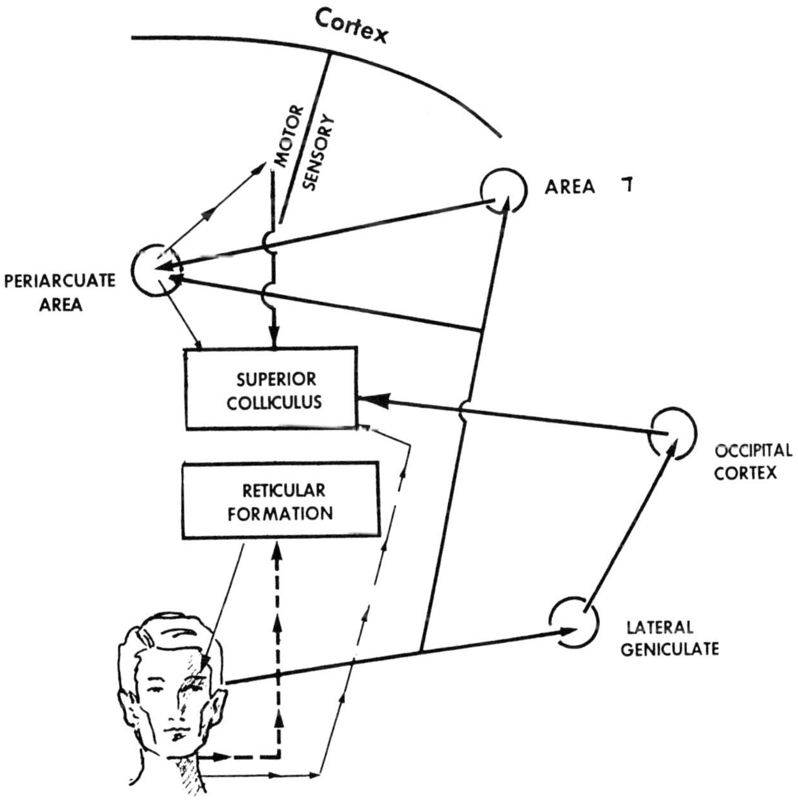

Figure 3.29. Visual—periarcuate—cortical interaction afferents from cervical area.

action of eyes, cortex, and superior colliculus provides a useful model of how neural tissue converts sensory information into a signal appropriate for motor control.

Kunzle and Akert(123) showed that there is a corticotectal tract from the frontal eye field (Brodmann's Area 8 also known as the periarcuate area), which projects to superficial and middle layers of the superior colliculus and is thought to participate in mechanisms related to saccadic eye movements.

The periacuate area projects to the motor cortex, and Weil and Lasser(124) have shown that approximately 55% of the crossed corticospinal tract fibers end in the cervical spine; some are obvious for limb and girdle control, but the majority end directly on alpha motor neurons to control or fine-tune head-neck movements.

CNS Descending Afferents to the Cervical Spine

Huerta and Harting(125) showed that the superior colliculus (tectospinal system) with its descending tract that crosses within the dorsal tegmentum and terminates within the gray matter of the cervical spinal cord plays an important role in head and eye movements.

Because there are topographic differences regarding the location of tectospinal neurons that project to different regions of the cervical spinal cord, a "motor map" within the superior colliculus is likely, with reference to eye, head, and body movements. The posterior lateral portion of the superior colliculus is the only zone that contains tectospinal cells that project upon the cervical enlargement. The posterior lateral zone received information regarding somatosensation from the contralateral lower visual field, so as to rapidly effect contraction of forelimb and axial musculature via the tectospinal pathway.

Still, proper orientation of the animal to such a stimulus requires not only movements of the forelimb and trunk, but also necessitates contraction of the neck musculature for movement of the head. Such movements are necessary for the cat to foveate the peripherally located stimulus. The motor connectivity necessary for such coordinated movements is present since neurons in the caudal superior colliculus project not only to the cervical enlargement, but to the upper cervical cord as well.

Rostral regions of the superior colliculus, containing a somatosensory representation of the face and a visual map of the central visual field, possess tectospinal neurons that project only to the upper cervical spinal cord gray matter. Because motoneurons within the upper neck cervical spinal cord innervate muscles of the neck, a stimulus falling within the central visual field could elicit a quick orienting response of the head via the tectospinal projection to upper cervical spinal cord levels. Likewise, tactile stimulation of the face could excite tectospinal neurons that, in turn, would stimulate motoneurons innervating muscles of the neck. Since stimuli falling within these regions of visual or somatosensory space could be easily foveated or oriented by merely turning the neck, tectospinal cells receiving sensory inputs from the central visual field and face region need only to project upon the upper cervical cord.

Peterson and Fukushima(126) showed that reticulospinal neurons projecting to the neck tend to cluster in the dorsal medullary reticular formation (including the pontis caudalis, gigantocellularis, and ventralis), while neurons projecting to thoracic or to lumbar levels are clustered progressively more ventral. The trajectory of reticulospinal axons with the cervical enlargement covers extensive areas of laminae VII, VIII, and IX and in some cases extends to both sides of the spinal cord. Stimulation studies show that the regions for neck and back motoneurons were more extensive than those from which limb motoneurons received excitation.

There is also reticulospinal inhibition, a monosynaptic inhibition of motoneurons supplying the dorsal neck muscles. The area includes the dorsal region posterior to the abducens nucleus, which also contains inhibitory burst neurons that inhibit abducens motoneurons during rapid eye movements to the contralateral side.

An important feature of spinoreticular and tectal neurons is that they are most readily excited by novel stimuli and cease to re-

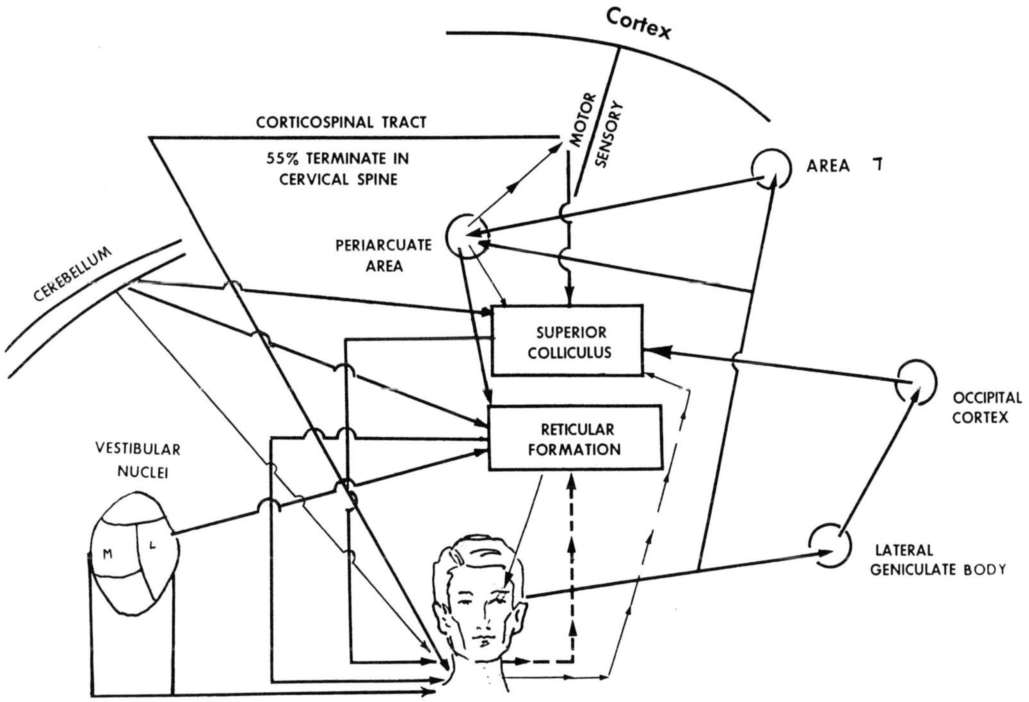

Figure 3.30. Efferents to cervical area. Visual—periarcuate—cortical interaction afferents from cervical area.

spond when the same stimulus is presented repeatedly. The presence of such habituation suggests that somatic visual sensory inputs to the reticular formation may be involved in the generation of alerting or orienting responses that are excited by novel stimuli.

A second class of inputs to the medial RF are those arising in the vestibular labyrinth, which relay in the vestibular nuclei and cerebellum. In addition to sensory and vestibular input, the RF receives direct excitatory input from central motor systems such as the periarcuate cortex and deep cerebellar nuclei.

The widely divergent excitatory action of the RF system and the extensive branching of its individual elements, along with the input it receives from areas of the CNS, suggests that the system is likely to function as a final premotor organizing center for those aspects or reflex and voluntary movement that produce activation of broad synergistic groups of muscles.

Schaffer et al(127) stated that when considering complexity of motor phenomena involved in eye-head coordination, it has to be expected that discharge patterns of brainstem neurons mediating such mechanisms cannot be uniform. Nevertheless, it is obvious that neurons of the left nucleus rectus medialis, units of the type II in the right reticular formation, and left vestibular nucleus cells of type I have several properties in common. Apart from their responsiveness to vestibular stimulation, the influence of neck proprioception is qualitatively similar. Neck proprioception exerts more distinct influences on reticular formation cells than on neurons of the vestibular nuceli. It can therefore be assumed that the reticular formation neurons are responsible for mediating tonic neck reflexes on the eyes as well as for the change in the beating field of nystagmus during different head positions.

Cells of the structures mentioned above are also excited with directionally specific characteristics during active head movements. Excitation and inhibition of discharge occur in an extremely clear manner during compensatory backward movement of the eyes. The discharge rate is usually very high from the onset of the return movement forward, which serves to stabilize the eyes in space and has the speed of the head movement. One can therefore assume a speed code to be present. This is already visible in neurons of the nucleus vestibularis medialis, which projects to the oculomotor nuclei via the medial longitudinal fasciculus.

Brink and colleagues(128) have shown that propriospinal neurons in and near C4 and L3–L4 transmit tonic neck signals to the cervical and lumbosacral enlargements, respectively. They presumably often carry vestibular signals as well, because earlier experiments demonstrated convergence of vestibular and neck input onto many neurons in the medial gray matter of C4(129) and L3–L4(130). Whether the propriospinal neurons make synapses with motoneurons is not known, although the evidence of others suggest that at least lumbar neurons do.

These long propriospinal neurons are modulated by various directions of neck rotation and can transmit these signals to different lumbar levels. These neurons are probably the same as the medial long propriospinal neurons with vestibular and reticular input recently described by Sasaki et al(131), who suggested they were involved in postural reactions. It can be expected that, like other cervical neurons, these cells will remain active after spinal section providing, perhaps together with propriospinal pathways originating from more caudal cervical levels, a route by which activity originating in the neck can reach the L3–L4 region and the lumbosacral enlargement. Despite this projection, it is very difficult to find L3–L4 neurons modulated by neck rotation in spinal cats, even though there are many spontaneously active neurons in these segments and many modulated neurons in C4. It must be assumed that the response of lumbar neurons is heavily dependent on supraspinal pathways. This may be due to two reasons. First, tonic neck signals in lumbar propriospinal neurons may be mainly generated by vestibulospinal and reticulospinal pathways, which are known to be modulated by neck rotation(132) and also to make synapses with lumbar propriospinal neurons(133). Second, lack of modulation in spinal cats may result from disfacilitation, due to the interruption of descending pathways, leading to lack of responsiveness to purely spinal inputs. Because many spontaneously active neurons were found at typical depths in L3–L4 in spinal cats, the first possibility seems the more likely one. Whatever is the explanation, the results demonstrate a striking difference in the importance of supraspinal structures for the response of cervical and lumbar neurons to neck rotation.

The results suggest that the tonic neck reflex is produced by a neural substrate. That is, the appropriate signal is carried by descending pathways and by propriospinal neurons acting both in series and in parallel. While at least cervical propriospinal neurons receive neck afferent input by intraspinal pathways, there is no evidence for or against the possibility that, deprived of supraspinal input, these neurons, by themselves, are sufficient to produce a normal reflex pattern even in the cervical enlargement(128). However, electrical stimulation of the C2 dorsal root ganglion, combined with transections of the neuraxis, suggests that supraspinal control is necessary to produce a normal pattern(134).

Visual Input to Cerebellum and Vestibular System

It could then be asked if visual stimuli affect the cerebellum and vestibular system. Baloh and Honrubia(135) suggested that the relationship between the head and the object in the environment may change in several ways. The object may move relative to the head, the head may move relative to the object, or the head and object may move simultaneously. The visual and vestibular signals interact synergistically to stabilize gaze during most natural head movements. If the neck is also turned, the neck-occular reflex participates in the compensatory movement. The effect produces better ocular stability than would be possible if each system worked alone. Occasionally, vestibular and visual signals conflict and one signal must override the other in order to maintain gaze stability. In these instances, the visually mediated ocular reflexes override the vestibulo-ocular reflex.

Maekawa and Natsui(136) showed that visual input to the vestibulocerebellum exists in the rabbit, and they stated that climbing fiber-mediated field potential was evoked in the ipsilateral flocculus following electric or visual stimulation of the retina.

These results were confirmed by Simpson et al(137) in research involving cats. Whole-field flash illumination was also effective in evoking field potentials and unitary Purkinje cell activity characteristic of climbing fiber activation. In cats, under barbiturate anesthesia, no visual-evoked mossy fiber field potentials were observed.

Maekawa and Takeda(138) observed visual signals mediated by mossy and climbing fibers to the dorsorostral quadrant of the flocculus. We may conclude from these data that a strict sensory separation into visual climbing and vestibular mossy fiber inputs does not hold throughout the entire vestibulocerebellum but it definitely exists in some of its subdivisions.

Ghelarducci et al(139) then provided convincing evidence for visual mossy fiber inputs to the rabbit flocculus, when they showed that sinusoidal movement of a slit light in front of the ipsilateral eye modified simple spike frequency in a sinusoidal fashion. In many of these Purkinje cells, vestibular stimulation in the dark also modified firing so that not only vestibular mossy and visual climbing fiber paths converged, but also both sensory inputs via mossy fibers.

Precht(140) added support to the above finding when he stated that it is apparent that vestibular and visual pathways of mossy and/or climbing fibers may converge in the vestibulocerebellum and are both able to influence firing of a given Purkinje cell.

Robinson(141) demonstrated that although Purkinje cell outflow to the vestibular nuclei is inhibitory, it can enhance or inhibit the vestibulo-ocular reflex.

Takemore(142) showed that, in animals with lesions of the floccule or inferior olive, the vestibulo-ocular reflex cannot be modulated by visual stimulation.

Precht(140) stated that the flocculus of the cerebellum receives vestibular information via mossy fiber pathways and to a lesser extent via visual information arriving in both the mossy and climbing fiber systems. In addition, neck proprioceptive input is channeled to the same cerebellar area. Thus, Purkinje cells of the flocculus receive information regarding head velocity, retinal image slip velocity, and head position with respect to body and space via these sensory channels. This information is used by the Purkinje cells in the control of their target neurons. The floccular output neurons project to those second order vestibular neourons that are the central link in the pathway connecting labyrinth and eye muscles, i.e., the VOR.

Figure 3.31 demonstrates the major anatomical connections that are likely to mediate visual control of eye movement via the olivocerebellar pathways.

Bergman(143) found that ganglion cells encoding information destined for the ipsilateral cerebellar flocculus send a predominantly contralateral projection to the pretectal nucleus and nucleus of the optic tract.

Collewijn(144) also found that the neurons of the nucleus of the optic tract are both directionally selective and velocity sensitive, discharging preferentially in response to large contour-rich, optokinetic stimuli moved in the posterior-anterior direction with respect to the viewing eye.

It was then demonstrated that the accessory optic nucleus also receives afferents predominantly from the contralateral retina and that the nucleus of the optic tract pretectal nucleus and the accessory optic project ipsilaterally to the dorsal cap of Kooy, the medial division of the inferior olive(145, 146). These climbing fibers, which originate from the dorsal cap, recross the brainstem to synapse in the contralateral flocculus(147).

A review by Wilson et al(148) showed that the flocculus also received mossy fiber vestibular inputs from the ipsilateral and contralateral semicircular canals and vestibular nuclei. At present, it is not certain how visual mossy fiber input reaches the flocculus. The vestibular nuclei project to the other regions of the cerebellar cortex and deep nuclei (fastigial especially). Neck receptors have also been shown to project to areas of the flocculus that receive labyrinthine and visual input.

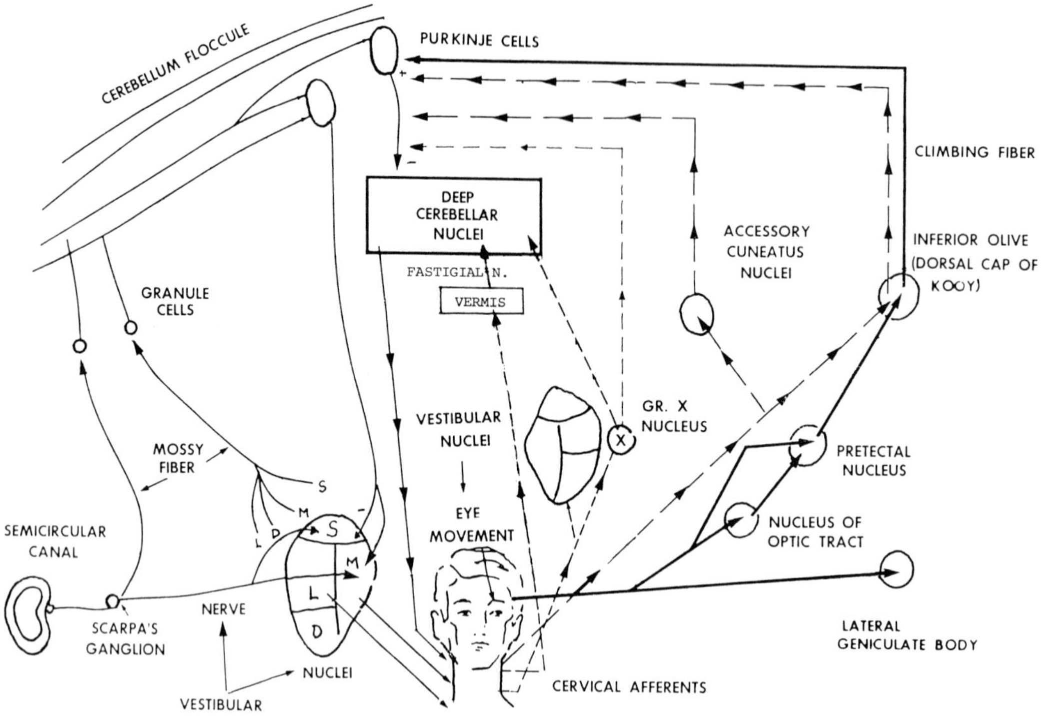

Figure 3.31. Visual interaction. Efferents to cervical area and afferents from cervical area.

The lateral vestibulospinal tract extends the entire length of the spinal cord but has short fibers that end only in the cervical cord. The medial vestibulospinal tract extends to the upper thoracic cord, with the majority of the fibers also terminating in the cervical cord. They establish monosynaptic contacts, and these contacts are inhibitory.

Bentivoglio(149) concluded that the majority of cerebellospinal fibers that originate from the medial and interpositus nucleus terminate both on interneurons and motoneurons in the contralateral upper cervical segments. Barmack(150) later used the above information to show how a stimulus that appears posteroanterior in the visual field of the left eye, would be functionally equivalent to direct exciting of the left vestibular nucleus via the left horizontal semicircular canal by rotation of the head to the left.

There is difficulty in analyzing and interpreting the activity of animals under various experimental conditions. Under such conditions it is virtually impossible to assess the true interpretation of the nervous system. In a freely moving behaving animal, any area will typically be receiving simultaneous signals from systems carrying voluntary motor commands, sensory information, and reflex responses elicited by changing exteroceptive and proprioceptive signals.

Zangemeister and Starr(102) concluded that the more intentionally governed head movement influences the eye and gaze patterns on different levels of the CNS. Head movement changes on a higher level with various experimental conditions (e.g., prediction, forced versus natural movements), and it acts on a lower level through its variant dynamic trajectories in the VOR and therefore on eye movement.

The absence of visually elicited eye movement prevents the acquisition of visually coordinated behavior, even if head and neck movements are intact. Eye movements, therefore, seem to be a necessary prerequisite for coordinated movements of the eye-head-neck. There are also certain reflex phenomena that are particular to cervical paraspinal muscles and these reflexes may affect eye-head-neck movement patterns(109, 110).

From the studies, it appears that the coordinated movement of eye-head-neck interaction toward a goal involves a number of parallel, independently active neural centers that initiate the movements. However, there is ongoing monitoring of these separate systems and via the visual VOR connections, they are finely integrated for proper sequencing, a smooth coordinated pattern for the achievement of that final position. The head and neck move as a unit, which makes sense when one considers the anatomy and segmentation of the area, but this still allows for a great degree of freedom.

There is, in part, a central program that is dependent on or made up of a number of neural centers such as the superior colliculus, periarcuate area, cortex, RF cerebellum or vestibular nerve. All project to the cervical spine, but information is necessary from the periphery (i.e., eyes, joints, neck muscles) into the neural centers for them to utilize or synthesize the information for that integrated action of the nervous system in facilitating synchronous movement.

Chiropractic Relevance

We know that one of the functions of the vestibular system that is strategically placed in the brainstem (medulla) is to help coordinate head and eye movement—cephalad—with that of postural tone and body movements—caudally.

Head and eye movements are monitored via the semicircular canals that are placed on either side of the head, converting the movement sensation (mechanical) into a neural impulse, which is transmitted via the nerves into the vestibular nuclei.

Caudally, via the vestibulospinal tract that ends on alpha motor neurons to extensor muscles along with the reticulospinal tract that also ends on extensor alpha motor neurons, these tracts help us to maintain our upright posture. Soechting and Berthoz(151) showed that by introducing perturbation into human subjects with eyes open and then closed, vision plays an important role in the control of postural reactions during sudden perturbation of stance.

I will briefly review studies that have addressed the anatomy and physiology of the upper cervical area. Manipulation of the area may affect these systems and this will explain many of our clinical observations.

Fitz-Ritson(152), in a review of the anatomy and physiology of the paraspinal musculature, outlined the complexity of the spindle arrays and the fact that the highest amount of spindles in the body are located in the paraspinal muscles in this area.

Bakker and Richmond(153), in their summary, state that "in intervertebral muscles, it may also be important to think of muscle spindles not simply as isolated entities, but as members of a complex information-gathering system."

Because the muscles of the cervical area are so richly supplied with muscle spindles that act as their sensors, any change in the muscles' proprioceptive input (tension, trauma) will provide the spinal cord, cuneatus, lateral cuneatus, and X-vestibular nuclei and cerebellum with a great deal and variation of afferent information. This will change the physiology of the system controlled by the centers thus affecting their output, i.e., eye movement and postural imbalances.

Age and chronic pathologies as shown by Jowett et al(154) can cause changes in paraspinal muscles. They showed that with age and disabling lesions of the spine, the multifidus muscle adopts an increasingly postural role as fast fibers atrophy and slow fibers predominate.

Barker and Milburn(155) showed that devascularization of muscle for 30 minutes led to rapid degeneration of the nuclear bag fibers. When normal blood flow was restored, regeneration of the intrafusal fibers began by day 3 and was most rapid among the remnants of the bag fibers. The regenerated spindles vary in structure, innervation, and hence function.

Wyke(156) draws attention to the fact that age or degenerative changes in the spinal joint affect the articular cartilage thus affecting the articular afferents into the CNS. This will affect the spinal reflexes and, of course, the entire CNS.

If we now review some of the studies that have addressed the cervical area, i.e., by trauma and/or injection, we will see that the signs and symptoms are many and varied. Igarashi et al(157), using monkeys, state that equilibrium disturbances may occur after neck lesions such as "whiplash"—flexion-extension injuries. Immediately after left C1–C2 dorsal root section, a reduction of the slow phase eye speed is a proper nystagmic parameter to study the neck proprioceptor contribution to oculomotor function. All animals after unilateral C1–C2 dorsal root section demonstrated moderate dysequilibrium confirming that neck injury can produce ataxia. deJong et al(158), using cats, monkeys, and humans, injected local anesthetics into unilateral neck muscles. They found that, following the anesthetic, there was presumably an interruption to the flow of afferent information from neck muscles and joint receptors. Ataxia in humans was associated with a broad-based, staggering gait, hypotonia of the ipsilateral muscles, falling, or tilting. Nystagmus was not induced in humans. The data demonstrate the dependence of neck afferents on the vestibular system and suggest that in the presence of previous vestibular lesions, neck joint or muscle disorders may be a cause of clinical vertigo or ataxia.

Hinoki et al(159) drew the following conclusions after clinical observations of traumatized patients with vertigo and lumbar pain. They noted that there was hypertonicity of the lumbar soft supporting tissues, and especially the lumbar erector muscles (i.e., overexcitement of the lumbar proprioceptors). They proposed this as a cause of vertigo due to whiplash injury. Equilibrium tests, after fixing the waist with a corset, were useful for detecting ataxia of lumbar origin. Their explanation of this phenomenon is that overexcitement of the lumbar proprioceptors and dysfunction of the brainstem and the cerebellum are closely related in bringing about vertigo due to whiplash injury. The lumbar proprioceptors, in particular, may be important, in close correlation with the cerebellum in producing vertigo of this type. After infiltration of procaine into tender sports in the lumbar soft supporting tissues, the dysequilibrium of the eyes, body, and cerebellar ataxia was relieved.

In addressing the significance of manipulative therapy to the cervical area, Gutmann and Vele(160) studied 27 adults with lumbar pain and sciatica as their chief complaints and found concomitant upper cervical disturbances (joint, muscle pathomechanics). EMG readings were performed on arms and legs in various muscle groups before and after the upper cervical manipulation. They found a minimum of 10% change in the EMG readings in 74% of the cases along with decreased low back pain and sciatica.

The reason this may occur is shown in a study by Miller et al(161) in which they placed spinal lesions at the C2–C3 level in monkeys, which cut the lateral vestibulospinal tract. This produced two major effects on the forelimb muscles: Background EMG activity was usually abolished in the triceps ipsilateral to the lesion, with partial loss of activity in the opposite limb. This draws our attention again to the vestibulospinal tract and its effect on extensor muscle tone.

Sandoz(62), in his discussion on mechanoreceptors, stated that they are responsible for the tonic neck reflexes and are located in the joints between occiput, atlas, and axis. With mechanical derangements of the upper cervical spine, these mechanoreceptors are capable of producing secondary derangements lower in the spine, pelvis, and even the extremities, by creating muscle tone imbalances between right and left sides.

A harmonious balance of the muscles around the cervical spine (entire body) seems to be necessary when one discusses the normal mechanics of the cervical spine. Simons(163) showed that in the sternocleidomastoid muscle, sensitive trigger points may produce, instead of referred pain, severe disturbance of equilibrium in which the patient will stagger and veer to the side of the lesion and may have blurring or "misty" vision, even vertigo and nystagmus. All of these symptoms have been relieved by treatment of the trigger points. The reason for this appears to be that the hypoglossal nerve (CN XI) has a section that projects into the spinal cord as far as cervical levels C3–C4, and the afferents from the sternocleidomastoid project into the spinal cord and into the brainstem nuclei as described above. Finally, there is the triginimal nuclei and tract (CN V) that synapses with α-motor neurons at the C1–C2 spinal levels, which helps us to understand why there may be temporomandibular joint dysfunction after whiplash injuries along with upper cervical spine pathomechanics.

A number of factors may affect how muscles function. We saw above how decreased blood supply can affect the muscles. Barker and Milburn(155) and Jowett et al(154) showed that aging has an effect on the muscles. When one investigates further the basic spinal stretch reflex (SSR), new data, as provided by Wolpaw(164), show that there are possibly two components to the stretch reflex—supra and segmental. Over weeks of training the SSR amplitude can be changed. He further showed that with the amplitude change, the antagonistic muscle was also affected, and these changes involve structural or biochemical change. These are the substrates for muscle memory or a learned motor (muscle) pattern(165).

CONCLUSION

The cervical spine, as mentioned by Bach-y-Rita(1a) and as outlined in the chapter, is of primary importance in the functioning of the entire body. Its potency can therefore not be overlooked in the treatment and rehabilitation of the entire locomotor system.

References

1. Gitelman R. The treatment of pain by spinal manipulation. In: Goldstein M, ed. The Research Status of Spinal Manipulative Therapy. National Institute of Neurological and Communicative Disorders and Stroke Monograph No. 15. Bethesda: United States Department of Health, Education and Welfare, 1975.

1a. Bach-y-Rita P, ed. Recovery of function: theoretical consideration for brain injury rehabilitation. Baltimore: Univ. Park Press, 1980, pp 39–45.

2. Fitz-Ritson D. The anatomy and physiology of the muscle spindle and its role in posture and movement: a review. J Can Chiro Assoc 1982;25(6): 144–150.

3. Kendal E, Schwartz J, eds. Principles of neural science. (New York: Elsevier/North Holland, 1980, pp 284–304.

4. Mountcastle VB, ed. Medical physiology V1, Part VII. Neural control of posture and movement. C23–32. St. Louis: C V Mosby 1980, pp 669–892.

5. Bakker D. Richmond F. Abrahams V. Central projections from cat suboccipital muscles: a study using transganglionic transport of horseradish peroxidase. J Comp Neurol 1984;228:409–421.

6. Bakker D, Richmond F. Muscle spindle complexes in muscles around upper cervical vertebrae in the cat. J Neurophysiol 1982;48:62–74.

7. Richmond F, Abrahams V. Morphology and enzyme histochemistry of dorsal muscles of the cat neck. J Neurophysiol 1975;38:1312–1321.

8. Richmond F, Abrahams V. Morphology and distribution of muscle spindles in dorsal muscles of the cat neck. J Neurophysiol 1975;38:1322–1339.

9. Richmond F, MacGillis D, Scott D. Muscle fiber compartmentalization in cat splenius muscle. J Neurophysiol 1985;53:868–885.

10. Brink E, Jinnai K, Wilson V. Patterns of segmental monosynaptic input to cat dorsal neck motoneurons. J Neurophysiol 1981A;46:496–505.

11. Wyke B. Neurological aspects of low back pain. In: The lumbar, spine and back pain. Jayson M, ed. New York: Grune & Stratton, p 189–256.

12. Haldeman S. The neurophysiology of spinal pain syndromes. In: Modern developments in the principles and practice of chiropractic. Haldeman S, ed. New York: Appleton-Century-Crofts 1981, pp 119–142.

13. Newton R. Joint receptor contributions to reflexive and kinesthetic response. Physiother Can 1982;62:22–29.

14. Wyke B. Neurology of the cervical spinal joints. Physiother Can 1979;65(3):72–76.

15. Schomburg T, Steffens H. Facilitation interaction between cutaneous afferents from low threshold mechanoreceptors and nociceptors in segmental reflex pathways to alpha motoneurons. Brain Res 1983;260:131–134.

16. Dvorak J, Dvorak V. Neurologie der wirbelbogengelenke. Man Med 1982;20:70–84.

17. Terrett A, Vernon H. Manipulation and pain tolerance. Am J Phys Med 1984;63(5):217–225.

18. Siegel J, Tomaszewski K. Behavioral organization of reticular information studies in the unrestrained cat. I. Cells related to axial, limb, eye and other movements. J Neurophysiol 1983;50:696–716.

19. Brink E, Jinnai K, Wilson V. Pattern of segmental monosynaptic input to cat dorsal neck motoneurons. J Neurophysiol 1981;46:496–505.

20. Bilotto G, Schor R, Uchin Y, Wilson V. Localization of proprioceptive reflexes in the splenius muscle of the cat. Brain Res 1982;238:217–221.

21. Mergner T, Nardi G, Beckle W, Deecke L. The role of canal-neck interaction for the perception of horizontal trunk and neck rotation. Exp Brain Res 1983;49:198–208.

22. Kenins P, Kikillus H, Schomburg E. Short and long-latency reflex pathways from neck afferents to hind limb motoneurons in the cat. Brain res 1978;149:235–238.

23. Peterson B, Bilotto G, Fuller J, Goldberg, J Leeman G. Interaction of vestibular and neck reflexes in the control of gaze. In: Progress in oculomotor research. Fuch AF, Becker W, (eds). New York: Elsevier/North Holland, Inc 1981, pp 335–342.

24. Bakker D, Richmond F, Abrahams V. Central projections from cat suboccipital muscles: a study using transganglionic transport of horseradish peroxidase. J Comp Neurol 1984;228:409–421.
25. Fitz-Ritson D. The direct connections of the C2 dorsal root ganglia in the Macaca Irus monkey: relevance to chiropractic therapeutics. J Manipulative Physiol Ther 1985;8(3):147–156.
26. Murakami S, Kato M. Central projections of nuchal group I muscle afferent fibers of the cat. Exp Neurol 1983; 79:472–487.
27. Boyle R, Pompeiano O. Response characteristics of cerebellar interpositus and intermediate cortex neurons to sinusoidal stimulation of neck and labyrinth receptors. Neurosci 1980;5:285–292.
28. Chan Y, Manzoni D, Pompeiano O. Response characteristics of cerebellar dentate and lateral cortex neurons to sinusoidal stimulation of neck and labyrinth receptors. Neurosci 1982;7:2993–3011.
29. Sherrington CS. Note on the spinal portion of some ascending degenerations. J Physiol (Lond) 1931;14:255–302.
30. Collier J, Buzzard EF. The degeneration resulting from lesions of posterior nerve root and from transverse lesions of the spinal cord in man: a study of twenty cases. Brain 1903;26:559–91.
31. Ranson SN, Davenport HK, Doles EA. Intramedullary course of the dorsal root fibers of the first three cervical nerves. J Comp Neurol 1982;54:1–12.
32. Pass LJ. Anatomic and functional relationship of nuc. dorsalis (Clarke's column). Arch Neurol Psychiatry 1933;30:1025–1045.
33. Corbin KB, Hinsey JC. Intramedullary course of the dorsal root fibers of each of the first four cervical nerves. J Comp Neurol 1935;63:119–126.
34. Corbin KB, Lhamon WT, Petit DW. Peripheral and central connections of the upper cervical dorsal root ganglia in the rhesus monkey. J Comp Neurol 1937;66:405–414.
35. Yee J, Corbin KB. The intramedullary course of the upper five cervical dorsal root fibers in the rabbit. J Comp Neurol 1939;70:297–304.
36. Chang HT, Ruch TC. Organization of the dorsal columns of the spinal cord and their nuclei in the spider monkey. J Anat 1947;81:140–149.
37. Escolar J. The afferent connections of the 1st, 2nd and 35rd cervical nerves in the cat. An analysis by Marchi and Rasdolsky methods. Neurology 1948;89:79–92.
38. Torvik A. Afferent connections to the sensory trigeminal nuclei, the nucelus of the solitary nuclei and adjacent structures. An experimental study of the rat. J Comp Neurol 1956;106:51–142.
39. Sprague JM. The distribution of dorsal root fibres on motor cells in the lumbosacral spinal cord of the cat, and the site of excitatory and inhibitory terminals in monosynaptic pathways. Proc R Soc B. 1958;149:534–556.
40. Grant G, Rexed B. Dorsal spinal root afferents to Clarke's column. Brain 1958;18:567–576.
41. Kerr FW. Structural relation of the trigeminal spinal tract to upper cervical roots and the solitary nucleus in the cat. Exp Neurol 1961;4:134–148.
42. Hand PJ. Lumbosacral dorsal root termination in the nucleus gracilis of the cat. Some observations on terminal degeneration in other medullary sensory nuclei. J Comp Neurol 1966:126:137–156.
43. Sterling P, Kuypers HG. Anatomical organization of the brachial spinal cord of the cat. The distribution of dorsal root fibres. Brain Res 1967;4:1–15.
44. Liu CN. Afferent nerves to Clarke's and the lateral cuneate nuclei in the cat. Arch Neurol Psychiatry 1956;75:67–77.
45. Igarashi M, Alford B, Natanabe T, et al. Role of neck proprioceptors for the maintenance of dynamic bodily equilibrium in the squirrel monkey. Laryngoscope 1969;79:1713–1727.
46. Brodal A, Walberg F, Blackstad TH. Termination of spinal afferents to inferior olive in cat. J Neurophysiol 1950;3:431–454.
47. Mizuno N. An experimental study of the spiro-olivary fibers in the rabbit and the cat. J Comp Neurol 1966;127:267–292.
48. Boesten AJ, Voogo J. Projections of the dorsal column nuclei and the spinal cord on the inferior olive in the cat. J Comp Neurol 1975;161:215–238.
49. Berkley KJ, Worden IG. Projections to the inferior olive of the cat. Comparisons of input from the dorsal column nuclei, the lateral cervical nucleus, the spino-olivary pathways, the cerebral cortex and the cerebellum. J Comp Neurol 1978;180:237–252.
50. Buisseret-Delmas C. An HRP study of the afferents to the inferior olive in cat. Arch Ital Biol 1980;118:270–286.
51. Richmond FJR, Courville J, Saint-Cyr JA. Spino-olivary projections from the upper cervical spinal cord: an experimental study using autoradiography and horseradish peroxidase. Exp Brain Res 1982;47:239–251.
52. Bakker D, Richmond F, Abrahams V. Central projections from cat suboccipital muscles: a study using transganglionic transport of horseradish peroxidase. J Comp Neurol 1984;228:409–421.
53. Cowan WM, Gottlieb DI, Hendrickson AE, et al. The autoradiographic demonstration of axonal connections in the central nervous system. Brain Res 1972;37:21–51.
54. Rexed B. The cytoarchitectonic atlas of the spinal cord in the cat. J Comp Neurol 1952;96:415–496.
55. Burton H, Loewy A. Descending projections from the marginal core layer and other regions of the monkey spinal cord. Brain Res 1976;116:485–491.
56. Emmers R, Akert K, eds. A sterotaxic atlas of the brain of the squirrel monkey (Saimiri Sciureus). 1963. Madison: University of Wisconsin Press pp 90–98.
57. Manocha S, Shantha T, Bourne G, eds. A stereotaxic atlas of the brain of the Cebus monkey (cebus apella). Oxford, England: Oxford University Press 1968; 78–90.
58. Shriver JE, Stein BM, Carpenter MB. Central projections of spinal dorsal roots in the monkey. I. Cervical and upper thoracic dorsal roots. Am J Anat 1968;123:27–74.

59. Szabo J, Cowan Wm. A stereotaxic atlas of the brain of the Cynomolgus monkey (macaca fascicularis). J Comp Neur 1984;222:265–300.
60. Anderson FD. Distribution of dorsal root fibers in the cat spinal cord. Anat Res 1960;136:154.
61. Olszewski J. On the anatomical and functional organization of the trigeminal nucleus. J Comp Neurol 1950;92:401–413.
62. Dunn J, Marzke H. Central distribution of the dorsal root of the first cervical nerve of the marmoset monkey. Anat Res 1967;157:357.
63. Rexed B, Brodal A. The nucleus cervicals lateralis. J Neurophysiol 1951;14:399–407.
64. Brodal A, Rexed B. Spinal afferents to the lateral cervical and nucleus in the cat. J Comp Neurol 1953;98(2):179–207.
65. Ha H, Liu CN. An anatomical investigation on the lateral cervical nucleus of the cat. Anat Res 1961;139:234.
66. Ha H, Liu CN. Spinal afferents to lateral cervical nucleus and their terminals. Anat Res 1962;142:237–238.
67. Ha H, Liu CN. Synaptology of spinal afferents in the lateral cervical nucleus of the cat. Exp Neurol 1963;8:318–327.
68. Boivie J. Thalamic projections from lateral cervical nucleus in monkey. A degeneration study. Brain Res 1980;198:13–26.
69. Morin F, Kitai S, Portnoy N, Demirjian C. Afferent projections to the lateral cervical nucleus: a micro electrode study. Am J Physiol 1963;204:667–672.
70. Kitai S, Ha H, Morin F. Lateral cervical nucleus of the dog: anatomical and microelectrode studies. Am J Physiol 1965;209:307–311.
71. Blomquist A, Flink R, Bonsher D, et al. Tectal and thalamic projections of dorsal column and lateral cervical nuclei: a quantitative study in the cat. Brain Res 1978;141:335–341.
72. Hirai N, Hongo T, Sakai S. Cerebellar projection and input organizations of the spinocerebellar tract arising from the central cervical enlargement in the cat. Brain Res, 1978;157:341–345.
73. Imai Y, Kusama T. Distribution of the dorsal root fibers in the cat. An experimental study with the Nauta method. Brain res 1969; 13:338–359.
74. Matsushita M, Ikeda M. The central cervical nucleus as cells of origin of a spinocerebellar tract arising from the cervical cord: a study in the cat using horseradish peroxidase. Brain res 1975;100:412–417.
75. Matsushita M, Hosoya Y, Ikeda M. Anatomical organization of the spinocerebellar system in the cat, as studied by retrograde transport of horseradish peroxidase. J Comp Neurol 1979;184:81–106.
76. Wiksten B. The central cervical nucleus in the cat III. The cerebellar connections studied with anterograde transport of 3-leucine. Exp Brain Res 1979;36:175–189.
77. Cummings JP, Petras JM. The origin of spinocerebellar pathways. I. The nucleus cervicalis centralis of the cranial cervical spinal cord. J Comp Neurol 1977;173:655–692.
78. Wiksten B, Grant G. The central cervical nucleus in the cat. IV. Afferent fiber connections. Exp Brain Res 1983;51:405–412.
79. Abrahams VC, Anszee G, Richmond FJ, Rose PK. Neck muscle and trigeminal input of the upper cervical cord and lower medulla of the cat. Can J Physiol Pharmacol 1979;58:642–651.
80. Carleton SC, Carpenter MB. Afferent and efferent connections of the medial, inferior and lateral vestibular nuclei in the cat and monkey. Brain Res 1983;278:29–51.
81. Takahashi O, Takeuchi Y, Matsushima R. Direct connections of primary afferent fibers with central cervical nucleus neurons projecting to the cerebellum in the cat. Brain Res 1985; 328:390–395.
82. Hirai N, Hongo T, Sasaki S, Yoshida K. The neck and labyrinthine influences on cervical spinocerebellar tract neurons of the central cervical nucleus in the cat. Prog Brain Res 1979;50:529–536.
83. Mountcastle V, ed. Medical physiology. 14th ed. St. Louis: The CV Mosby Company, Vol I., 1980; pp 839–845.
84. Oscarsson O. Functional organization of the spino- and cuneo-cerebellar tracts. Physiol Rev 1965;45:495–522.
85. Carpenter MB, Stein BM, Shriver JE. Central projections of spinal dorsal roots in the monkey II. Lower thoracic, lumbosacral and coccygeal dorsal roots. Am J Anat 1968;123:75–118.
86. Walker AE, Weaver TA. The total organization and termination of the fibers of the posterior columns in macaca mulatta. J Comp Neurol 1942;76:145–58.
87. Kuypers JM, Tuerk JD. The distribution of the cortical fibres within the nuclei cuneatus and gracilis in the cat. J Anat 1964;98:143–162.
88. Brodal A, Pompeiano O. The vestibular nuclei in the cat. J Anat 1957A;91:438–454.
89. Walberg FD, Bowsher D, Brodal A. The termination of primary vestibular fibers in the vestibular nuclei in the cat. An experimental study with silver methods. J Comp Neurol 1958;110:391–405.
90. Pompeiano O, Brodal A. Spino-vestibular fibres in the cat. An experimental study. J Comp Neurol 1957;108:353–382.
91. Brodal A, Angaut P. The termination of spinovestibular fibers in the cat. Brain Res 1967;5:494–500.
92. Johansson H, Silfvenius H. Connections from large, ipsilateral hind limb muscle and skin afferents to the rostral main cuneate nucleus and to the nucleus X region in the cat. J Physiol 1977;265:395–428.
93. Fitz-Ritson D. Neural control of eye, head and neck movement. Future directions for the chiropractic profession. J Manipulative Physiol Ther 1984:251–260.
94. Wilson V, Maeda M, Franck J, Shimazu H. Mossy fibre neck and second order labyrinthine projections to cat flocculus. J Neurophysiol 1976;39:301–310.
95. Matsushita M, Hosoya Y. The location of spinal projection neurons in the cerebellar nuclei (cerebellospinal tract neurons) of the cat: a study with the horseradish peroxidase technique. Brain Res 1978;142:237–248.

96. Fukushima K, Peterson B, Uchino Y, Coulter J, Wilson V. Direct fastigiospinal fibers in the cat. Brain Res 1977;126:538–542.
97. Batton R, III, Jayaraman A, Ruggiero D, Carpenter M. Fastigial efferent projections in the monkey: an autoradiographic study. J Comp Neurol 1977;174:281–306.
98. Wilson V, Uchino Y, Susswein A, Fukushima K. Properties of direct fastigiospinal fibers in the cat. Brain Res 1977;126:543–546.
99. Shaw M, Baker R. Direct Projections from vestibular nuclei to facial nucleus in cats. J Neurophysiol 1983;50:1265–1280.
100. Vidal P, Roucoux A, Berthoz A. Horizontal eye position-related activity in neck muscles of the alert cat. Exp Brain Res 1982;46:448–453.
101. Takeuchi Y, Nakano K, Uemura M, Matsuda K, Matsushima R, Mizhno N. Mesencephalic and pontine afferent fiber system to the facial nucleus in the cat: a study using the horseradish perioxidase and silver impregnation techniques. Exp Neurol 1979;66:330–342.
102. Zangemeister W, Starr L. Active head rotations and eye-head coordination. Ann NY Acad Sci 1981;374:540–559.
103. Biguer B, Jeannerod M, Prablanc C. The coordination of eye, head and arm movements during reaching at a single visual target. Exp Brain Res 1982;46:301–4.
104. Bizzi E, Polit A, Morasso P. Mechanisms underlying achievement of final head position. J Neurophysiol 1976;39(2):435–44.
105. Dichgans J, Bizzi E, Morasso P, et al. Mechanisms underlying recovery of eye-head coordination following bilateral labyrinthectomy in monkeys. Exp Brain Res 1973;18:548–62.
106. Bizzi E, Chappe W, Hogan N. Mechanical properties of muscles: implications for motor control. Trends Nfuro Sci 1982;5:395–8.
107. Wilson V, Precht W, Dieringer N. Responses of different compartments of cat's splenius muscle to optokinetic stimulation. Exp Brain Res 1983;50:153–6.
108. Bilotto G, Schor R, Wilson V. Localization of proprioceptive reflexes in the splenius muscles of the cat. Brain Res 1982;238:217–21.
109. Vidal P, Roucoux A, Berthoz A. Horizontal eye position related activity in neck muscles of alert cat. Exp Brain Res 1982;46:448–53.
110. Ezure K, Fukushima K, Wilson V. Compartmentalization of the cervicocolic reflex in cat splenius muscle. Exp Brain Res 1983;51:397–404.
111. Berthoz A, Anderson J. Frequency analysis of vestibular influence on extensor motor neurons. II. Relationship between neck and forelimb extensions. Brain Res 1971; 34:376–380.
112. Esure K, Sasaki S. Frequency response analysis of vestibular-induced neck reflex in the cat. I. Characteristics of neural transmission from horizontal semicircular canal to neck motoneurons. J Neurophysiol 1978;41:445–458.
113. Esure K, Sasaki S, Uchino Y, Wilson V. Frequency-response analysis of vestibular-induced neck reflex in cat. II. Functional significance of cervical afferents and polysynaptic descending pathways. J Neurophysiol 1978;41:459–471.
114. Peterson B, Bilotto G, Goldberg J, Wilson V. Dynamics of vestibulo-ocular, vestibulocollic and cervicocollic reflexes. Ann NY Acad Sci 1981;374:395–402.
115. Barlow D, Freeman W. Cervico-ocular reflex in the normal adult. Acta-Otolaryngol 1980;89:487–496.
116. Hikosara O, Maeda M. Cervical effects on abducens motoneurons and their interaction with vestibulo-ocular reflex. Exp Brain Res 1973;18:512–530.
117. Peterson B, Goldberg J, Bilotto G, Fuller J. Cervicocollic reflex: its dynamic properties and interaction with vestibular reflexes. J Neurophysiol 1985;5(1):90–109.
118. Gentalucci M, Scandolara C, Pigarev I, et al. Visual responses in the postarcuate cortex (area 6) of the monkey, that are independent of eye position. Exp Brain Res 1983;50:414–68.
119. Mountcastle V, Motter B. The functional properties of the light-sensitive neurons of the posterior parietal cortex studied in waking monkeys: foveal sparing and opponent vector organization. J Neurosci 1981;1(1):3–26.
120. Godschalk M. Lemon R, Kuypers H. Behaviour of neurons in monkey periarcuate and precentral cortex before and during visually guided arm and hand movements. Exp Brain Res 1981; 44(1):113–6.
121. Kubota K, Funahash S. Direction specific activities of dorsolateral prefrontal and motor cortex pyramidal tract neurons during visual tracking. J Neurophysiol 1982;47(3)362–76.
122. Berson D, Mcllwain J. Visual cortical inputs to deep layers of cat's superior colliculus. J Neurophysiol 1983;50(5):1143–53.
123. Kunzle H, Akert K. Efferent connections of cortical area 8 (frontal eyefield) in macaca fascicularis: a re-investigation using the autoradiographic technique. J Comp Neurol 1977;173: 147–64.
124. Weil A, Lasser A. A qualitative distribution of the pyramidal tract in man. Arch Neurol Psychiatry 1929;2:495–510.
125. Huerta M, Harting J. Tectal control of spinal cord activities: neuroanatomical demonstration pathways connecting the superior colliculus with the cervical spinal cord grey. In: Kuypers H, Martin G, eds. Progress in brain research No. 57, descending pathways to the spinal cord. New York: Elsevier Biomedical Press, 1982.
126. Peterson B, Fukushima K. The reticulospinal system and its role in generating vestibular and visumotor reflexes. In: Sjolund B, Bjorklund A, eds. Brain stem control of spinal mechanisms. Proceedings of the 1st Eric K. Fernstrom symposium. New York: Elsevier Biomedical Press, 1982.
127. Schaffer K, Meyer D, Zierau H. Neural activity pattern in different brain stem structures during eye-head movements. In: Granit R, Pompeiano O, eds. Reflex control of posture and movement. New York: Elsevier Biomedical Press, 1979.
128. Brink E, Suzuki I, Timerick S, Wilson V. Tonic neck reflex of the decerebrate cat: a role for propriospinal neurons. J Neurophysiol 1985;54:978–987.
129. Wilson V, Ezure K, Timerick S. Tonic neck reflex

of the decerebrate cat: response of spinal interneurons to natural stimulation of neck and vestibular receptors. J Neurophysiol 1984;51:567–577.

130. Suzuki I, Timerick S, Wilson V. Body position with respect to the head or body position in space is coded by lumbar interneurons. J Neurophysiol 1985;54:123–133.

131. Sasaki S, Alstermark B, Lundberg A, Pinter M. Descending control and functional role of long C3–C4 propriospinal neurons reflex organization of the spinal cord and its descending control. Canberra, Australia. 1983; Abstracts 2,7.

132. Pompeiano O, Manzoni D, Srivastava U, Stampacchia G. Convergence and interacitonof neck and muscular vestibular inputs on reticulospinal neurons. Neuroscience 1984;12:111–128.

133. Vasilenko D, Kostyukov A. I Brain stem and primary afferent projections to the ventromedial group of propriospinal neurons in the cat. Brain Res 1976;117:141–146.

134. Nakajima K, Maeda M, Ishii S, Miyazaki M. Neuronal organization of the tonic neck reflex. Equilibrium Res 1981;40:195–201.

135. Baloh R, Honrubia V, eds. Clinical neurophysiology of the vestibular system. Philadelphia: F A Davis Co., 1979, pp 1–11.

136. Maekawa K, Natsui T. Climbing fiber activation of Purkinje cells in rabbits' flocculus during light stimulation of the retina. Brain Res 1973;59:417–20.

137. Simpson J. Precht W, Llinas R. Sensory separation in climbing and mossy fiber inputs to cat vestibulo-cerbellum. Pfleugers Arch Eur J Physiol 1974;351:183–93.

138. Maekawa K, Takeda T. Mossy fiber responses evoked in the cerebellar flocculus of rabbits by stimulation of the optic pathway. Brain Res 1975;98:590–5.

139. Ghelarducci B, Ito M, Yagi N. Impulse discharges from floccular Purkinje cells of alert rabbits during visual stimulation combined with horizontal head rotation. Brain Res 1975;87:66–72.

140. Precht W, ed. Neuronal operations in the vestibular system. In: Studies of the brain function. New York: Springer-Verlag, Vol 2,1978.

141. Robinson DA. Adaptive gain control of vestibulo-ocular reflex by the cerebellum. J Neurophysiol 1976;39:954–69.

142. Takemore S. Visual suppression test. Ann Otol Rhinol Laryngol 1977;86:80–5.

143. Berman N. Connection of the pretectum in the cat. J Comp Neurol 1977;174:227–54.

144. Collewijn H. Direction-selective units in the rabbit's nucleus of the optic tract. Brain Res 1975;100:489–508.

145. Giolli R, Guthie M. The primary optic projections in the rabbit. An experimental degeneration study. J Comp Neurol 1969;136:99–126.

146. Hoffman K, Behrend K, Schoppmann A. A direct afferent visual pathway from the nucleus of the optic tract to the inferior olive in the cat. Brain Res 1976;115–150–3.

147. Hoddevik G, Brodal A. The olivocerebellar projection studied with the method of retrograde axonal transport of horseradish peroxidase V. The projections to the flocculonodular lobe and the paraflocculus in the rabbit. J Comp Neurol 1977;176;269–80.

148. Wilson V, Melvill-Jones G, eds. Mammalian vestibular physiology. New York: Plenum Press, 1979.

149. Bentivoglio M. The organization of the direct cerebellospinal projections. In: Kuypers H, Martin G, eds. Progress in brain research No. 57. Decending pathways to the spinal cord. New York: Elsevier Biomedical Press, 1982, pp 279–291.

150. Barmack N. Immediate and sustained influences of visual olivocerebellar activity on eye movment. In: Talbott RE, Humphrey DR, eds. Posture and movement. New York: Raven Press, 1979, pp 127–129.

151. Soechting J, Berthoz A. Dynamic role of vision in the control of posture in man. Exp Brain Res 1979;36:551–561.

152. Fitz-Ritson DE. Therapeutic traction. A review of enurological principles and clinical applications. JManipulative Physiol Ther 1984;7(1):39–49.

153. Bakker DA, Richmond FJR. Muscle spindle complexes in muscles around the upper cervical vertebrae in the cat. J Neurophysiol 1982; 48(1):62–74.

154. Jowett R, Fidler M, Troup D. Histochemical changes in the multifidus in mechanical derangements of the spine. Orthop Clin North Am 1975;6(1):145–61.

155. Barker D, Milburn A. Development and regeneration of mammalian muscle spindles. Sci Prog 1984;69:45–64.

156. Wyke B. Neurology of the cervical spinal joints. Physiotherapy 1979;65(3):72–76.

157. Igarashi M, Miyata H, Alford B, Wright W. Nystagmus after experimental cervical lesions. Laryngoscope 1972;82:1609–21.

158. de Jong PT, de Jong VB, Cohen B, Jongkees L. Ataxia and nystagmus induced by injection of local anesthetics on the neck. Ann Neurol 1977;1:240–246.

159. Hinoki M, Hine S, Ushio N, et al. Studies on ataxia of lumar origin in cases of vertigo due to whiplash injury. Equilibrium Res 1973;3(1):141–152.

160. Gutmann G, Vele F. The joints of the upper cervical spine and their effects upon motor sterotypes. From Manuelle Medizin und ihre wissenschaftlichen Grundlagen. Wolff H, Trier D eds. Verlaf fur physikalische medizin, Heide borg, 1970.

161. Miller AD, Roossin P, Schor R. Roll tilt re after vestibulospinal tract lesion. Exp Br 1982;48:107–112.

162. Sandoz RN. Some reflex phenomena with spinal derangements and adju Swiss Chiro Assoc 1981;7:45–6

163. Simons DG. Muscle pain syndro J Phys Med 1976;55(1):15–4

164. Wolpaw J. Adaptive plastic spinal stretch reflex (SSR): opment. Brain Res 1983

165. Wolpaw J, O'Keefe J. A primate spinal stretch two-phase process. J (11):2718–2724.

4 Normal Mechanics of the Upper Cervical Spine

Adrian S. Grice, M.Sc., D.C., F.C.C.S.(C)

The cervical spine is the most mobile section of the vertebral column. The postural righting reflexes, which arise from the apophyseal joints particularly in the human, are the major regulators of the body's posture and locomotor dynamics(1). The relationship of posture and locomotion to the upper cervical region can be approached from a number of points of view. In this chapter, the biomechanical aspects of this relationship will be emphasized.

It has long been recognized that upright posture, characterized by bipedal support of the heavily muscled, large pelvic ring, supporting two independent large shoulder girdles on the thinly curved "S" column of the lumbar and thoracic spine, and the support of the comparatively heavy cranium on the smaller cervical column, typifies a structure which is inherently unstable. This underlies the axiom that the human body is built for mobility, not stability. These and similar observations led Tobias in 1982(2) to call "man, the tottering biped"; Feldenkrais(3) to draw the analogy of the body's postural system to "three inverted pyramids," and Johnston(4), in 1960, to develop concepts and measurements of the "pyramidal man" embodied in his postural anlaytical system. These postural measurements showed not only a posterior pinal gravity line at the lumbar region, but equently a decompensated anterior ceral head carriage (Fig. 4.1, *a* and *b*).

comparative review of the cervical omy in the quadruped and biped arements reveals that, with horizontal ral head carriage, the nuchal ligment quadruped is highly developed with a well-demarcated nuchal ridge. The cervical spinous processes are long and well developed, forming long levers for ligamentous attachment and muscular action. In man, the upright weight of the head is normally carried more directly over the cervical spine so that the center of gravity of the skull is just anterior to the base of

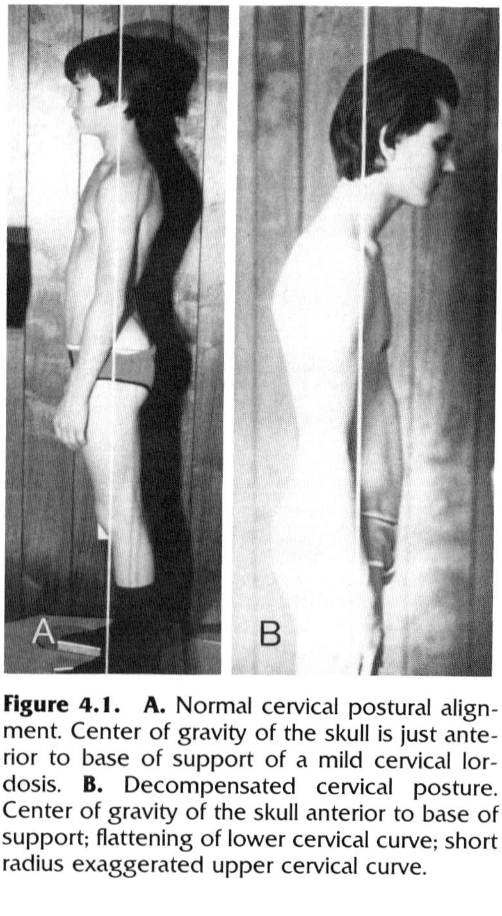

Figure 4.1. A. Normal cervical postural alignment. Center of gravity of the skull is just anterior to base of support of a mild cervical lordosis. **B.** Decompensated cervical posture. Center of gravity of the skull anterior to base of support; flattening of lower cervical curve; short radius exaggerated upper cervical curve.

support, therefore the tension on the nuchal ligmament and spinous processes, as well as on the cervical musculature, is reduced. As a result, the nuchal ridge is less marked and the cervical spinous processes are shorter. The multiple layers of muscle provide for a wide range of motion in all orthogonal axes. In the human spine the C2 spinous process remains the largest with the second cervical vertebra characteristically the most predominant. The normal cervical lateral curve should be one of a mild lordosis, which is thought to be protective of the skull and brain as well as of the vertebral and intervening joints by providing a dampening effect on the shock of axial deceleration(5) (Fig. 4.2., *a* and *b*).

It is obvious that the cervical column, on the basis of anatomical and functional observations, lends itself easily to a subdivision into upper and lower regions. One must be mindful, however, that as discussion on the upper cervical spine proceeds, in relationship to biomechanics, diagnosis, symptoms, and treatments, that such a division is arbitrary. The biomechanics and neurophysiology of the upper cervical spine form part of an integrated system with the body as whole.

Historically, the chiropractic perspective has emphasized the statics of spinal function, with great emphasis, especially in the upper cervical spine, placed on bony alignment in the neutral position. More recently, the dynamic function of the spine has come to be appreciated along with concepts of motor patterning of function. These aspects of upper cervical spinal function will occupy the greatest emphasis in this chapter.

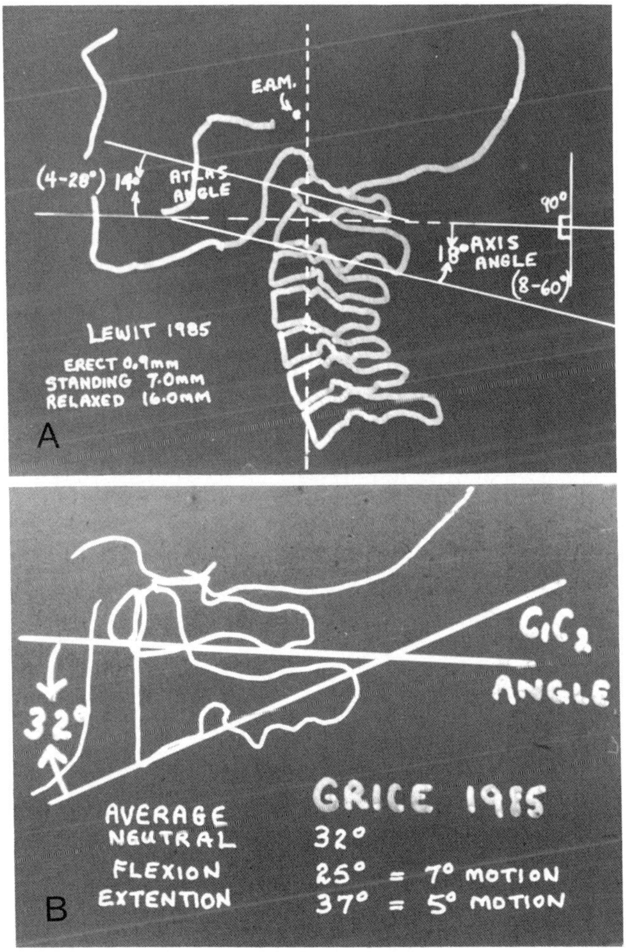

Figure 4.2. **A.** Static alignment of the upper cervical spine, lateral view. **B.** Sitting C1, C2 angle (author's own study): average, 32°; average flexion, 25°, resulting in 7° motion; average extension, 37°, resulting in 5° motion.

Static support and dynamic function of the upper cervical spine depend upon (a) intrinsic factors—spinal ligaments, osseous structures (in particular the joint facings), and the intervertebral disc (C2–C3), and (b) extrinsic factors—the muscular structures which are comprised of a complex deeper layer of suboccipital muscles, sometimes called the suboccipital complex muscles, and a superficial layer of large postural muscles. The stiffness offered by the soft tissues of the spine has been calculated to be in the order of 2 kg and provides enough intrinsic support to maintain the relative shape of the spine(6). We must also be aware that the spine deprived of its muscles and external ligaments will still have dynamic behaviors which are a function of the osseous configurations. The structure-governs-function, and function-governs-structure axioms are, therefore, particularly interesting when one evaluates the upper cervical region.

The ligamentum nuchae is one of the most important supporting structures of the cervical spine, in particular, of the upper cervical segments. This structure is active mainly at the limits of joint motion, particularly of forward flexion. However, the attachment of many muscles to the ligamentum nuchae makes it a more dynamic and active ligament for the support and the control of cranial movements, since muscle tonus change can alter the tension of the ligament.

NORMAL MECHANICS

Segmental biomechanics will be discussed according to the following critera: (a) range of motion; (b) pattern of motion; (c) axis of motion. Throughout the discussion a correlation will be maintained between specific anatomical structures and the specific joint functions that they influence and/or control.

Occiput-Atlas

Flexion/Extension

The most important motion between occiput and atlas is in the sagittal plane producing flexion and extension (Fig. 4.3.).

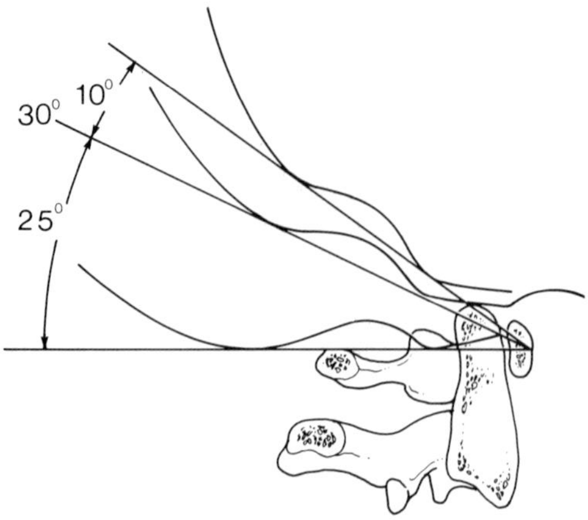

Figure 4.3. Flexion-extension range of motion between occiput (C0) and atlas (C1).

Steindler(6) reviews some of the historic literature on this flexion/extension range of motion: Mollier (1899), 20–35°; Virchow (1909), 20–28°; Strasser (1913), 35°; and Knese (1948–50), 21.7°. He states that the greater movement is in extension, and that during this motion the extent of gliding movement is 10 mm. White and Panjabi(7) cite a range for total flexion and extension of 13°. According to Hohl(8) the C0–C1 joints are restricted to a flexion/extension motion with a range of 15°. Fielding's(9) cineroentgenographic study reports a range of motion as flexion, 10°, extension, 25°. Arlen(10) reports a total of 14.84° with +5.31° variation. Conley(11), when reporting a marking system for the upper and lower cervical spine, reported on three sample cases showing flexion of 1°, 7°, and 5° with extension of 12°, respectively. Werne and Munksgaard(12) have made one of the most significant contributions to our understanding of the upper cervical region in observations from both postmortem and radiographic studies. Their postmortem studies on six males and eight females (ages 19–82, average age of 51.2) showed a flexion/extension range from 18 to 41° with an average of 29.8°. On 104 radiographic studies, the range was 9 to 39.5° with an average of 23.4°. Movement between C1–C2 was ascribed to be from 3.5 to 32.5° with an average of 13.4° total flexion/extension. Their studies showed no significant difference between the sexes and no sig-

Radiographic Studies of C0–C1 Motion

	Flexion		Extension	Range
Werne, 1957		13.4°		3.5°/32.5°
Fielding, 1957	10°		25°	
Hohl, 1964		15.0°		
Braakman and Penning, 1971		30.0°		
Lane, 1971	−6.6°		11.4°	
Conley, 1974	1°,7°,5°		12°,7°,12°	
Arlen, 1978	14.8°		13.2°	±5° and 6°
Lewit, 1985		15°		
Henderson, 1985		−0.6 mm −1.1 mm		

Figure 4.4. Radiographic studies of C0–C1 motion.

nificant difference in the ages of the subjects. Lewit(13) reviewed some of the literature in this field and his summary was that 13° of extension and 10° of flexion were representative of motion between C0 and C1. It is obvious that these authors studying the range of motion in the cervical region have produced figures that have a wide range in the one simple movement of flexion and extension (Fig. 4.4). To understand these observations, recognition must be given not only to the range of motion observed but also to the patterns of motion possible in this region.

Jones(14) presented observations regarding flexion in the cervical spine in two distinct patterns of motion: (1) chin retraction followed by cervical flexion; and conversely, (2) flexion of the cervical spine followed by chin retraction. With chin retraction, he observed that the cervical spine first moved backward, i.e., the cervical lordosis straightened, then the upper cervical spine moved forward into flexion. With marked chin retraction, the midcervical segments angulated forward. As flexion of the cervical spine proceeds, a flattening of the cervical spine follows and a lordotic reversal may take place. With cervical flexion followed by chin retraction, greater motion is seen in the lower cervicals, the midcervicals show less angulation, and the upper cervical spine extends (C0–C1 particularly).

Grice(15) suggested that this pattern of motion accounts for the apparent fixation and reversal of motion often seen in the upper cervical region. Using a standard flexion/extension stress film study done in full flexion without chin retraction, Grice and Injeyan (author's data) made further observations on this topic confirming the pattern of motion during C0–C1 flexion. It was reported that during early cervical flexion with chin retraction, the upper cervical segment C0–C1 has a range of about 10 degrees, while reversal of or extension of occiput takes place with full cervical flexion with or without chin retraction unless the patient is very young in which case, in our opinion, the ligamentum nuchae is very flexible or extensible.

Werne and Munksgaard(12) and Braakman and Penning(16) made further observations that confirm this pattern of motion. Their observations deal largely with flexion between C0 and C2 demonstrating that the total range of motion is greatly enhanced during chin retraction. With neck flexion and extension, the measurements between the occiput and odontoid angles in neutral flexion and extension were reported. These angles were 101° neutral, 106° flexion, and 95° extension, producing a total range of 11° of motion. Next, the angles of flexion and extension with chin retraction and jaw jutting forward were measured, showing angles of 116° flexion and 85° extension, demonstrating a total range of 31°—a significantly higher range of motion.

Some authors have taken the position that little or no movement takes place between C0 and C1 during cervical flexion. What are the mechanisms that produce this observation? Jackson(17) points out that normally, gross forward flexion of the cervical spine should be limited only by the chin striking the sternum. In the physiologically mobile individual, as the chin strikes the sternum, extension at the occiput normally takes place because the lower cervicals allow continued neck motion. This would be demonstrated on x-ray as a lack of C0-C1 motion since the occiput extends when full flexion is reached. A second mechanism was previously discussed when observing the function of the ligamentum nuchae. This ligament receives the attachment of many muscles (notably the splenius capitus), which help to stabilize the cervical spine and assist in connecting the cervical segments into a functional posturally dynamic unit. With the gradual degeneration of posture, and the resultant forward carriage of the head, this ligament and the supporting muscular attachments become shortened. When these posterior elements are shortened, normal forward flexion of the cervical spine would result in an extension movement of occiput as these structures "brake" the forward inclination of occiput producing a posterior rotation on the atlas. This is frequently observed as a normal finding(18, 19). In these cases, the range of cervical flexion is then limited not by the chin abutting the sternum, but by the resistance of the posterior elements which have undergone adaptive shortening and contracture, as a result of altered static posture, which now may be limited in their reversibility and may be considered normal for that individual (Fig. 4.5). Lane(20) reported that 35 of 50 subjects showed this C0–C1 posterior arch malposition in flexion and 16 of 17 normal asymptomatic volunteers demonstrated this alignment during "reading posture."

The use of cineradiographic analysis by Jones(21) and Fielding(8) allows for the most precise determination of the maximum point of occiput-atlas flexion, since under these circumstances the position of maximum flexion of these joints can be seen. A review of Fielding's study confirms that his observations were most probably made in the chin retraction position of flexion, which allows the maximum range of motion, resulting in a reported angle of C0–C1 flexion as 10°. The proper use of chin retraction in plain film studies can demonstrate a normal range of motion with the extension range up to 25°, as reported (Fig. 4.4).

Rotation/Lateral Flexion

Pure rotation between C0 and C1 is considered by most authors as nonexistent (Fig. 4.6). Werne(12) and Hjortsjo(22) suggested that only biaxial motion of the C0–C1 joint could take place. Their discussion compared the joints to eggs lying in tablespoons, and concluded that rotation could take place only in a longitudinal axis and with rocking between the "tip" and the "handle." Henka(25) determined the axis of motion by sagittal and frontal sections of the joint. The transverse axis, he suggested, was through the center of the mastoid, and the sagittal axis through a point two to three inches superior to the dens. Various other authors(7, 16, 24) have located the axis of motion in a very similar position. The anatomy of the area would suggest that pure rotation cannot occur; however, a combined lateral flexion and rotation may occur. Steindler(21) describes the condyles forming a 55–60° angle with the anterior of the condyles being 21 to 25 mm apart and the posterior 30 to 34 mm apart (Fig. 4.7). In the lateral plane, the anterior curve of the condyle has a radius of 13 mm; the posterior curve has a radius of 21 mm, with frequent assymetries right to left (Fig. 4.8). This angulation of the condyles would suggest no single arc of motion but rather a sliding or rocking combined rotation motion. Werne(12) experimentally attempted to confirm the combined or coupled movement at C0–C1 and C1–C2 on rotation and as he expected, with the occiput fixed, rotation of the trunk produced lateral flexion. Illi(25) has a more clinically valuable method of explaining rotation between C0 and C1 (Fig. 4.6). He explains that the occipital condyle is larger than the atlas lateral mass and rotation is permitted because of this discrepancy in size, but that because of the angle and shape of the condyles, it is obvious that lateral motion is required during rotation. We can also see again that there is no single axis of motion permitted. Kapandji(24) is of the opinion that rotation amounts to 3° in the C0–C1 region. With 3° of lateral flexion, Werne(12) found 8° of lateral flexion between C0 and C1 with an axis of motion 2 cm superior to the apex

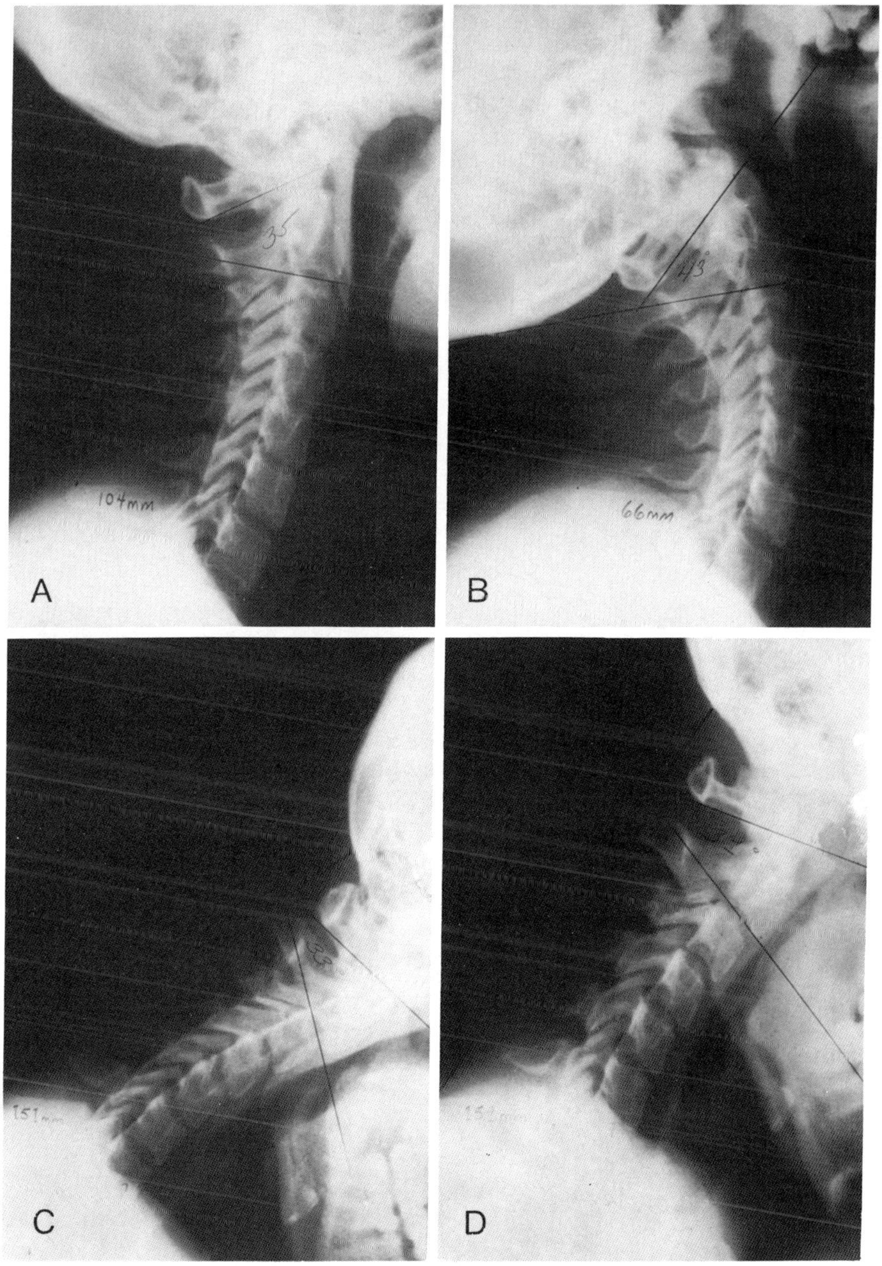

Figure 4.5. **A.** Neutral cervical lateral ligamentum nuchae measurement from occiput to C7 spinous, 104 mm. **B.** Extension: normal upper cervical extension ligament measurement, 66 mm. **C.** Full cervical flexion: ligament measurement, 151 mm; normal lower cervical flexion, reduced upper cervical motion of C0–C1–C2. **D.** Chin retraction cervical flexion: ligament measurement, 151 mm; flexion of lower cervicals present, gliding and tipping, with normal upper cervical motion of C0–C1–C2.

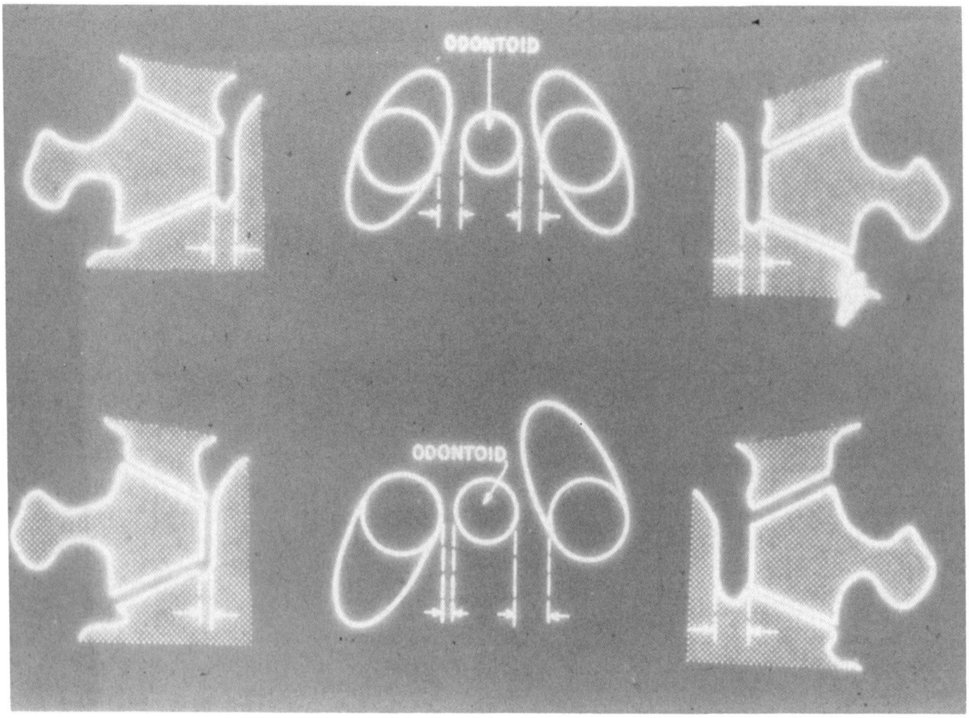

Figure 4.6. Schematic depiction of occiput, C1 and odontoid shows how larger occipital condyle allows rotation of C1 lateral masses and, because of angulation of condyles, produces coupled lateral flexion. (Left rotation of C0 produces right lateral flexion of C1).

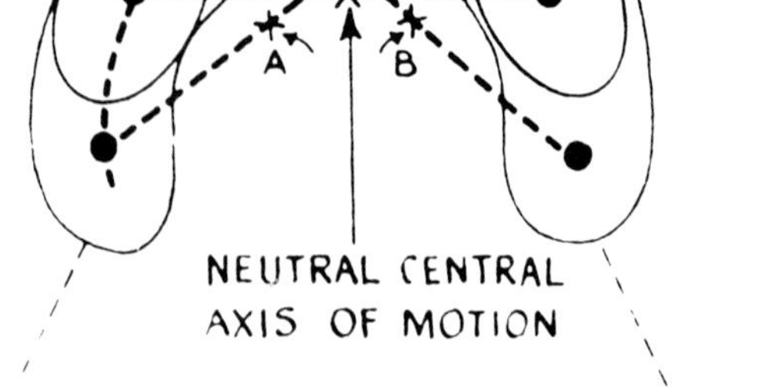

Figure 4.7. Schematic depiction shows angle of C0 condyles normally 55–60°, anterior condyles 21–25 mm apart, posterior condyles 30–34 mm apart. Arc of motion established by each condyle with centroid A. No single axis of motion exists. Rotation and lateral flexion must be coupled motions.

of the odontoid. Braakman and Penning(17) suggest a 5° range of motion in lateral flexion (Figs. 4.9 and 4.10).

Lewit and Krausova(26) and Lewit(13) report lateral flexion between C0 and C2 of 5.5° and suggest part of this motion was between C0 and C1.

Werne reported lateral flexion only as a combined or coupled motion. This pattern of motion has been discussed by several authors and from these discussions, some idea of the pattern of motion can be established.

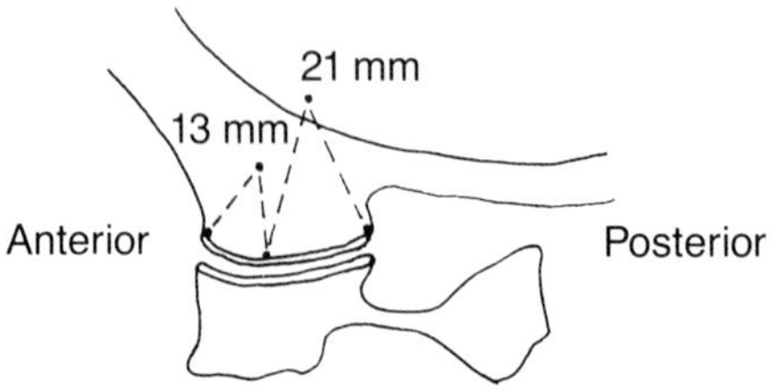

Figure 4.8. C0 condyle. Anterior and posterior slope 13 and 21 mm radius, respectively.

C0–C1 Lateral Flexion Motion ± Rotation

	Lateral Flexion	Rotation
Kapandji, 1974	3.0°	3.8°
Werne, 1957	8.0°	Combined
Braakman and Penning, 1971	5.0°	
Baake, 1931	5.0°	
Lewit, 1985	5.5°	C0–C2 Combined
Dvorak, 1984	4°	

Figure 4.9. C0–C1 lateral flexion motion ± rotation.

Hohl and Baker(27) demonstrated radiographically that with lateral flexion of only 15°, rotation of the axis takes place. Lewit(13) and Jirout(28, 29) stated that lateral flexion was absolutely dependent on rotation and lateral flexion, which starts at the craniocervical region, begins with rotation of C2.

Atlas-Axis

Flexion/Extension

Motion in the sagittal plane at C1–C2 has been reported as smaller that that of C0–C1 (Fig. 4.11). White and Panjabi(7) report a flexion/extension range of 10°. Prantl(30)

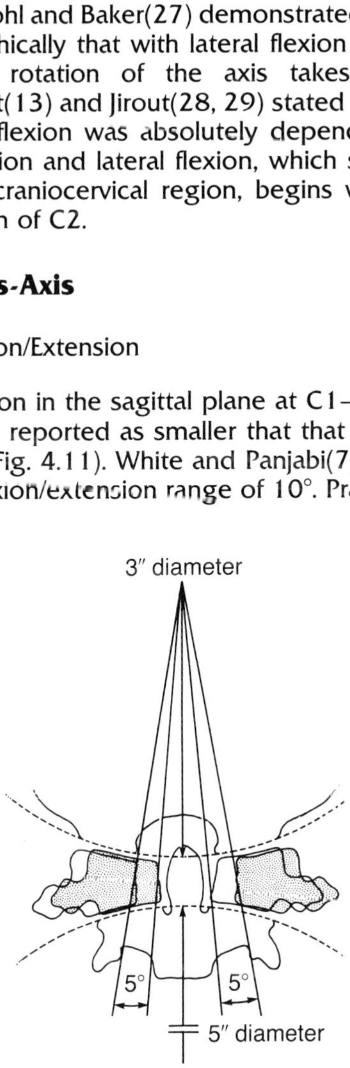

Figure 4.10. Five degrees of lateral flexion take place between C0 and C1 using the arc of the condyles to form a center of motion. C0 condyles form an angle of 132° radius, approximately 3 inches.

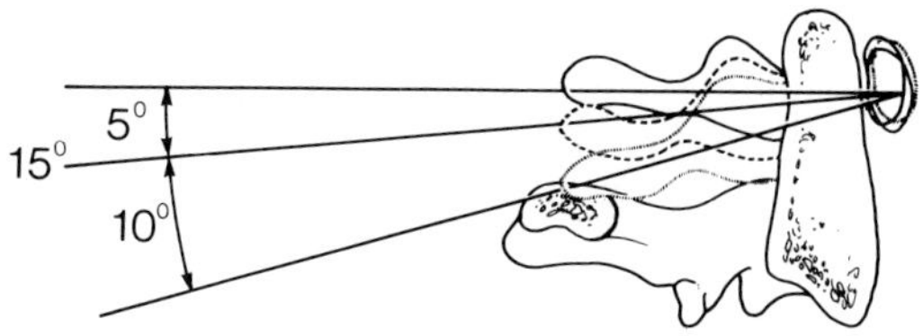

Figure 4.11. Flexion-extension range of motion between atlas (C1) and axis (C2).

recently reported on the use of clinical radiographic methods of evaluating the range of motion in the cervical region—the Buette-Bauml (1959) overlay method as well as the Arlen, (1978) method. He concludes that the C1–C2 range of sagittal motion is from 12 to 21°. Arlen(31) reported 5.94°+4.53° and 4.36+3.5° of C1–C2 flexion and extension, respectively. Hohl(8) suggests a normal flexion/extension of 15°. Fielding(9) reported a range of 15° with 5° flexion and 10° of extension using cineradiography as his method of study. Poirier and Charpy(32) reported a range of 11° while Werne and Munkggaarde(12) reported 11° with a range of 2 to 21.5°. Lewit(13) reported a range of motion of 15° flexion and extension, the latter figure being the most commonly reported in the normal range of motion. Braakman and Penning(16) report up to 35° of movement while Grieve(33) reports about 8° of flexion, 10° of extension (Figs. 4.12 and 4.13).

The pattern of motion between C1 and C2 is largely controlled by osseous elements, i.e., the shape of the articulations and the movement of the anterior arch of the atlas around the odontoid process. This motion is a rocking, gliding motion between the C1 and C2 facets and a gliding motion between the odontoid and anterior arch of atlas. Several opinions on the normal shape of the axis and atlas facets seem

C1–C2 Motion: Literature Review and Opinion

	Flexion	Extension	Range
White and Panjabi, 1978	10.0°		
Cailliett, 1964	5°	10°	
Grieve, 1981	8°	10°	

Figure 4.12. Literature review and opinion. C1C2 motion.

Radiographic Studies of C1–C2 Motion

	Flexion		Extension	Range
Werne, 1957		11.0°		2–21.5°
Fielding, 1957	5°		10°	
Hohl, 1964		15.0°		
Braakman and Penning, 1971		35.0°		
Arlen, 1978	5.9°		4.3°	±4.5:3.5°
Aho, 1955		13.6°		9–20°
Lewit, 1985		15.0°		
Grice, 1985	7.0°		5.0°	1–11°:2–14°
Henderson, 1985	Male	Female		
	7.9 mm	8.9 mm		

Figure 4.13. Radiographic studies. C1C2 motion.

to be presented. Kapandji(24) describes the axis superior facet as convex and the atlas inferior facet as convex, the final shape arising from the hyaline cartilage structures that form these convexities. Other authors agree(7, 12, 27, 34–41).

Fielding(9), however, describes the superior facet of the axis as convex and the inferior facet of atlas as flat. This latter description is more in keeping with observations and descriptions by anatomical authors(7, 42–47) who often describe the inferior facet of C1 as concave. These contours of the atlas and axis facets would produce a rocking/gliding motion during flexion and extension that could easily be upset by altered muscle tone. Werne(12) discusses the movement of the anterior arch of atlas on the dens. In retroflexion (extension), the arch slides upward, and in anteflexion (flexion), the anterior arch slides downward, the average motion being 1.4 mm. When corrected for radiographic magnification, this motion appears much greater. Kapandji(24) relates a mechanism and an anatomical relationship that allowed no gaping of the anterior arch and the dens during flexion and extension. These theoretical observations do not agree with what appears to be seen in radiographic motion studies (Fig. 4.14). Werne in radiographic and autopsy studies also confirmed that on

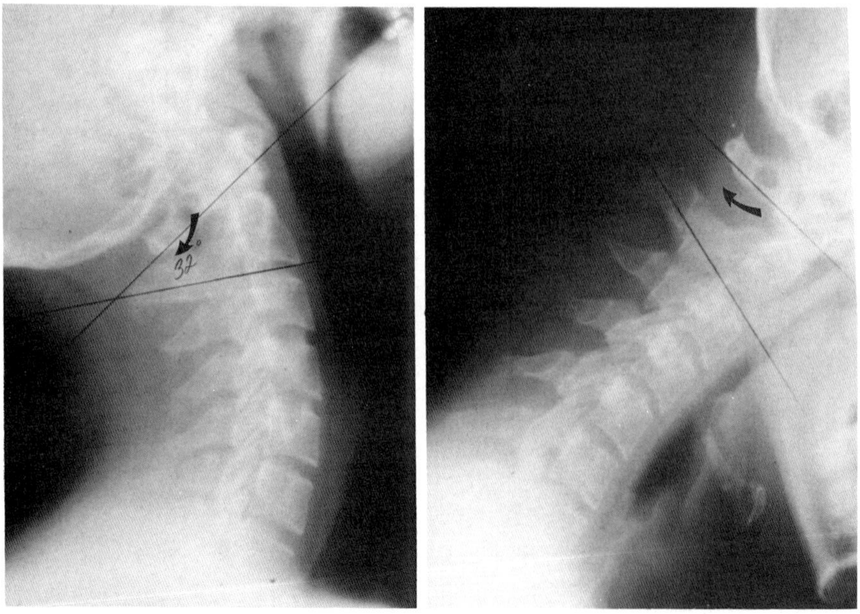

Figure 4.14. Anterior arch of atlas in flexion and extension. Mild elastic separation from odontoid (see *arrows*).

flexion, cranial gaping took place. In his postmortem studies, little or no transverse translation was observed; however, slight vertical translation appeared possible when C1 and C2 were in the neutral position. The normal gaping that occurs suggests that the yieldability of the transverse ligament during flexion and extension, in certain pathologies and traumas, may be excessive.

Rotation/Lateral Flexion

Rotation between C1 and C2 is the major motion in the upper cervical region and constitutes 45–50% of the total range of cervical rotatory movement (Figs. 4.15 and 4.16).

Hohl and Baker(27) describe the range as 45° to each side. Their lateral and oblique x-ray studies showed considerable offset between the C1 and C2 facets during this motion. Anteroposterior films with rotation showed narrowing of the joint space which was caused by superimposition of the superior C1 facet on the inferior C2 facet and rotation of the C2 spinous process. They further point out that because the joints are convex in shape, the C2 vertebra moves inferiorly during rotation and therefore narrowing of the C1–C2 joint space is seen radiographically.

Fielding(9), in cineradiographic studies, measured rotation of the whole cervical spine of up to 90° and C1–C2 rotation as 50% or 45°. His observation was that C0–C1 moved as a unit on C2 up to 50% of the rotation, then the C2 spinous process begins to rotate, followed by the rest of the cervical spine with decreasing amounts of rotation.

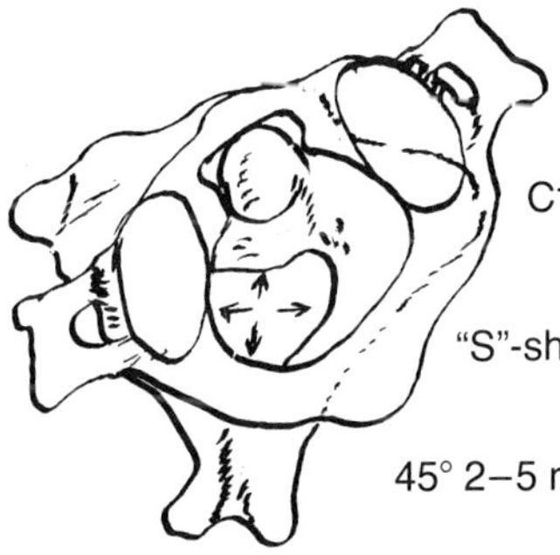

Figure 4.15. C1C2 rotation. Spinal canal is "S" shaped at 45°; there is 2–5 mm of occlusion.

Rotation of C1–C2 Segment

	Rotation	Lateral Flexion
Hohl, 1967	45°	Combined facets offset
Fielding, 1957	45°	
Selecki, 1969	45°	
Dvorak, 1984	40–50°	
Braakman and Penning, 1971	30°	

Figure 4.16. Rotation. C1–C2 segment.

Selecki(48) further observed this pattern of rotation (based on cadaver studies) and states that the first 0 to 30° of rotation occurs solely between C1 and C2 and further rotation up to 45° produces motion in the rest of the cervical spine. This observation is more in keeping with the palpation findings seen in the clinical practice of this author.

Dvorak and associates(49) site a range of 40–50° or 50° total cervical rotation. Lewit(13) also comments on the pattern of rotational motion. His observations are that rotation starts at C1–C2 and continues up to about 25°. At this point, rotation occurs from C3–C7 in succession, i.e., from cranial to caudal at which time this motion is accompanied by lateral flexion, simultaneously including a passive motion between C0 and C1 previously discussed.

Jirout(50–52) discusses a synkinesis of C1 and C2 during lateral flexion. Lewit(13) has further developed Werne's observations(53). Werne purported that rotation of C2 during lateral flexion was due primarily to the influence of the ligaments. Lewit, on the other hand, placed emphasis on the shape of C2–3 articulating facets as well as of the condyle (C2 wedge shape and the cuneiform shape of C1) therefore resulting in displacement and shift of C1 and C2 (Figs. 4.17 and 4.18). Lewit's study(54) on 38 healthy subjects showed an average of 3.6 mm of motion between the basion relative to the tip of the odontoid. Krausova and Lewit's study(55) showed 4.5 mm of motion between C0 condyles and C1 lateral mass with 2.5 mm of motion between C1 and C2 dens, with final rotation of the C2 spinous away from side of lateral bending on average of 23.9 mm. Lewit reported a number of altered biomechanical move-

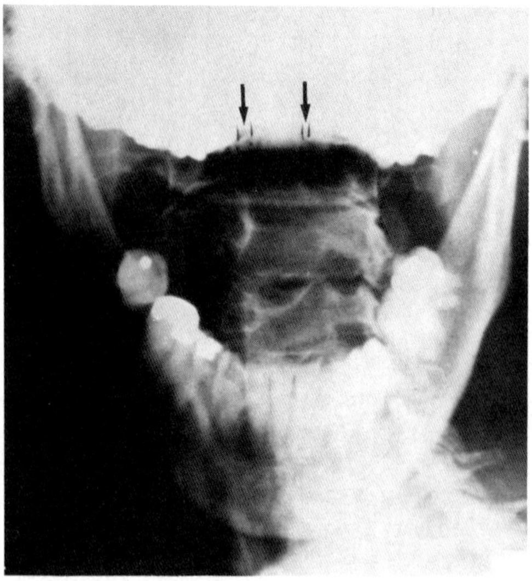

Figure 4.17. Right posterior rotation of cervical spine produces left lateral flexion of C1 (see *arrows*).

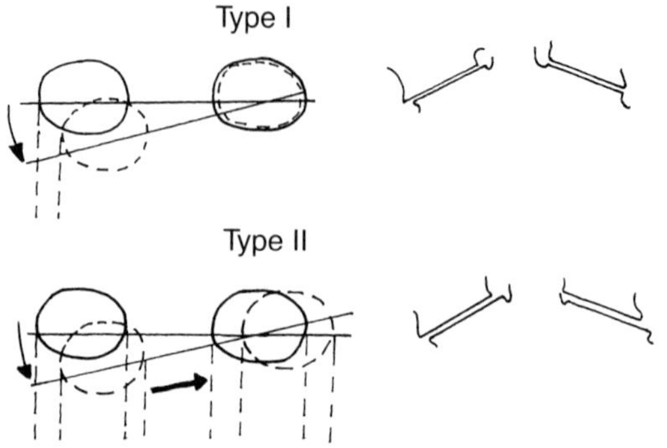

Figure 4.19. *Top,* type I normal motion. Lateral flexion to the left, C1–C2 left articular surfaces offset, right articular surface aligned. *Bottom,* type II. Both left and right articular surfaces offset (see text).

ments, which will be dealt with later, in these healthy subjects.

Hohl and Baker's radiographic study(27) showed that only 15° of lateral flexion/rotation of the axis takes place and, as further lateral flexion occurs, lateral displacement of the atlas and axis occurs. Jirout's study(52) of 372 younger patients showed several patterns of motion during lateral flexion. The type I (Fig. 4.19) pattern, which is considered the normal motion, consists of a displacement of the articular surfaces on the side of lateral flexion and alignment on the opposite side. In Jirout's opinion, this is due to posterior displacement of the articular surfaces on the side of lateral flexion and was seen in the majority of cases. The type II pattern is a displacement of both articular surfaces and was seen in the next highest number of cases. Type III, lateral offset, occurred only on the opposite lateral flexion. In type IV, no displacement occurs in either articular surface (Fig. 4.20). Jirout points out that adequate rotation of C2 is necessary during lateral flexion regulating this motion. Aberrant muscle action will cause the observed type II, III, or IV motion. The axis of motion for rotation at

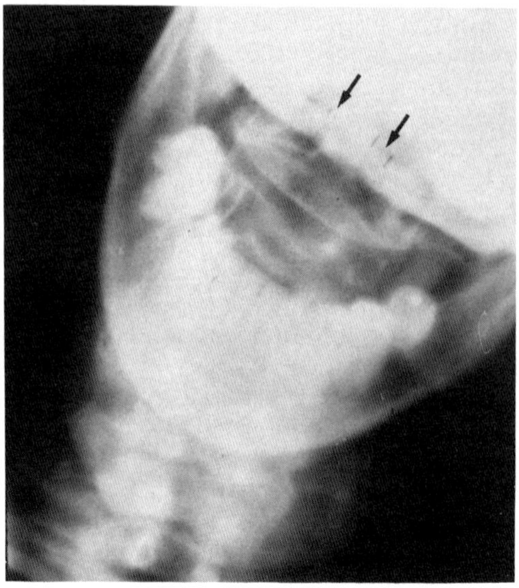

Figure 4.18. Right lateral flexion of cervical spine produces right lateral shift of C1–C2.

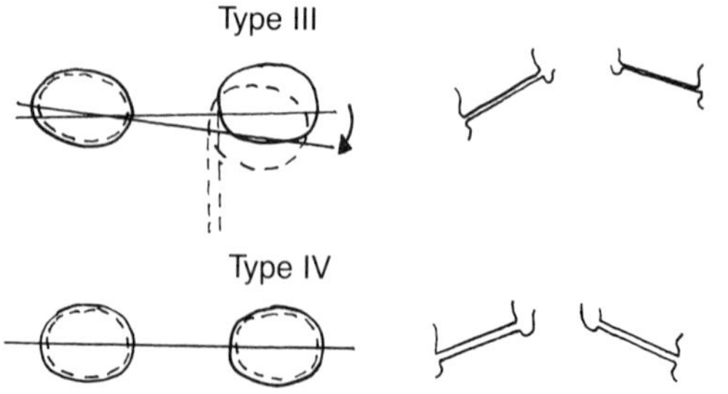

Figure 4.20. *Top,* type III. Left lateral flexion offset only on right facet. *Bottom,* type IV. No motion of articular facets on lateral flexion (see text).

C2 during lateral flexion is in the region of the contralateral facet. During abnormal restriction of C2 rotation, displacement of axis against C1 to the side opposite rotation occurs.

The rotational dynamics at C1–C2 have several implications that must be considered clinically relevant during corrective therapy. First, rotation results in lateral displacement of C1–C2. Selecki(48) showed that rotation of 30° caused some displacement of a rubber container (meant to represent the spinal cord and its coverings) on the side away from the direction of rotation. This rotation caused a reduction in the anteroposterior plane as well as a lateral moulding of the container into an "S" shape. As rotation continued to 45°, this appearance was enhanced with a reduction in the anteroposterior plane of 2–5 mm (Fig. 4.15).

These changes would not interfere with the contents of the spinal within physiological limits, but excessive rotation, ligamentous laxity, and/or pathomechanical motion may contribute to subtle trauma at this level and become very important in rotational adjustment for the upper cervical region. Selecki further studied the vertebral artery noting that rotation of 30° caused some kinking of the contralateral vertebral artery, i.e., rotation to the right caused narrowing of the left vertebral artery. This kinking progressed up to 45°, i.e., to the normal limit of motion. Additional rotation (beyond the normal range, which resulted in trauma to specimen) produced kinking or occlusion of both arteries. His observation was that rotation caused kinking and stretching of the artery by forward displacement of the atlas on the axis due to the fact that these arteries travel between C1 and C2 transverse foramen. Although a loop exists at full rotation, stretching of the artery inevitably results.

In a manipulation of C1–C2 for rotation, the clinician should rotate the spine to 30° and then produce mild lateral flexion, e.g., 3–5° at the C1–C2 junction. This should produce optimal biomechanical rotational correction and should be less traumatic than full cervical rotation, which has the possibility of stretching vital structures there.

PATTERNS OF MOTION OF THE WHOLE UPPER CERVICAL COMPLEX

It is convenient to divide a discussion of the integrated motion patterns into that of flexion/extension of C0–C1–C2 and rotation/lateral bending of C0–C1–C2. A synthesis of much of the literature, including the work of Fielding, Braakman and Penning, Kapandji, and Jirout allows us to describe the typical and normal integrated actions of this region.

During the early stages of flexion, the Co–C1–C2 range of motion is complete. This motion is maximal when chin retraction occurs and the lower cervical range of motion is restricted. As full flexion occurs in the cervical spine, the ligamentum nuchae is stretched to its full extent and the occiput is pulled into extension, therefore limiting the apparent motion between C0–C1 and C2.

Rotation and lateral flexion are controlled by the musculature attached to the occiput. During rotation, the occiput is driven on C2 and the rest of the cervical spine, with C1 being drawn with the occiput forming a kind of intermediate linkage. During lateral flexion the muscles on the convexity contract eccentrically to lower the occiput, which, as the occipital condyle on the concave side descends on the C2 lateral articulation, produces rotation of C2 spinous process to the convexity. The motion forces ipsilateral tipping of C1 because of the wedge-shaped pincer action of C0–C2 articulations. Again the atlas has an intermediate rotational linkage. To illustrate this, then, during right lateral flexion, the occiput tends to rotate posterior on the left while C2 rotates posteriorly on the right. C1 assumes an intermediate linkage position largely in a passive manner. These patterns of motion can be easily disturbed by aberrant muscle tensions leading to abnormal biomechanics or joint fixations. This intermediary role of C1 provides an ideal contact point for correcting many biomechanical aberrations and fixations and clearly is the reason why many techniques have developed around the C1 vertebral segment.

References

1. Wyke BD. Neurology of the cervical spinal joints. Physiotherapy 1979;65:72–76.
2. Tobias PV. Man the tottering biped: the evolution of his erect posture. In: Garlick D, (ed.) Proprioception posture and emotion. CPME 1982.
3. Feldenkrais M. Body and mature behaviour. International. Univ Press Inc Third I.U.P., 1975.
4. Johnston LC. Three dimensional spinal analysis: the key to statistical research and public service. Digest Chiro Econ 1967;10(2):18–19.
5. Morris JM. Spinal mechanics. In: Spinal deformities and neurological dysfunction. Chou SN Seljeskog EL eds. New York: Raven Press, 1978:25–40.
6. Steindler A. Kinesiology of the human body. 3rd ed. Springfield, IL: Charles C Thomas, 1970:141–47.
7. White AA, Panjabi MM. The clinical biomechanics of the spine. Philadelphia: Lippincott, 1978.
8. Hohl M. Normal motions in the upper portion of the cervical spine. J Bone Joint Surg 1964; 46:1777.
9. Fielding JW. Cineroentgenography of the normal cervical spine. J Bone Jt Surg 1957;39A:1280.
10. Arlen A. Biometriche Rontgen-Funkhonsdiagnostik der Halswarbelsaule, Fischer, Heidelburg (Schriftenreiche Manuelle Medizin Bds), 1979.
11. Conley RN. Stress evaluation of cervical spinal mechanics. J Clin Chiro (3) special ed, 1974.
12 Werne S, Munksgaard E. Studies in spontaneous atlas dislocation. Acta orthop scand (Suppl)13, 1957.
13. Lewit K. Manipulative therapy in rehabilitation of the locomotor system. Wellington: Butterworths, 1985:78.
14. Jones MD. Cineradiographic studies of the normal cervical spine. Calif Med 1960;93;293–296.
15. Grice AS. Preliminary evaluation of 50 saggital cervical motion radiographic examinations. J Can Clin Assoc 1977;21(1):33–34.
16. Braakman R, Penning L. Injuries of the cervical spine. Excerpta Med London, 1971.
17. Jackson R. The cervical syndrome. 34th ed. Springfield, IL: Charles C Thompson, 1966.
18. Henderson DJ, Dormon TM. Functional roentgenometric evaluation of the cervical spine in the sagittal plane. J. Manipulative Physiol Ther 1985;8:(4)219–227.
19. Howe J. Cineradiographic evaluation of normal and abnormal cervical spinal function. J Clin Chiro Ed 1972;2:76–88.
20. Lane G. Cervical spine: its movement and symptomatology. J Clin Chiro Arch Ed 1971;1:128–145.
21. Jochumsen OH. The curve of the cervical spine. ACA J Chiro, 1970, p.49.
22. Hjortsjo E. (cit Broman-Hjortsjo) Studier over kaklemekaniken Gleerup. Lund 1954.
23. Henka W. Die Bewegung Zwischen Atlas und Epistropheus zt8chr.f.rat Med III Reihe bdz. Leipzig und Heidelberg, 1958.
24. Kapandji IA. The physiology of the joints. Vol. 3. The trunk and vertebral column. London: Churchill Livingstone, 1974.
25. Illi FWH. Highlights of 45 years of experience and 35 years of research. Presented at European Chiropractic Union Convention, May, 1971.
26. Lewit K, Krausova L. Mechanismus and bewegungsausmass in den kopfgelenken bei passwen bewegungen. Zeitschrift fur Orthopadie undire Grenzgehiete, 103, 323.
27. Hohl M, Baker HR. The atlanto axial joint. J Bone Jt Surg 1964;46:(8):*1739–1752.*
28. Jirout J. Die Rolle der Axis bei der Seitneigung der halswerbelsulle und die "latente skoliose". Furtschritte auf dem Gebet der Rontgenslrahler 1968, 109:74–81.
29. Jirout J. The rotational component in the dynamics of the C2–3 spinal segment. Neuroradiology 1979; 17:177.
30. Prantl K. X-ray examination and functional analysis of the cervical spine. Manual Medicine 1985;2:5–15.
31. Arlen A. Mebuerfahren Zur Erfassung von Statik and Dynamik der Halswirbelsaule. Manuelle Medizin 1978:16:(1)4.
32. Poirier P, Charpy A. Traite d'anatomie humaine 1:74–89, Paris:1926.
33. Grieve G. Common vertebral joint problems. New York: Churchill Livingston, 1981.
34. Bunton RW, Grennan DM, Palmer DG, de Silva RTD. Lateral subluxation at the atlas in rheumatoid arthritis. Br Med J Radiol 1978, Dec S1:*963–67.*
35. Epstein BS. The spine: a radiological text and atlas. 4th ed. 1976. Philadephia: Lea & Febiger.
36. Gates D. Correlative spinal anatomy. Lakemont GA: CSA Printing & Bindery 1977.
37. Gray A, Lewis W. Anatomy of human body. Philadelphia: Lea & Febiger, 1973.
38. Hadley LE. The Spine. Springfield, IL: Charles C Thomas, 1964.
39. Humphry G. Treatice on the human skeleton. Cambridge: MacMillan & Co, 1858.
40. Wackenheim A. Roentgen diagnosis of the craniovertebral region. Berlin: Springer-Verlag, 1974.
41. Wortzman G, Dewar FP. Rotational atlantoaxial subluxation. Radiology 1968;90:479–484.
42. Grieve G. Common vertebral joint problems. New York: Churchill Livingston, 1981, p.3.
43. Lockhart RD, Hamilton GF, Fyfe FW. Anatomy of the human body. London: Faber and Faber Ltd, 1959, p.68.
44. Romanes GJ. Cunningham's manual of practical anatomy. Vol 3. Head and neck and brain. 14 ed, New York: Oxford University Press, 1979.
45. Rothman RJ, Simeone FA. The spine. Vol 1. Toronto: WB Saunders Co, 1974; p.24.
46. William PL, Warwich R. Gray's anatomy, 35 ed. Edinburgh: Longman, 1973, p.235.
47. Woodburne, Russell. Essentials of human anatomy. 7 ed. New York: Oxford University Press, 1983, p.295.
48. Selecki BR. The effect of rotation of the atlas on the axis: experimental work. Med J Austr. 1969, p.1012.
49. Dvorak J, Dvorak V, Schneider W. Manual medicine. Berlin: Springer-Verlag, 1984.
50. Jirout J. Patterns of changes in the cervical spine on lateral flexion. Neuroradiology 1971;2:164.

51. Jirout J. The effect of molization of the segmental blockade on the sagittal component of the reaction on lateroflexion of the cervical spine. Neuroradiology 1972;3:210.
52. Jirout J. Changes in the atlas-axis relationship on lateral flexion of the head and neck. Neuroradiology 1973;6:215–218.
53. Werne S. The possibilities of movement in the craniovertebral joints. Acta Orthop Scandinav 1959;28:165–173.
54. Lewit K. Pain arising in the posterior arch of the atlas. Eur Neurol 1977;16:263–269.
55. Krausova L, Lewit K: The mechanism and the measuring of the motility in the craniocervical joints during lateral inclinations. Acta Univ Carolinae Med Suppl 1965;21:123–126.

2 Applied Chiropractic Section: Pathomechanics and Clinical Management

5 Pathomechanics of the Upper Cervical Spine

Adrian S. Grice, M.Sc., D.C., F.C.C.S.(C)

In the previous chapter the normal statics and dynamics of the upper cervical spine were discussed with some reference to the normal patterns of motion. Pathomechanical behaviors of the upper cervical region result from

(a) abnormalities of osseous structures;
(b) abnormalities of endpoint limiting factors—ligaments;
(c) abnormalities of active motion by muscle activity.

Pathomechanics can be classified as follows:

(a) congenital or anatomical abnormality of osseous or soft tissues;
(b) ligamentous instability due to disease or trauma;
(c) muscular dysfunction due to disease, trauma, or faulty postural adaptation (contracture) or muscular physiological hypertonicity;
(d) neurological abnormality—disease state or abnormal patterning of function resulting in physiological changing.

Dynamic motion palpation, clinical tests of regional mobility, and functional radiography are important tools in the analysis of upper cervical dysfunction. In radiographic studies, the standard flexion/extension views with due regard for the normal biomechanical patterns of motion will give important pathomechanical information about upper cervical spinal function as well as of the intrinsic and extrinsic factors that may contribute to altered mobility. The recommended technique for the analysis of normal motion of the upper cervical region flexion and extension involves the patient assuming chin retraction and partial flexion of the cervical spine and chin elevation and extension of the cervical spine during the x-ray study.

If further evaluation of the biomechanics of the upper cervical spine is warranted, lateral flexion films in the anteroposterior (AP) open-mouth position will depict normal or abnormal rotation and lateral flexion mechanics of C0–C1 and C1–C2.

Jirout(1) showed that fixation in one plane may not be manifested in another plane. Therefore, for a thorough understanding of the upper cervical biomechanics, a number of views may be necessary. A thorough physical and motion palpation examination is important in deciding which dynamic radiographic study is most important for each case. Once the normal mechanics of the upper cervical spine are appreciated, pathomechanical behaviors can be defined in terms of hypomobility, hypermobility, or an aberrant motion pattern. Even though the individual actions at each of the three upper cervical joints are complex and governed by a variety of muscular components, it is most useful clinically to describe the patterns of hypomobility or fixation in relation to specific or individual muscles. Certainly aberrant mobility or fixation can occur due to ligamentous shortening or capsular changes, but muscular structures are more responsive to neurological change

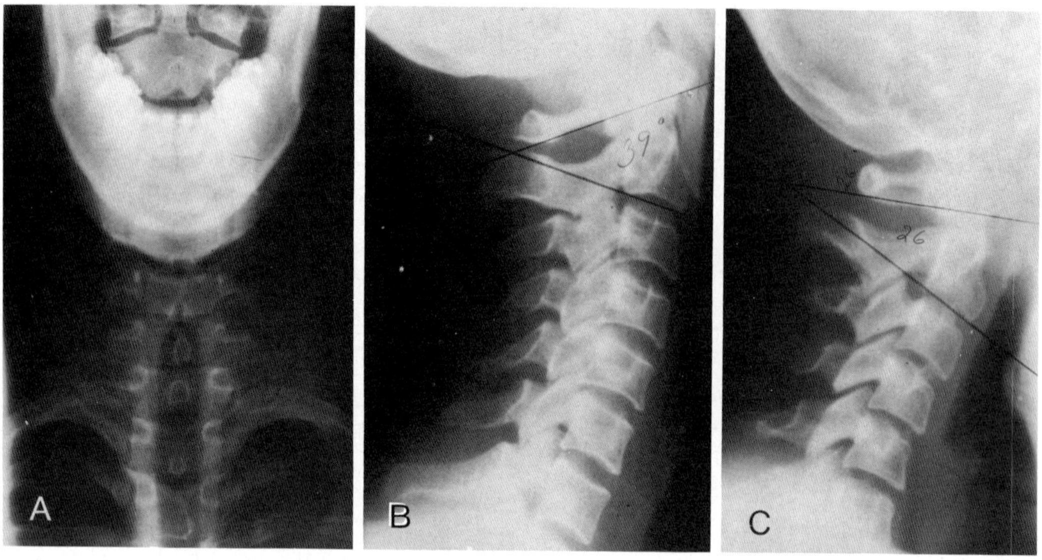

Figure 5.1. **A.** AP view showing neutral position of C2, right lateral shift of C1. **B.** Neutral lateral view shows anterior superior atlas C0–C1–C2 spacing should be equal. **C.** Neutral occipital extension posterior arch of C1 superior C0–C2 posterior approximation.

and to adjustive procedures(2). Alteration of muscle tone is the earliest cause of aberrant biomechanics or pathomechanics. Many of the aberrant reflexes bombarding the CNS that affect our general health come not only from joint proprioceptors but from those receptors in muscle. Changes in muscle tonus or harmony of muscle interaction produce changes in active and passive motion of the affected joints. The normal center of motion can be altered resulting in altered stress and strain on ligaments or osseous structures leading to compensatory hypermobility of segments above or below. Ligaments respond by either elongation or contracture. Cartilage may respond by alteration in collagen type, reduced repair, or destruction. Repeated mechanical stress has a direct effect on osseous tissue, resulting in deformation, sclerosis, exostosis and joint space narrowing, or cartilage wear and tear(3).

In tomographic studies, Illi demonstrated that degenerative changes at C1–C2 were much more common than plain film studies have revealed. It was his opinion, based on the incidence of aberrant statics and dynamics in the area, that many autonomic and painful symptom complaints had their origin at this level (personal communication).

Static and dynamic malalignment of the upper cervical spine has been recognized as important clinically by chiropractors since the beginning of our profession (Fig. 5.1, *A–C*). B. J. Palmer developed an entire system of treatment around this concept of abnormal joint position.

Dankemeyer and Rothmeier(4) were among the first to report in medical literature that when the atlas-axis interodontoid space was assymetrical, it did not necessarily mean that a luxation was present but rather it might be related to abnormal lateral tipping of the head, i.e., abnormal biomechanics. Traumatic case histories caused them to recognize that malpositioning of C1–C2 could resolve as normal function restored. Paul and Moir(5) reported that rotation of C2 on an AP film produced the appearance of lateral displacement, which they explained by projection magnification.

Coutts(6) had pointed out previously that if the displacement was bilateral, pathology or fracture could be suspected. Paul and Moir(5) also reported on a study of 9 so-called normal cases. Three showed a neutral assymetry, while two showed assymetry in lateral flexion with no significant change in the space with rotation of the head. Watkins(7) concurred with this finding that rotation produced no change in interodontoid space, which is a normal observation during lateral flexion.

Townsend and Rowe(8) were of the opinion that paraspinal muscle spasm in response to inflammation flattened the cervical spine and pulled C1 forward on C2, possibly creating hypermobility at this level or at C2–3 in flexion and extension. This type of "spasm-induced subluxation" will be discussed later as a pathological entity. Lewit(9) discussed hypermobility of the upper cervicals in flexion and related this pathomechanical phenomenon to the intrinsic factor of the ligaments, mainly the transverse ligament. He reported 22 of 41 patients with this hypermobility who also had anteflexion headaches. These patients were predominantly younger patients. He went on to report, however, that 93 of 95 patients with head and neck injuries showed hypomobility (restricted motion) at the cranio-cervical junction—another cause, he felt, of aberrant stress on ligaments.

PATHOMECHANICS: MUSCULAR PATTERNS

C0–C1 Flexion-Fixation: C0–C2 Flexion-Fixation

This may be produced bilaterally by any or all of the occipital extensors. Segmental (C0–C1) fixation is produced by hypertonicity of the rectus capitus posticus minor or the superior oblique (Fig. 5.2*A*). Fixation between C0 and C2 could be produced by hypertonicity of the rectus capitus posticus major (Fig. 5.3, *A* and *B*). Regional fixation of occiput flexion related to the entire cervicothoracic spine may involve any of the long occipital extensors including the trapezius, semispinalis capitus, longissimus capitus, splenius capitus, and sternocleidomastoid (Fig. 5.2*B*).

Unilateral involvement of any of these muscles creates a combination of occipital flexion fixation as well as restriction of rotation/lateral bending.

Statically, a bilateral involvement of these muscles is typically characterized by posterior nodding of the occiput (extension), a distortion pattern seen in the decompensated state of posture with an anterior neck carriage. Spasm and suboccipital tenderness are often noted on digital palpation of the occiput. Precise localization of tenderness and trigger points will help to ascertain more precise diagnosis of the specific myofascial attachments of each muscle and the probable causative muscle groups involved.

Lateral Flexion/Fixation: C0–C1–C2 Complex

Segmentally, this can be produced by hypertonicity of the rectus capitus lateralis (Fig. 5.4, *A–C*). Unilateral involvement of the occiputal extensors previously discussed, especially the splenius and semispinalis capitus, the long postural muscles, or the rectus capitus posticus major, produces excessive rotation of C2 spinous process during lateral flexion and can produce a static rotational misalignment of C2. The levator scapula and the splenius cervicus, if hypertonic, restrict normal C2 spinous rotation to the convexity (hypomobility). The levator scapula is involved particularly when arm movements are required or when a weight is carried in the hands. This muscle is not active for normal neck motions but in those occupations in which the arms are held up for long periods, these muscles undergo fatigue and strain (typists, computer operators, etc.). The splenius cervicis in poor postural situations or following trauma may become hypertonic and result in the pathomechanics described above.

Lateral flexion is absolutely dependent on C2 spinous rotation to the convexity(10). The semispinalis capitus, the scalenus anterior, the splenius cervicis, and possibly the sternocleidomastoideus muscle can alter these rotational mechanics by excessive activity on the convex side of lateral flexion. Jirout(11) in his study of 372 cases, classified upper cervical lateral flexion (see preceding chapter). No rotation was found in type II (offset of both lateral masses) (see Fig. 5.4*B*) 60.5% of the time and 68% of the time in type IV (no offset on either lateral mass). As we recall, it was Jirout's contention that during normal lateral flexion, the axis of rotation of C2 is on the articular facet on the side opposite the lateral flexion. Fixation of the upper cervical

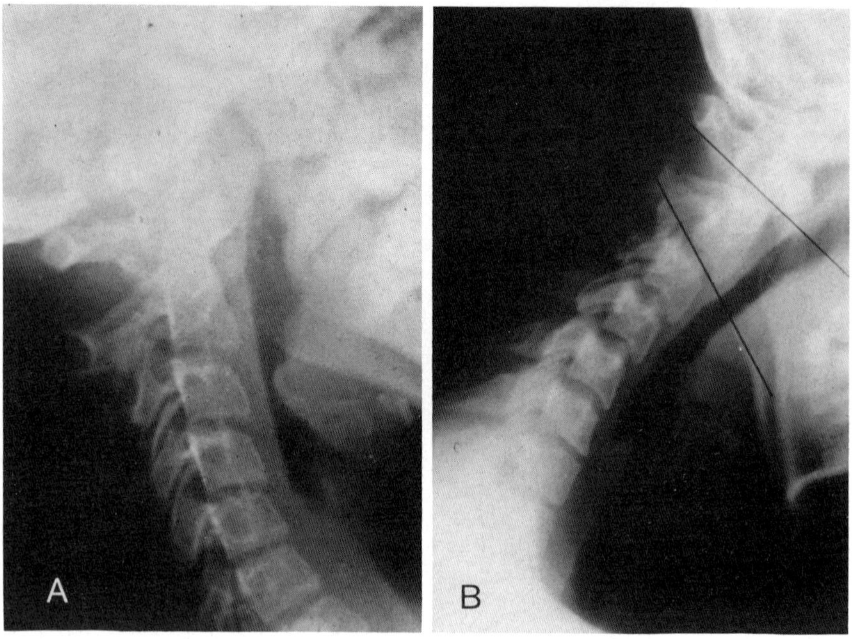

Figure 5.2. *A.* Marked fixation of COC1 in flexion, COC2 normal motion. C1 appears to be in excessive flexion. Suboccipital complex muscles probably involved. **B.** Chin retraction showing marked midcervical flexion with fixation of COC1. Splenius capitus may be involved.

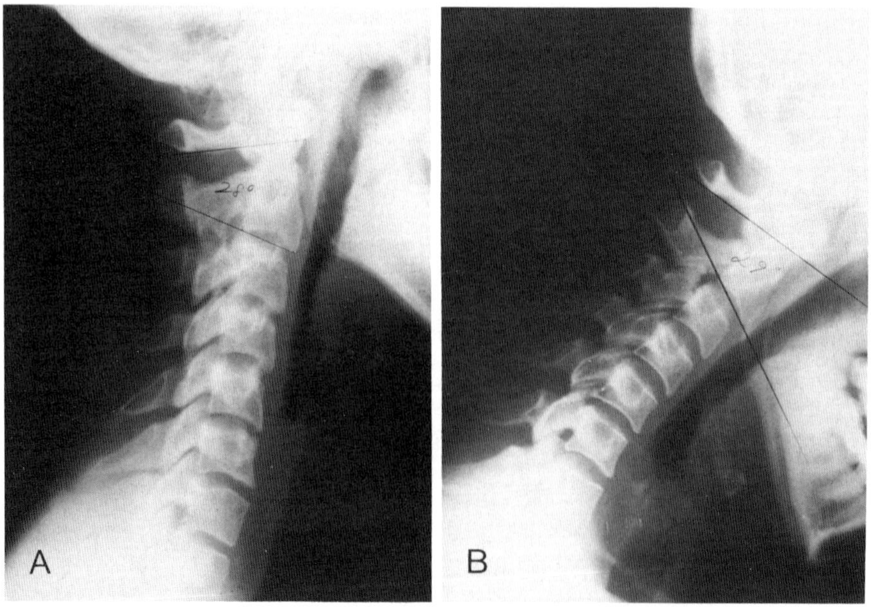

Figure 5.3. Neutral cervical view shows loss of normal cervical curve in normal CO–C1–C2 position. **B.** Flexion view shows normal lower cervical motion. Limited motion between COC1C2.

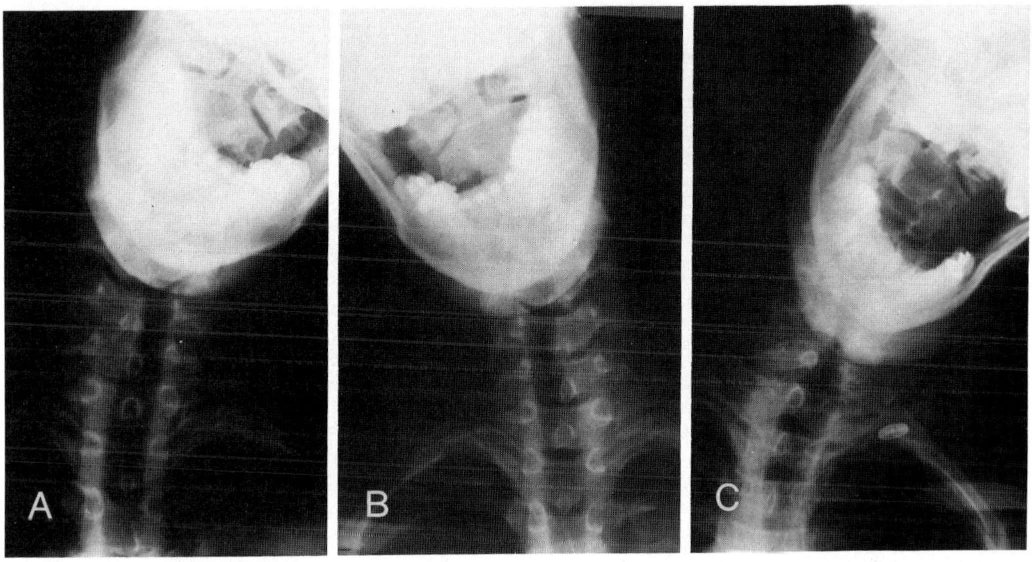

Figure 5.4. **A.** Right lateral flexion view shows normal widening of right interodontoid space, C1 right shift, mild overhanging of C1 lateral mass. (Mild spurring evident.) Note normal spinous rotation of C2 to the convexity. Atlas lateral masses, Jirout type I. **B.** Left lateral flexion shows narrowing of left interodontoid space, no lateral shift of atlas, no overriding of facets characteristic of complete lateral flexion rotation fixation of C0–C1–C2. C2 spinous normal rotation. Atlas lateral mass, Jirout type IV. Reversed rotation of lower cervicals suggests large postural muscles: semispinalis capitus, sacrospinalis. **C.** Right lateral flexion shows mild right widening of interodontoid space with overriding of opposite facet: Jirout type III. Author suggests rotation dynamics increased lateral flexion, dynamics reduced. Normal lower cervical C2 below spinous processes.

complex (physiological or pathological) may result in excessive or blocked lateral flexion at C1–C2 and involves the coupled motion of rotation, which is structurally bound. The tertiary motion of ventral or dorsal tilting during lateral flexion is often persistent following this motion (forced or otherwise) and may be the type of fixation that results in loss of joint play characteristically seen on motion palpation(12).

C0–C1 Extension Fixation

This is a far less common fixation that may involve rectus capitus anterior or the longus colli group of anterior cervical musculature. Clinically, this aberrant finding is seen in traumatic injuries involving hyperflexion (Fig. 5.5, *A* and *B*, and 5.6*A*).

C1–C2 Flexion Fixation

Hypertonicity of the extensor muscles such as inferior oblique, levator scapula, and splenius cervicis may restrict atlas flexion on axis. Unilateral involvement will usually be accompanied by fixations in rotation and lateral bending. Static findings indicate a malposition of atlas in extension. This subluxation was commonly referred to as an "anterior superior atlas" (Figs. 5.1*B* and 5.7, *A* and *B*).

Rotational Fixation

Pure rotational action does not occur and is instead synkinetically linked to lateral flexion and gliding. Unilateral involvement of the inferior oblique and/or the levator scapula muscles typically produces one of the most common fixations of the upper cervical complex, i.e., a reduction of atlantoaxial rotation and lateral tipping. Static findings associated with this fixation involve a rotational misalignment, tenderness over the posterior arch, and trigger points in the affected hypertonic muscles. Tenderness over the atlantoaxial joint (i.e., deep capsular ligaments) is also typical.

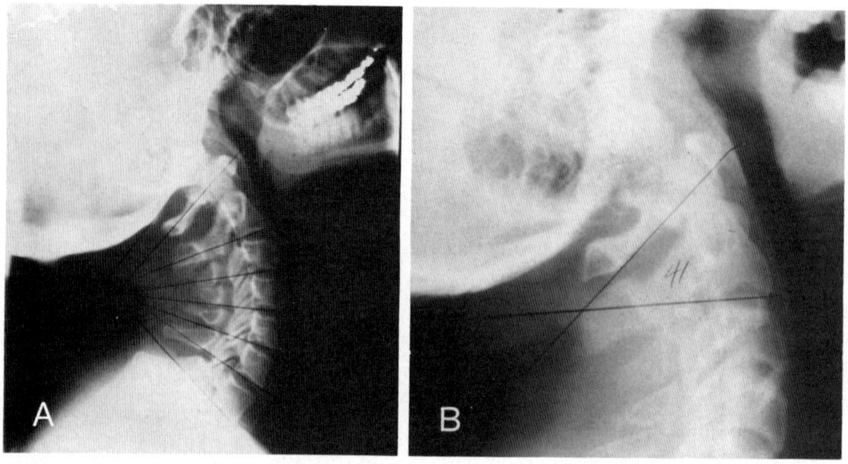

Figure 5.5. **A** and **B.** Cervical spine shows extension of midcervicals but C1 does not move posterior to C7 and this would indicate S.A. or longus colli involvement. Poor extension of occiput in this position suggests R.C.A. involvement as well.

Wortzman and Dewar(13) reported rotational dysfunction of C1–2 following relatively minor trauma, i.e., whiplash or head blows causing cervical muscle pain and or headache. The head posture was one of rotation with the head tilted away from the side of rotation. Rotation x-rays showed assymetrical function or C1–2 blockage of motion. As we have seen in normal x-ray-depicted mechanics, for example: right rotation will cause the left lateral mass to widen, the right to narrow, the left interodontoid space to narrow, the right to widen; the left C1–2 articulation widens and the right narrows. Failure of these changes to occur suggests fixation.

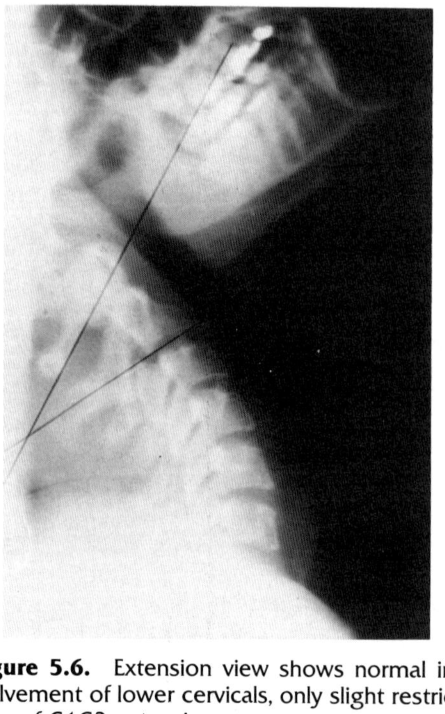

Figure 5.6. Extension view shows normal involvement of lower cervicals, only slight restriction of C1C2 extension.

C2–C3 Flexion/Extension Fixation

The classical pattern of hypertonicity of posterior (extensor) musculature causing fixation of flexion (i.e., tipping and gliding) and conversely, the involvement of the anterior musculature (i.e., scalenus anticus) causing extension fixation are seen at C2–C3. The muscles involved have been discussed; however, for flexion fixation, the deep multifidus muscle should be mentioned also (see C1–C2 rotation in preceding chapter) (Fig. 5.8, *A* and *B*).

C2–3 Rotation/Lateral Bending Fixations

The uncovertebral joints in the cervical spine (C2–C3) can become fixed and typically manifest a restriction of lateral bending. The muscles mentioned above plus the longisimus cervicis (sacrospinalis group) are commonly involved. Jirout(14) points out the importance of aberrant rotation at C2–

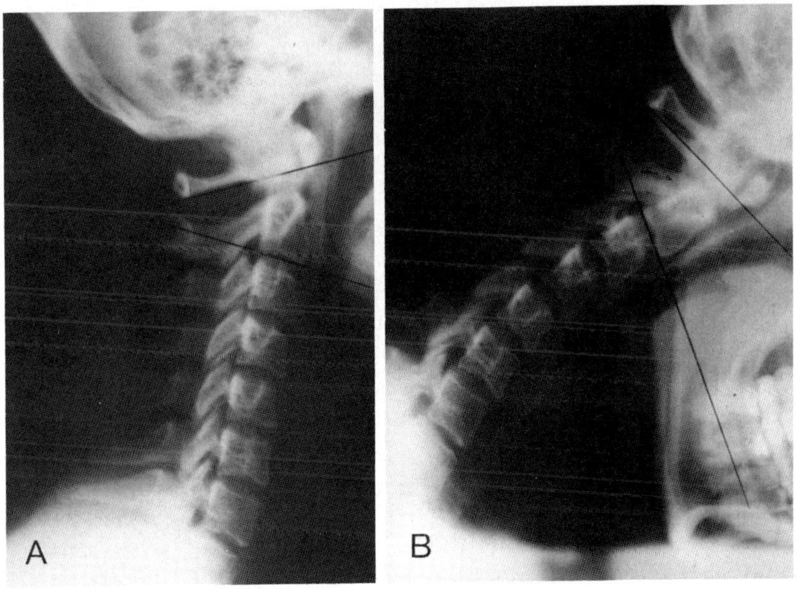

Figure 5.7. **A.** Neutral cervical lateral view shows loss of cervical curve with a mild anterior superior atlas malposition. **B.** Cervical flexion view shows unilateral involvement causing fixation of C0–C1 and tipping of atlas. C2 neutral lateral C1 shows tipping and fixation.

3 in relationship to headache and cervical pain and draws attention to the fact that these segments form an intermediate between the primarily rotational function of C1–C2 and the primarily flexion/extension function of C3–C4. The author notes that clinically, counterrotational fixations at these levels are common findings, i.e., a C1–C2 fixation on the right, and a C2–C3 fixation on the left.

CLINICAL CONSIDERATIONS OF PATHOMECHANICS

While this chapter has focused on the pathomechanics of the upper cervical spine, it

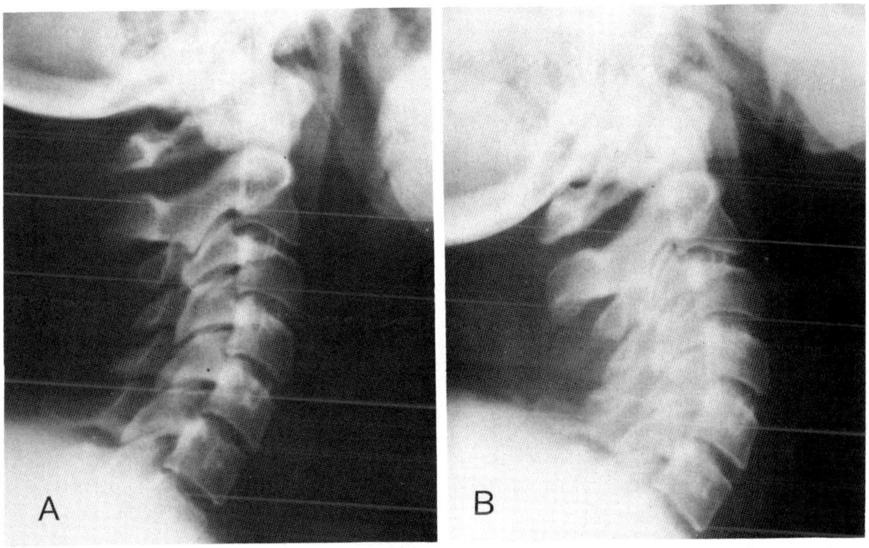

Figure 5.8. **A.** Neutral lateral view shows structural change of C2–C3 facet with sclerosis and gouging. **B.** Poor cervical extension fixation of C2–3. No posterior tipping.

is of interest to note that Lewit(15), in a discussion and presentation of cases of Ménière's disease and Barre-Lieou syndrome, stated that although the classic consideration is that this disease is a form of labyrinthitis, a large majority of cases are related to functional disturbances of the upper cervical spine. Careful clinical testing, monitoring of aberrant function, and pre- and posttrials of manipulation can offer important correlations of symptoms to aberrant cervical function. Pre- and postpalpation following manipulative therapy are also important to monitor interrelated biomechanical affects. For example, Watkins(16), Gillet and Liekens(16), and Gillet(17, 18) have drawn our attention to the fact that aberrant thoracic mechanics, i.e., "thoracic subluxation," can produce fixations at the C0–C1 or C0–C2 levels. One should be reminded that the term subluxation in chiropractic literature often includes a concept of minor static displacement or dynamic dysfunction of a motion segment, i.e., fixation or dyskinesia, and also includes consideration of hypermobility (Fig. 5.9 and Refs. 19–21). In medical parlance, the concept of subluxation usually refers to a gross instability or hypermobility that falls short of dislocation. The problem arises, however, as some researchers become more adept at recognizing spinal dysfunction. Abel(22), in his discussion of radiographic techniques of examination of the cervical spine, recommends a minimum of five views with a complete examination consisting of 11 views. One of the views recommended is a basilar view (often utilized by chiropractic upper cervical practitioners) which can demonstrate a much more subtle degree of static subluxation. In his opinion, 2 mm of disrelationship of the occipitoatlantoid joints represent a subluxation that may be reduced but may remain unstable (an opinion shared by chiropractors but often held up to ridicule). He goes on to state, however, that C1 subluxation is fairly common in traumatic situations and is often accompanied by fractures. Since the symptoms following cervical trauma are often due to soft tissue damage or compromise, the clinician must be cautioned that aberrant mechanics, subluxation, and fractures may give rise to very similar symptom pictures.

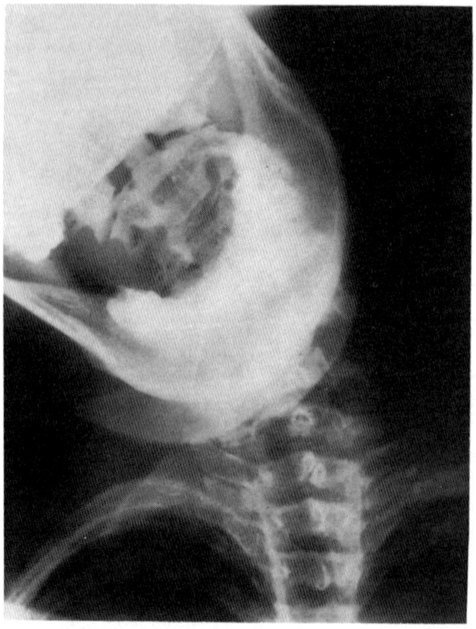

Figure 5.9. Left lateral flexion view shows excessive widening of interodontoid space and excessive overhanging of C1–C2 lateral masses (+2 mm). Mild spurring evident. C2 rotation also limited. C2 spinous deviation poor.

It should also be recognized that birth and early childhood may be the source of many adult spinal dysfunctions—both major, such as subluxation, or minor, such as in fixation or dyskinesia. Twisting and flexion of the neck with and without forceps can duplicate the injury we call "whiplash." Towbin(23) noted that abnormal fetal positions can subject the infant to intolerable forces. Abel(22) emphasized that in the neonate, 25% of the baby's weight is in the head and that haphazard lifting or movements can produce flail-like stress on the neck. He goes on to discuss spinal cord palsy being treated and prevented by early detection of these instabilities that may be caused by birth trauma, fractures, or other acquired traumas.

The arthritides can also lead to biomechanical instability of the upper cervical segments often called atlantoaxial subluxation (AAS). Yochum and Rowe(24) reviewed the literature relating to AAS listing rheumatoid arthritis, Still's disease, ankylosing spondylitis, psoariatic arthritis, Reiter's syndrome, degenerative joint disease, gout, systemic lupus, lipoid dermatoarthritis, septic arthritis, and infections producing inflammation as possible causes. Buehler and Sandman(25) not only listed a number of specific causes but divided the etiology into two basic causes: *(a)* involvement of the transverse ligament resulting in ligament laxity or tearing due to trauma; and *(b)* erosion, malformation, trauma, or reabsorption of the dens.

Yochum and Rowe's review of the literature defines the normal measurement of the atlantodental interspace (ADI) as 1–3 mm. The spinal canal at this level should be at least 22 mm wide. In children, the ADI should be no greater than 4 mm. Greenberg(26) reported the observation that this space decreases with age because of the loss of the articular cartilage. The incidence of AAS in rheumatoid arthritis has not been reported but Robinson(27) reported on an abstract by Sharp and Purser who reported 5 of 78 rheumatoid arthritis patients with significant subluxation.

Regarding the role of spinal anomalies, Carella(28) reported that over 50% of patients with headache symptoms showed x-ray findings of anomalies. These anomalies were found mainly at the C1 level, resulting in aberrant statics and dynamics of not only the upper cervical region but also the lower cervical area. Wackenheim(29) reported C0–C1 "functional block as an important cause of occipital neuralgia or headache," a common observation made by chiropractic clinicians. Watkins(30) studied flexion of C0–C1 and felt that C0–C1 approximation was normal and in cases where C0–C1 separated, he found more head pain symptoms. (This phenomenon was discussed in the preceding chapter.) Dalseth(31) was critical of radiograph studies showing hypomobility and stated that in his experience, assymetry of the craniovertebral region was common and hypomobility was found in healthy subjects and may be a normal function of a joint. Chiropractors and other clinicians who regularly correct these aberrant functions highly disagree that aberrent statics and dynamics, no matter how common, are normal. Much work remains to correlate the clinical significance of joint function symptoms and correction. Aho and colleagues(32) found an interesting fact in relationship to C1–2 flexion mobility, i.e., a normal group showed a 9–20° range of motion. In a second group with mild pathology the range of motion was 5–12°. They further observed in the early stages, it was only the motion studies that demonstrated the pathology.

CONCLUSION

One of the assumptions underlying the chiropractic diagnostic paradigm is that hypomobility in one segment or in one compartment of a spinal motion segment will lead to aberrant and then excessive mobility of other segments or compartments of the same segment. Excessive stress on musculoligamentous tissues can lead to pain, inflammation, proliferative reactions and protective spasms, and altered neurological reflex patterns. Betge(33) attempted to correlate the clinical findings of tenderness, static x-ray findings, motion palpation, and cineradiography in 50 cases. His analysis concluded that cineradiography for the cervical spine was 57% better than palpation for tenderness, 52% better than static x-ray, and 42% better than motion palpation. The clinician must learn to correctly diagnose the individual patterns of motion dysfunction and static malposition presented by each patient. The superimposition of potential congenital anomalies, degenerative changes, and in the rare case, surgical alteration makes a precise and individual diagnosis of pathomechanics imperative. In fact, this type of diagnosis is the hallmark of the chiropractic approach to the vertebral column. In order to accomplish this, a thorough understanding of the normal statics and dynamics of the upper cervical mechanism must be appreciated and the function of the upper cervical region must be placed into the context of the entire cervical column, the spine and, in fact, of the entire patient in a wholistic fashion. With this understanding in mind, dynamic motion palpation, specific diagnostic tests, radiographic examinations (static and dynamic stress films), and cineradiography can give the clinician some appreciation of the aberrant biomechanics—its cause and effect. A rational approach to correction, rehabilitation, and prevention can then be instituted, and an objective, immediate measurement or retest can be offered. Once the process of pathomechanics is understood and recognized, simple masking or altering of symptoms is insufficient, and the development and application of therapy that restores normal function, reverses pathomechanics, when possible, and prevents recurrence becomes the treatment of choice.

Spinal manipulation, selective therapeutic exercise, selective physiotherapeutic procedures, and mechanotherapy procedures are proving to be the treatment of choice, and further studies and careful application will enhance the health of our patients.

References

1. Jirout J. Correlations of the functional disturbances in the cervical spine as seen roentgenographically in frontal and sagittal projections. ACTA Univ Carol Med Suppl 1965;21:128–9.
2. Grice A. Muscle tone change following manipulation. J Can Chiro Assoc 1975;184:29.
3. Jirout J. Studies on the dynamics of the spine. Acta Radiol 1956;46:55–60.
4. Dankmeyer J, Rothmeier BJ. The lateral movement in the atlanto axial joints and its clinical significance. Acta Radiol 1943;24:44.
5. Paul LW, Moir WW. Non-pathological variations in relationship of the upper cervical vertebrae. Am J Roentgenol 1949;62:519–24.
6. Coutts MB. Atlanto-epistropheal subluxations. Arch Surg 1934;29:297–311.
7. Watkins RJ. Upper cervical mechanics. J Can Chiro, Vol 2, Spring 1969, pp. 132–145.
8. Townsend EH, Rowe ML. Mobility of the upper cervical spine in health and disease. Paediatrician 1952;10:507–513.
9. Lewit K. Ligament pain and anteflexion headache. Eur Neurol 1971;5:365–378.
10. Krausova L, Lewit K. The mechanism and the measuring of the mobility in the craniocervical joints during lateral flexion. Acta Univ Carol Med Suppl 1965;21:123–126.
11. Jirout J. Changes in the atlas-axis relationship on lateral flexion of the head and neck. Neuroradiology 1973;6:215–218.
12. Jirout J. Persistence of synkinetic patterns of the cervical spine. Neuroradiology 1979;18:167.
13. Wortzman G, Dewar F. Rotary fixation of the atlantoaxial joint: rotational atlantoaxial subluxation. Radiology 90:479–487.
14. Jirout J. Comments regarding the diagnosis and treatment of dysfunctions in C2–3 segment. Manual Med 1985;2:16–17.
15. Lewit K. Ménière's disease and the cervical spine. Virbelsaule in Faschungun Praxis 1963;26:92.
16. Gillet H, Liekens M. Belgian research notes. 3rd ed Brussels: H. Gillet, 1963.
17. Gillet H. Belgian research notes. 10th ed, Huntington CA: Motion Palpation Institute, 1973.
18. Gillet H. Typical upper dorsal fixation. J Clin Chiro Arch 1973;3:168–171.
19. Howe J. The chiropractic concept of subluxation and its roentgenological manipulation. J Clin Chiro. Rad, Sept/Oct 1973.
20. Watkins RJ. Subluxation terminology. J Am Chiro Assoc 1968;2:65–70.
21. Watkins RJ. What do you mean subluxation? Bull Euro Chiro Union, 1972;21(2):39–41.
22. Abel MS. Occult traumatic lesions of the cervical vertebrae. St Louis: Warren A Green Inc, 1970.
23. Towbin A. Spinal cord and brainstem injury at birth. Arch Path 1964;77:620.
24. Yochum T, Rowe L. Arthritides of the upper cervical complex. In: Aspects of Manipulative Therapy. Glascow E, Twomey L, Skull E, Kleynhans A, Idezak. R, eds. 2nd ed. London: Churchill Livingstone, 1985.
25. Buehler MT, Sandman TD. Anterior atlanto-axial subluxation: clinical and radiographic depiction. J Manipulative Physiol Ther, 1978;1(4):223–227.
26. Greenberg AD. Atlanto-axial dislocations. Brain 1968;91:655–684.
27. Robinson HS. Rheumatoid arthritis-atlanto-axial subluxation and its clinical presentation. Can Med Assoc J 1966;1:94.
28. Carella A. Slight anomalies of the atlas: their pathogenetic meaning. Neuroradiology 1972;3:224–227.
29. Wachenheim A. Functional atlanto-occipital block. Neuroradiology 1971;3:80–81.
30. Watkins RJ. Upper cervical mechanics. J Clin Chiro, Vol. 1971;2(2):132–145.
31. Dalseth I. Anatomic studies of the osseous craniovertebral joint (technical material). Man Med 1974;6:3–10.
32. Aho A, Vartiainen O, Salo O. Segmentary anteroposterior mobility of the cervical spine. Ann Med Intern Fem 1955, pp.287–299.
33. Betge G. The value of cineradiographic motion studies in the diagnosis of dysfunctions of the cervical spine. J Clin Chiro 1979;2(6):40–44.

6 Motion Palpation of the Upper Cervical Spine

Bruce Fligg, D.C.

UPPER CERVICAL TECHNIQUE

With the developing scientific knowledge base over the recent past, (Fig. 6.1) and the increasing acceptance of the orthopedic-biomechanical model in the practice of chiropractic (Fig. 6.2), there has been a greater emphasis placed on the development of skills that can detect and/or determine the state of a patient's health status relative to these models (Fig. 6.3). Motion palpation, an art in the detection of a patient's pathomechanical state, has therefore gained a wider acceptance in the practice of chiropractic. Numerous authors have written articles identifying the various motion palpation procedures(1–5); unfortunately, only a few have conducted inter-examiner reliability studies that have helped to establish the efficacy of this skill(6–8). Nevertheless, this skill, because it relies on the subtlest tactile information, allows the examiner to develop an intimate appreciation for the pathomechanical state of a set of spinal motion segments prior to manipulation. Overall, these skills plus the other "clinical" tools of the clinical decision-making process (Fig. 6.4) allow us to more proficiently manage a patient's health care condition.

Table 6.1
Objectives of Motion Palpation

General	Specific
Pathomechanical patterns	Adjustment selection
Coupled motion	Segment level (major vs. minor)
Quality and quantity of motion	Angle (line) of thrust
Integrity of intrinsic and extrinsic elements	Amplitude of thrust
	Effectiveness of adjustment

The objectives of motion palpation are listed in Table 6.1. The following is an overview of the general objectives. It is well established that the spine will often subluxate in specific pathomechanical patterns. The use of motion palpation as well as plumbline analysis provides excellent examination methods to determine these pathomechanical patterns. Another well-established phenomenon is that of coupled motion within a motion segment. The concepts of static malposition and directional fixation of the subluxation complex are fairly well understood. It is therefore equally important that we understand the significance of these coupled or synkinetic motions. Specific motion palpation procedures have been devised to determine the nature of these motions. Another objective of mo-

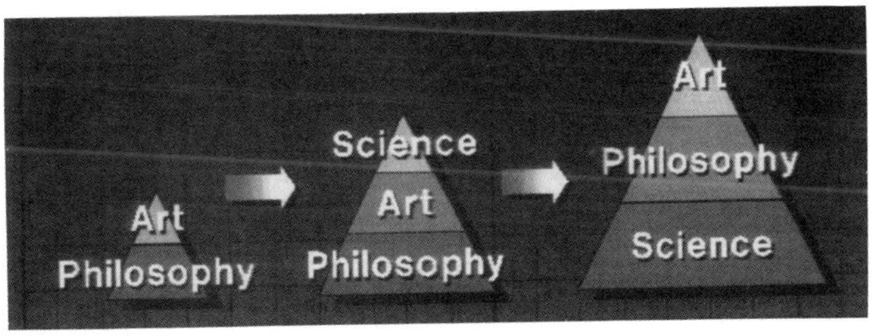

Figure 6.1. Scientific developments in the chiropractic profession. Note the proportion of the triangle that is now occupied by the section of *Science*. It would appear that our philosophy and our art in order to survive must be consistent with known scientific rationale.

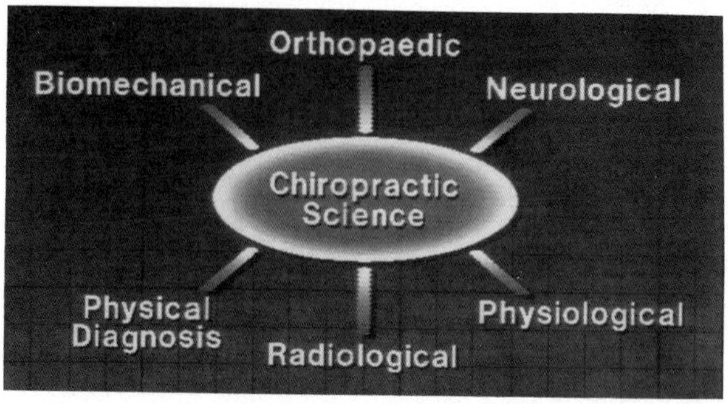

Figure 6.2. Sciences relative to chiropractic. The biomechanical model is merely one model of several that the chiropractic profession utilizes in describing the scientific rationale of its practice.

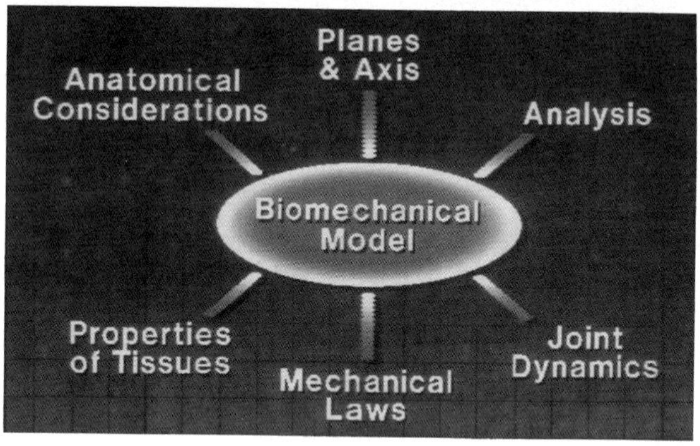

Figure 6.3. Various components of the biomechanical model. Motion palpation falls under the category of *Analysis* and therefore is the major diagnostic tool used in determining the state of the biomechanical aspect of a patient's health.

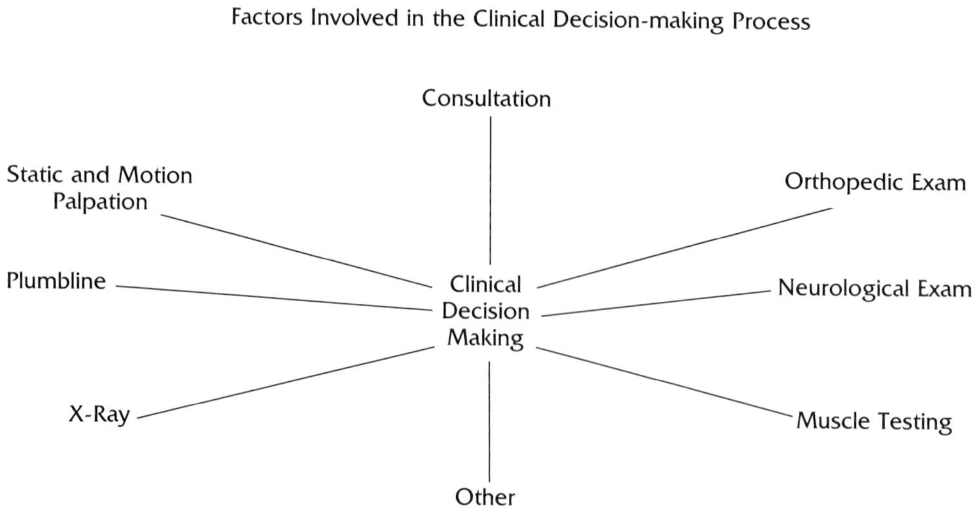

Figure 6.4. Various aspects involved in the clinical decision-making process. Motion palpation is one important element involved in this overall clinical decision-making process. It should be realized, however, that motion palpation is the main tool in identifying the fixation component of the subluxation complex.

tion palpation is to determine the quantity of motion that exists within a motion segment. It is extremely important to determine this quantity of motion especially when determining the extent of utilizing the long levers for removing tissue slack and creating a pivotal point in the act of spinal adjustment. It is also important to realize that hypermobile segments should not be manipulated and should be protected in the setup of a manipulation to ensure that only the hypomobile segment is affected. Motion palpation is probably one of the best palpatory skills enabling us to identify the integrity of the intrinsic elements (ligaments, capsular structures, etc.) as well as the integrity of the extrinsic elements (muscle, tendon, muscle tendinous junctions).

The greatest advantage of motion palpation, however, lies within the specific objectives. These objectives center around the actual application of the manipulation. Motion palpation procedures help us to select the specific manipulation and to identify the specific motion segments that require manipulating. They also establish the angle of thrust, the depth of thrust (amplitude), and most importantly, a tool for outcome assessment, the effectiveness of our manipulation. Ultimately, we must ensure that (1) the manipulation produced increased mobility at the motion segment specifically desired, and (2) the dysfunctional motion pattern has been corrected.

In order to accomplish these objectives, there are various approaches that the clinician can take. These various approaches are as follows: static joint challenge, end joint analysis, joint play, and dynamic motion palpation (Table 6.2). The selection of these procedures rests in the ability of the clinician to apply the appropriate motion palpation procedures according to the tolerance and nature of the patient's condition. For example, a patient presenting with an acute torticollis cannot tolerate many of the dynamic motion palpation procedures. The nature of the patient's condition and the restricting tolerances make static joint challenge the more ideal motion palpation approach. As the patient's condition improves, joint play and end joint analysis can be included as part of the examination procedure. Later in the management of the problem, as the condition passes out of the inflammatory stage, dynamic motion palpation procedures can be applied. Consider the case of a young muscular patient presenting with headaches in which the examiner merely uses static joint challenge to evaluate the state of the joints prior to manipulation. Because this patient's condition is probably in the early dysfunction stage, which implies the loss of muscle harmony, significant clinical information will be missed unless end joint, joint play, and expecially the dynamic motion palpation procedures are included in the examination.

There are eight main motion palpation tests used to examine the upper cervical spine.

For example, the eight tests do not include static joint challenge nor do they include motion palpation procedures in an antigravity situation. Often the antigravity position (supine) provides an important comparison when attempting to establish the role of the muscular component in the subluxation complex. Therefore, some of

Table 2
Types and Objectives of Motion Palpation

Type	Analysis
Static spinal joint challenge	A type of joint play. Tests for involuntary capsular movements in a static position. Usually applied prone for lumbars and thoracics, supine for cervicals. Utilizes the short levers, i.e., TVPs, spinous, articular pillars, mamilaries.
Joint play	Tests for involuntary capsular movements. Mennel (2) first described these procedures as they applied to extremities.
End joint analysis	Tests for integrity of the elastic barrier (capsular and ligamentous structures), largely developed by Gillet and Liekens (3).
Dynamic motion palpation	Examines the functional characteristics of the joint, i.e., coupled motions, quantity and quality of motion, pathomechanical patterns. (according to Grice and Gitelman) (4, 5).

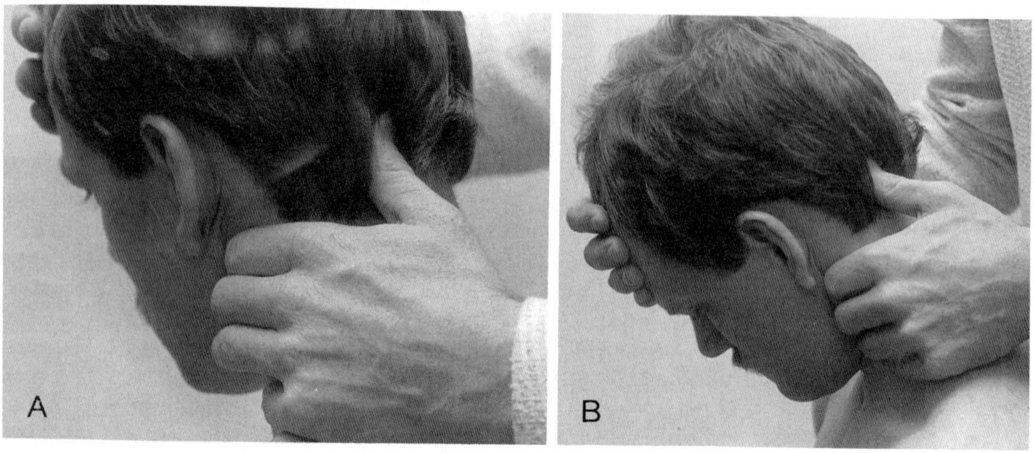

Figure 6.5, A and B. Motion palpation procedure utilized to examine occipital flexion involving the large semispinalis capitus muscle. It is important with this procedure to isolate the flexion with the indifferent hand to the upper cervical region. Often it is necessary for the patients to assist in the initial motion and they should be instructed to draw their chins into their chests.

the following procedures should be applied in this position. Many times these motion palpation procedures in the antigravity position become the mobilization procedures during the initial phases of the treatment program.

MOTION PALPATION PROCEDURES

Occiput-Atlas Joint

Test 1

Occiput Flexion (Figs. 6.5–6.7). There are two procedures that help determine the presence and extent of occiput flexion on atlas. The first deals with the control of occiput flexion by the long cervical-occipital-thoracic muscles such as semispinalis capitus. This test is very similar to the anterior glide motion palpation procedure of the cervical spine. To test for occipital flexion, the contact hand is placed such that the index and second fingers have an anterior contact around atlas and axis, while the thumb contact is on the occipital rim just lateral to the midline (see Figs. 6.5 and 6.6). The indifferent hand, which is placed on the patient's forehead, controls the motion of flexion. It is important that only the upper cervical region is flexed while testing

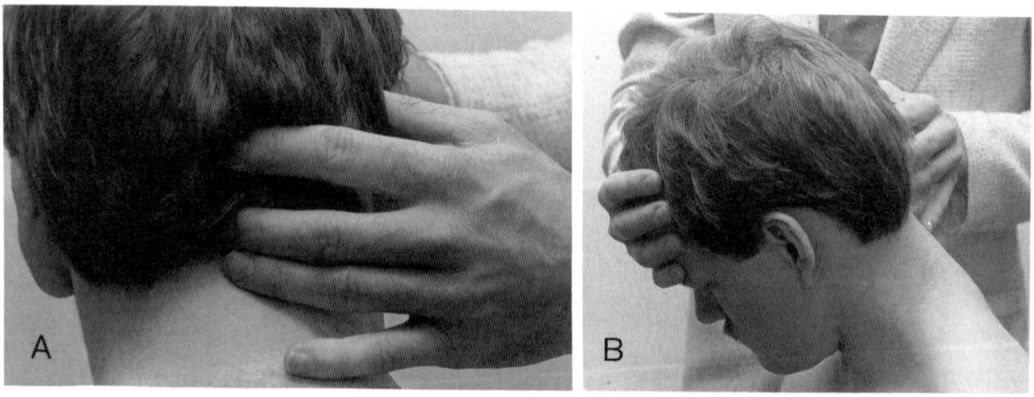

Figure 6.6, A and B. Motion palpation procedure used to examine occipital flexion relative to the atlas and axis. Again it is important to isolate the flexion with the indifferent hand to the upper cervical region. The second finger during the flexion procedure should be palpating the posterior arch of atlas in order to determine its position relative to the occipital rim and the spinous of axis.

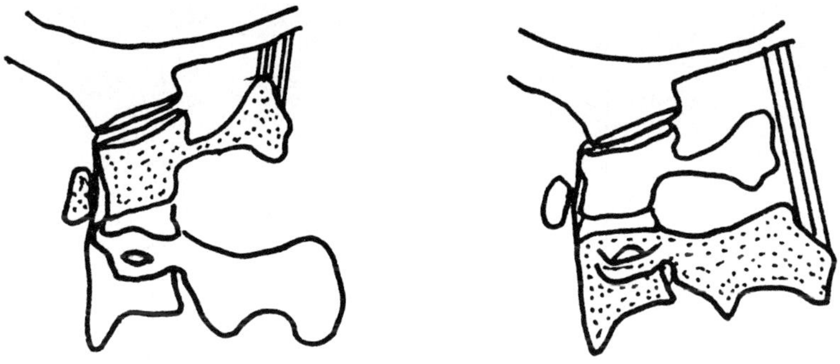

Figure 6.7, A and B. Two possible flexion fixations palpated using the procedures described in Figures 6.5 and 6.6 **Figure 6.7A,** occipital flexion fixation relative to atlas involving the rectus capitus posterior minor muscle. **Figure 6.7B,** occipital flexion fixation involving C-2 and the rectus capitus posterior major muscle. Also note that these flexion fixation patterns can be correlated with functional cervical flexion x-rays.

for this motion instead of producing lower cervical flexion as well. This is accomplished by producing a chin-retraction motion. With this procedure, the contacting thumb on the occipital rim presses cephalad as the occiput is flexed on atlas. A small springing end joint sensation should be palpated, indicating occipital flexion. However, if a fixation should be present, a loss of this springing motion is palpated as a resistance against the thumb. Many times if the semispinalis capitis muscle is implicated, a trigger point is palpable and radiates pain to the lateral aspects of the temple and parietal regions. It should also be noted that upper thoracic fixations often occur as a result of this fixation pattern.

A second test to check for upper cervical flexion is one in which the three-finger contact as seen in Fig. 6.6 is taken. Here, the index finger contacts the occipital rim, the second finger contacts over the space of the posterior arch of atlas, and the third finger contacts over the spinous process of axis. Again, the indifferent hand is placed on the patient's forehead and controls the motion of flexion. This flexion motion should again be isolated to the upper cervical region. The three fingers will palpate the relationship between occiput, atlas, and axis

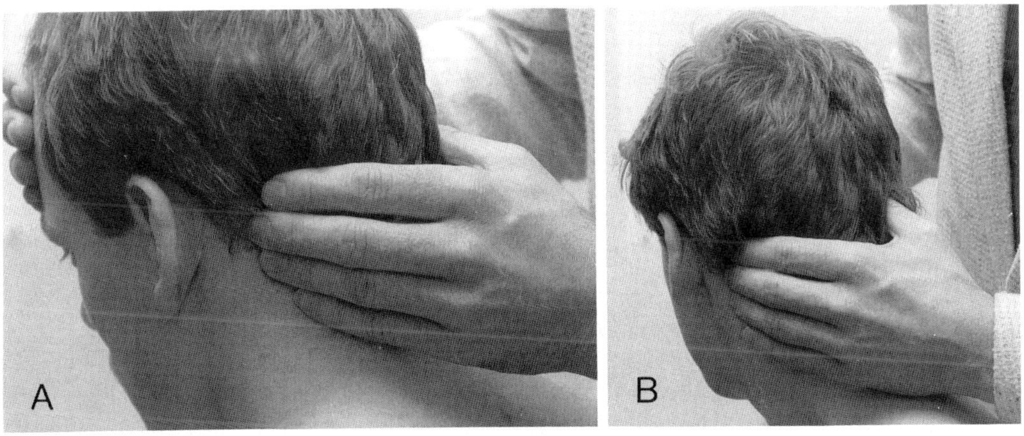

Figure 6.8, A and B. Procedure utilized to analyze the anterior rotation component of the occiput. The large splenious capitus muscle eccentrically controls this motion. Note that the first three fingers of the doctor's contact hand are placed on the posterior aspect of the mastoid process. As the occiput is rotated away from the contact hand, the fingers palpating on the mastoid produce an end-joint challenge.

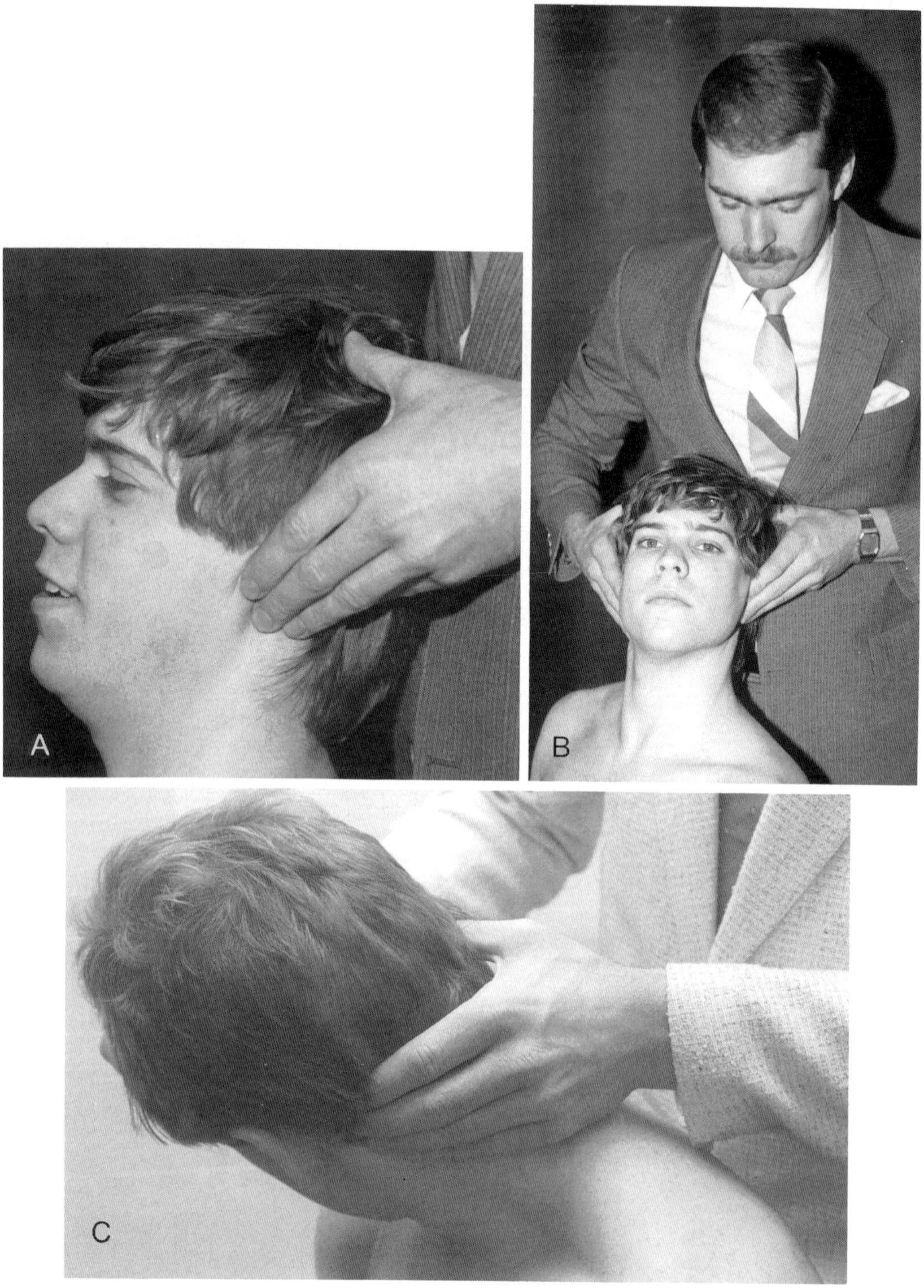

Figure 6.9. A and B. Motion palpation procedure to test for posterior rotation. The main long muscle that can limit this motion is the SCM muscle. Particular attention should be paid to the positioning of the occiput. Note the small amount of upper cervical flexion (occiput on atlas). This small motion preloads the sternocleidomastoid muscle and thereby makes it easier to distinguish a posterior fixation.

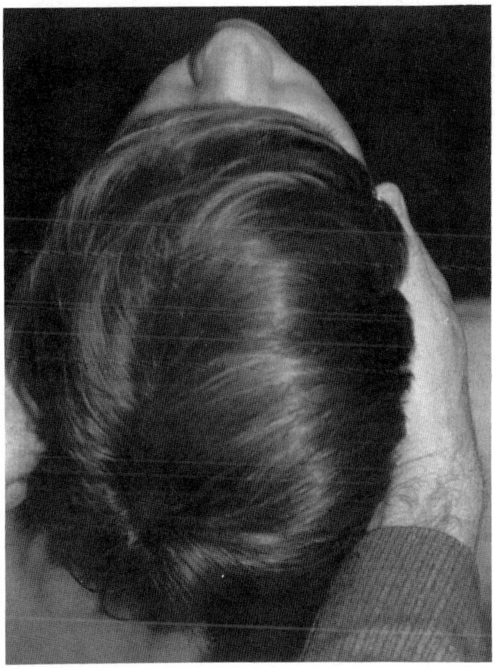

Figure 6.10. Normal upper cervical extension as viewed by the examiner from above. With normal extension, the nose and chin remain in the midline position.

during flexion. This will help to determine the effect of the suboccipital muscles such as rectus capitus posticus major and minor. Should the minor muscle be involved, the atlas will be palpated closer to the occipital rim during forward flexion whereas if the major muscle is implicated, the posterior arch will be palpated closer to the spinous of C-2 (Fig. 6.7).

Test 2

Occipital Rotation (Figs. 6.8–6.9). There are two basic procedures that help to determine the amount of occipital rotation. One procedure establishes the amount of anterior rotation while the other procedure establishes the amount of posterior rotation.

Anterior Rotation (Fig. 6.8). It should be noted that there is a small amount of occipital rotation that takes place. It is under the control of large muscles such as splenius capitus. Anterior rotation of the occiput is palpated in a similar fashion to the anterior rotation motion palpation of the cervical spine. Instead of the three fingers contacting the articular pillars of the cervical region, the three fingers are placed posterior to the mastoid process on the con-

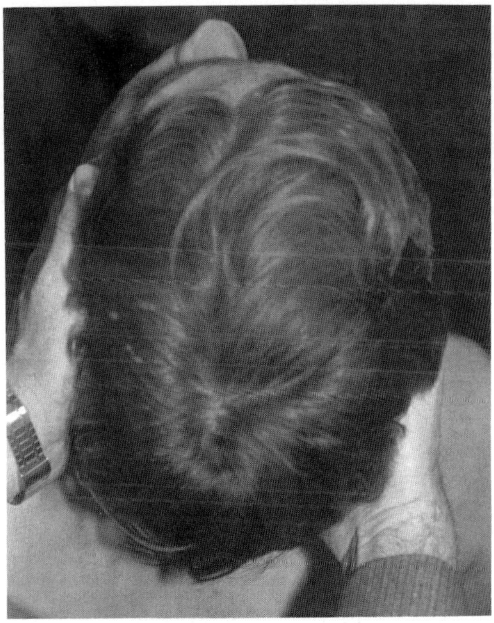

Figure 6.11. Abnormal cervical extension. Note the deviation of the nose and the chin away from the side of the sternocleidomastoid involvement (right side).

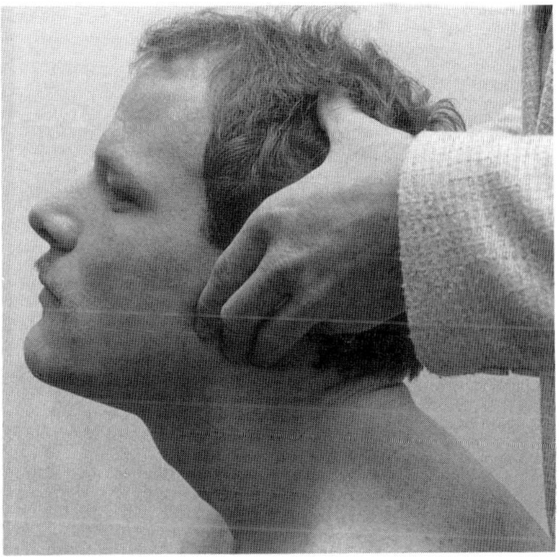

Figure 6.12. Motion of occiput extension on atlas. The finger contacts establish the movement of the atlas relative to the mastoid and mandible and compare this movement bilaterally. Note the isolation of extension motion to the upper cervical region.

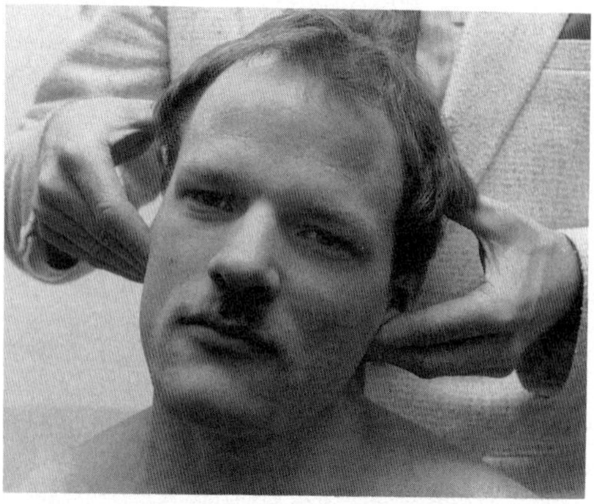

Figure 6.13. Occiput lateral flexion on atlas. It is important that the lateral flexion be isolated to the upper cervical region and therefore limited to a maximum of 25°. This three-finger contact is described in Figure #6.16.

tralateral side to the doctor/patient positioning (Fig. 6.8). The thumb of the contact hand is placed on the ipsilateral side of the occiput and helps in controlling occipital rotation along with the indifferent hand, which is placed on the patient's forehead. The patient's head is then rotated away from the contact hand. To further stress the muscular component, the patient's neck can be flexed and then rotated away from the doctor's contact hand.

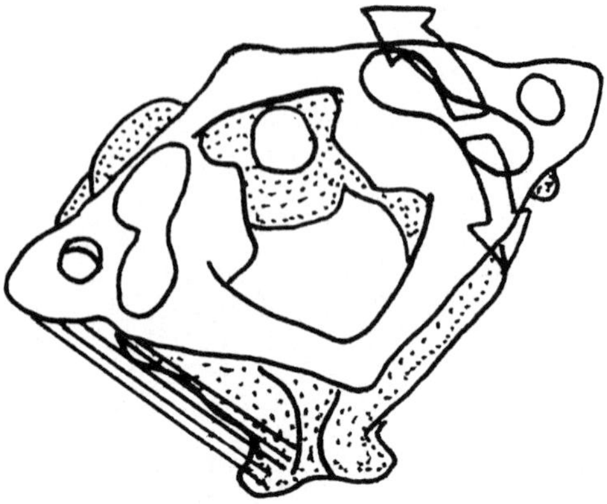

Inferior oblique

Figure 6.15. Atlas rotational malposition of left rotation. Our motion palpation findings would indicate a right rotational fixation, i.e., inability of the atlas to rotate right. The inferior oblique on the *left side* is indicated as being the major holding element contributing to this fixation/malposition. Often there is a hypermobility on the opposite side to the fixated joint as illustrated by the *arrows* on the *right side.*

If normal mobility is present, there is a small end joint "springing" sensation. A fix-

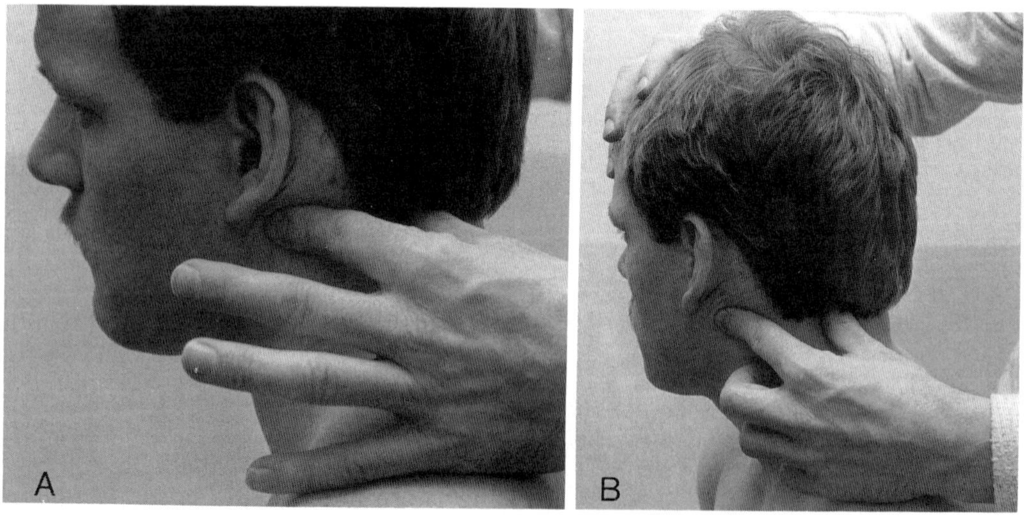

Figure 6.14. A and B. Contact hand and indifferent hand positioning for analyzing the rotation motion of atlas on axis. Note that the index finger of the contact hand is placed on the posterior lateral aspect of the transverse process of atlas just below the mastoid process. During the first 25° of rotation there is pure atlas rotation on axis, and therefore the axis should not be palpated as moving. This first 25° of rotation are considered a critical element in the overall biomechanics of cervical rotation.

ation would be palpated as a pressure resistance with the contact finger, indicating a loss of this springing sensation. In many cases, the splenius capitus muscle is involved and a trigger point can be located beneath the fingers that radiates pain to the vertex region. The doctor should also examine the upper thoracic region to see whether there are compensatory pathomechanical findings related to this occipital fixation.

Posterior Rotation (Fig. 6.9). This motion palpation procedure is similar to the posterior motion palpation procedures of the cervical spine that tests for the eccentric control of the scalenae muscles. The contact hand of the doctor is placed such that the first three fingers contact the anterior aspect of the patient's mastoid on the contralateral side to the patient-doctor positioning. The doctor, who is standing slightly behind the patient's shoulder on the contralateral side to the contact, leans the patient back slightly and flexes the patient's upper cervical region (occiput on atlas). Following this, the patient's head on the site of contact is rotated posteriorly and slightly superiorly. This not only tests for posterior rotation of the occiput on atlas but also tests for the elasticity of the sternocleidomastoid (SCM) muscle. Normal mobility should be palpated as a springing-

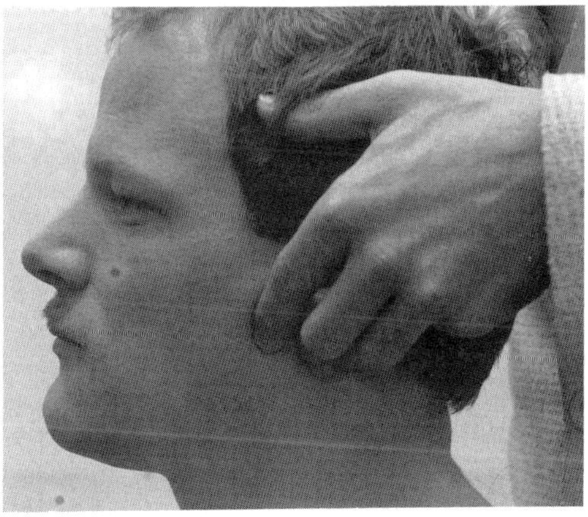

Figure 6.16. Three-finger contact positioning for establishing the relationship between mandible, transverse process, and mastoid. This contact is performed bilaterally, and the head movements are controlled largely by the thumbs and the heel of the hands bilaterally.

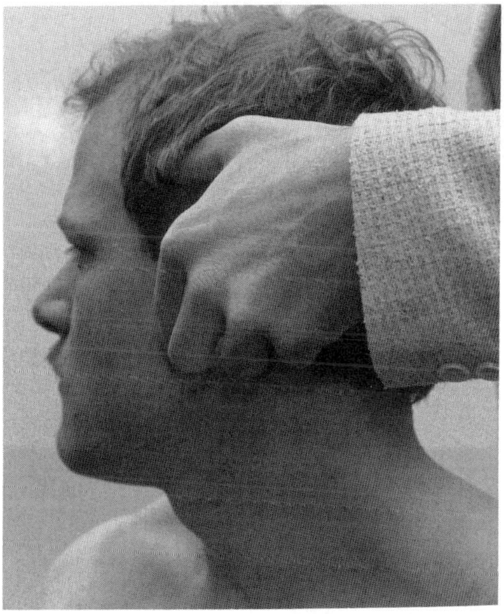

Figures 6.17. Motion palpation procedure used to identify the coupled motion action of atlas relative to occiput.

ness at the end range of motion. Fixation of this motion is felt as an increasing amount of pressure with a loss of the normal end joint feel. If one suspects a SCM involvement, the orthopedic testing of extension should be performed (Figs. 6.10 and 6.11). The patient's occiput will deviate as the muscle's inability to elongate occurs so that the chin and nose deviate from the midline. Also, it is advisable to palpate the SCM muscle for trigger points and motion palpate the sternoclavicular joint for pathomechanics related to its insertion (Fig. 6.9C).

Test 3

Occiput Extension (Fig. 6.12). The finger placement for this test is the same as that for the test of atlas coupled motion (see Fig. 6.16). The occiput is rocked in extension on atlas. This motion produces an opening in the space between the mandible and transverse process (TVP) contacts. The doctor should not only appreciate this opening bilaterally but should compare the symmetry of the opening. A loss of the opening bilaterally or a symmetrical difference in this opening suggests an inability of the occiput to extend on the atlas.

Test 4

Occiput Lateral Flexion (Fig. 6.13). The same three-finger placement is used as in the test of atlas coupled motion. This test is virtually the same as that used in the palpation of atlas lateral shift except that upon lateral flexion of occiput on atlas, the space between contacting fingers should widen as well. This opening is appreciated by the finger contacts on the side contralateral to the atlas shift. Failure to do so implicates involvement of the suboccipital muscles such as rectus capitus lateralis and superior oblique, or the long occipital extensors.

Test 1

Atlas-Axis Joint

Atlas Rotation on Axis (Figs. 6.14 and 6.15). As previously described, the atlas accounts for 50% of the overall range of cervical rotation, and half of this rotation takes place during the first 25° of cervical rotation. It is important to establish not only the overall mobility of this motion segment but also to determine where in the range of rotation a fixation might occur. This aspect is extremely important to establish when applying this to the manipulative procedure for it establishes how far to rotate the head and neck as a long lever when taking up the slack and creating a pivotal point for short lever thrusting. The motion palpation procedure used to determine this is seen in Figures 6.14A and 6.14B. Here the doctor uses a thumb-index finger contact on the contralateral side. The thumb is placed on the ipsilateral aspect of the spinous of C2 to the index finger contact on the posterior lateral aspect of the TVP of atlas. The indifferent hand is placed on top of the patient's forehead and assists in controlling the patient's head. The patient's head is then rotated away from the side of testing. As the head is rotated away, a separation is appreciated between the index finger and the thumb. This indicates normal mobility. However, if the spinous of C-2 presses in against the thumb in an attempt to rotate with the atlas, this is indicative of an atlas-axis fixation. It should be noted that the inferior oblique muscle is often implicated when abnormal rotation findings are palpated (see Fig. 6.15). This muscle can itself, through a trigger point, refer pain or indirectly by restricting the suboccipital triangle, create a suboccipital neuralgia.

When rotating the patient's head away, there is pure atlas rotation on axis during the first 25°. Past 25° the axis will be palpated as rotating. However, the atlas continues to rotate beyond the axis. It is important to establish where in the range of rotation this fixation occurs.

Test 2

Atlas-coupled Motion (Figs. 6.13, 6.16, and 6.17). The atlas is considered a compensatory hypermobile motion segment. The coupled motions of the atlas relative to occipital motion are necessary for certain neck righting and occipital righting postural reflexes. It is important then that we palpate to determine the nature of these coupled motion patterns. When selecting a manipulative procedure for the upper cervical region, these coupled motion patterns often direct the secondary thrust angles. For example, when applying a rotary atlas adjustment, a small amount of lateral thrust can be added with a cephalad or caudal component. Whether or not to add this lateral component from a cephalad or caudal direction is determined by our motion palpation findings of this coupled motion pattern. There are two motion palpation procedures that we utilize to palpate for this coupled motion. For these two procedures the finger placement is the same. The index finger is placed on the mastoid, the second finger is placed on the lateral aspect of the TVP of atlas, and the third finger is placed on the mastoid (Fig. 6.16). If the doctor's fingers are larger than the surface area allowable by the patient, the index finger can palpate the space between the mandible and atlas and the second finger can palpate the space between the atlas and mastoid. The doctor palpates bilaterally and controls the head motion by using counterpressure between the two fingers, the two-hand contact, and the thumbs that extend to the top of the head (Fig. 6.16).

Rotation. The patient's head is then rotated from side to side. As the occiput rotates to the right, the atlas makes a compensatory shift to the left and also tilts inferior on that side. The motion palpation finding for this normal coupled action is as follows: the TVP of atlas is more palpable by the second finger of the left hand as it shifts lateral during right rotation. It also becomes palpable closer to the mastoid process on the left side. Likewise, during right rotation on the right side, the index finger palpates the atlas shifting to the left and closer to the mandible. Both right and left side palpation findings suggest normal coupled motion.

Abnormal findings are palpated as follows: During right rotation, the second finger of the left hand does not appreciate the atlas shifting laterally and the TVP of atlas does not approximate the mastoid. Likewise, the right hand, second finger, does not palpate the atlas shifting to the left and the TVP moving closer to the contact finger on the mandible.

Lateral Flexion (Fig. 6.13). The second test to palpate for atlas compensatory motion is one in which the occiput is tilted in lateral flexion. It should be noted that the occiput should only be tilted 10–15°. The atlas makes a compensatory shift to the ipsilateral side and therefore, the second finger of the contact hand on the side of lateral flexion should palpate the atlas moving into it. Likewise, the contact hand on the contralateral side to lateral flexion feels the atlas moving away. In cases of pathomechanical motion, the atlas will travel with the occiput so that the second finger of the contact hand contralateral to the lateral flexion motion palpates the atlas more prominently.

References

1. Fligg DB. The art of motion palpation. J Can Chiro Assoc 1984;28(3):331–334.
2. Mennell SMcM. Joint pain, diagnosis and treatment using manipulative techniques. 1st ed. Boston: Little, Brown and Co, 1964.
3. Gillet H, Liekens M. Belgian chiropractic research notes. 11th ed. Huntington Beach: Motion Palpation Institute, 1983.
4. Grice A. A biomechanical approach to cervical and dorsal adjusting. In: Haldeman S, ed. Modern developments in the principles and practice of chiropractic. New York: Appleton-Century-Crofts, 1980:331.
5. Gitelman R. A chiropractic approach to biomechanical disorders of the lumbar spine and pelvis. In: Haldeman S, ed. Modern developments in the principles and practice of chiropractic. New York: Appleton-Century-Crofts, 1980:297.
6. Wiles M. Reproducibility and interexaminer correlation of motion palpation findings of the sacroiliac joint. J Can Chiro Assoc 1980;24(2):59.
7. Mior S, et al. Intra and interexaminer reliability of motion palpation in the cervical spine. J Can Chiro Assoc 1985;29(4):195–198.
8. Berestrom E, Courtis C. An inter- and intra-examiner reliability study of motion palpation of the lumbar spine in lateral flexion in the seated position. Eur J Chiro 1986;34:121–141.

7 Adjustive and Manipulative Techniques

Zoltan T. Szaraz, D.C.

Historically, the upper cervical spine constituted the fundamental philosophical beginning for the proliferation of various adjustive techniques.

D. D. Palmer's son, B. J., took the nerve impingement theory of his father to assert that only two vertebrae in the spine, the atlas and the axis, could be "subluxated," causing "interference to transmission of mental impulses"(1). This hypothesis resulted in his formation of the Hole in One (H.I.O.) chiropractic adjustive "system," incorporating analysis and correction, in which only the first or second cervical vertebra was adjusted.

Since then, a great many chiropractic techniques have developed, each with their own theories, methods of analysis, and corrections(2). Proliferation and diversification of upper cervical techniques may be contributed to early pioneers, followers of B. J. Palmer's School of Chiropractic, and the clinical recognition that adjustive procedures directed toward the upper cervical spine and the sacroiliac joint may have greater effects on general body postures than adjustments at other regions of the spine(3–7).

Clinically, the significance of the upper cervical spine has been identified as a major influencing factor in numerous clinical syndromes(8–12). The rationale, biomechanics, and neurophysiological effects of spinal manipulation have all been well documented(7, 13–18).

Soft tissue techniques are incorporated in the management of articular dysfunction as they have an important role not only in the generation of the articular dysfunction(19, 20) but also in the maintenance of the same(20, 21). Furthermore, the treatment of these soft tissues in "reflex syndromes"(13, 20, 22) leads to normalization of segmental dysfunction.

The author's intention is to provide a compendium of corrective procedures related to normalization and/or restoration of dysfunction of the occipitoatlantoaxial complex. It is not intended to cover all chiropractic techniques of the upper cervical area. That would be an onerous task.

The procedures that follow incorporate low force, repetitive mobilization techniques, soft tissue techniques, high velocity, short lever adjustive techniques, and corrective exercises. All descriptions apply to a right-sided lesion, unless otherwise noted (See Table 7.1).

MANIPULATIVE PROCEDURES

Occiput—Atlas Joint

Motion Palpation Finding:

- Lack of forward flexion of occiput on the cervical spine.
- Fullness and resistance against the palpating thumb at the insertion of spinalis and semispinalis capitis on occipital bone unilaterally or bilaterally.

Fixation. Flexion of occiput on the cervical spine unilaterally or bilaterally.

Muscular Involvement. Spinalis-semispinalis capitis unilaterally or bilaterally.

Adjustive Technique. The patient is in a supine position with the doctor in a low

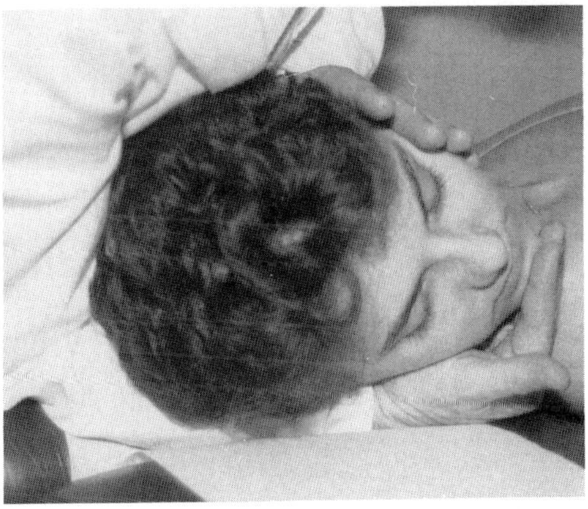

Figure 7.1. Correction for a right flexion fixation of the occiput on the cervical spine, implicating the semispinalis capitis muscle involvement.

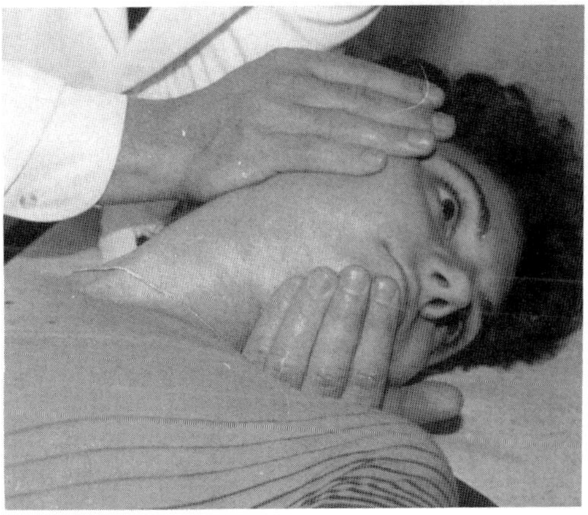

Figure 7.2. Correction for a combined fixation of occiput flexion and rotation on the same right side, implicating the splenius capitis muscle.

squatting position standing at the head of the table (Fig. 7.1). The doctor cups the patient's jaw with his right hand, while placing the middle of his contact forearm against the greater occipital protuberance. As the patient's head is rotated onto this forearm, the patient's chin is tucked in to provide maximal occiput flexion. The indifferent hand is then placed on the superior mastoid process and a firm hold is established between the down forearm and superior heel-of-the-hand contact. The doctor's contact forearm rests on the headpiece of the table parallel with the direction of the involved (down side) musculature. Maximal occipital flexion position is maintained while a long axis traction is applied toward the doctor. The thrust is a short amplitude impulse given at the height of traction along the inferior forearm.

Caution. The patient's head must be firmly held between the forearm and the indifferent hand so that at the time of the thrust the occiput and not the soft tissues move. No pressure, at any time, should be applied to the patient's jaw other than positioning the occiput in the maximal flexion.

Motion Palpation Finding:

- Restricted forward flexion and rotation of occiput on the cervical spine.
- Fullness and resistance against palpating finger at the insertion of the splenius capitis muscle into the mastoid process unilaterally.

Fixation. Forward flexion and rotation of occiput.

Muscular Involvement. Shortened or hypertonic splenius capitis unilaterally.

Adjustive Technique. The patient is in a supine position with the doctor in a low squatting position standing at the head of the table (Fig. 7.2). The indifferent hand cups the patient's chin and the patient's head is rotated onto the indifferent forearm, creating a lateral flexion pivot point for the occiput. Maximal flexion position of the occiput may be achieved by tucking the patient's chin in and laterally flexing the occiput over the down forearm until maximal tension is reached in the involved (up side) splenius capitis muscle. The contact hand with a palmar contact point is placed against the superior mastoid process. The doctor's contact forearm should be parallel with the involved musculature. Long axis traction is then applied with the contact hand in a cephalad direction exaggerating the lateral flexion position of the occiput over the passive, indifferent forearm. A dynamic, short amplitude thrust may be given at the height of traction to provide additional stretch to the muscular elements involved in the lesion.

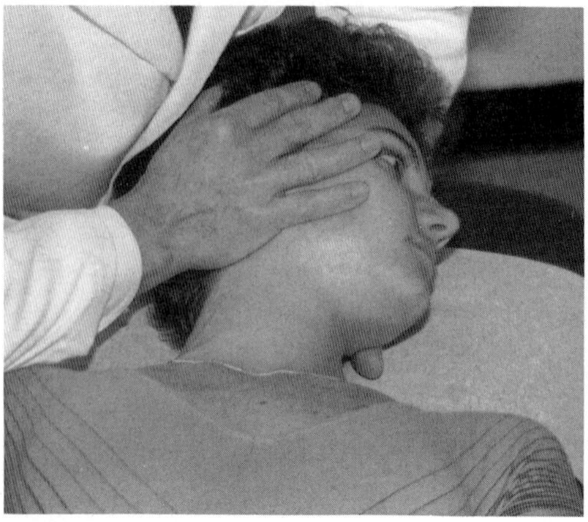

Figure 7.3. Correction of a rotary type fixation of occiput on atlas.

Motion Palpation Finding:

- Lack of anterior rotation of occiput on atlas.
- Lack of separation of space between transverse process (TVP) of atlas and mandible.

Fixation. Rotation.

Muscular Involvement. Short, suboccipital muscles (obliquus capitis superior).

Adjustive Technique

The patient is in a supine position while the doctor is in a low squatting position at the head of the patient, on the side of the lesion (Fig. 7.3). The patient's head is rotated onto the indifferent cupped hand, fingers firmly secured against rim of occiput to provide sufficient traction. Contact is taken with pisiform on mastoid process, fingers pointing toward patient's face. As soon as the contact is taken, provide sufficient cephalad traction while rotating occiput guided by contact hand. When the exact point of fixation is reached, long axis traction is applied. The rest of the contact hand should be straight, forearm pointing into the direction of occipital rotation. The thrust is a short amplitude impulse given under traction along the occipital condyles.

Caution. If the occiput is at the point of fixation and the long axis traction is appropriate for the build of the patient, only a slight dynamic thrust needs to be given at this point to affect the superior articular facet. If too much force is used, excessive rotation will result with possibility of injury to the soft tissues.

Motion Palpation Finding:

- Lack of lateral shifting of the occiput at the end of lateral flexion range (capsular or articular) in our example toward the left. Similarly, if muscular components are involved, the atlas will not shift toward the concavity (right), preventing reciprocal occipital shift.

Fixation. Lateral flexion.

Muscular Involvement. Short, suboccipital muscles on the contralateral side (e.g., rectus capitis posterior minor or major (RCPM), obliquus capitis superior (OCS).

Adjustive Procedure. The patient lies supine while the doctor is in a low squatting position at the head of the patient on the side of the articular-capsular lesion (Fig. 7.4). Rotate the patient's head onto cupped indifferent hand with fingers firmly secured against rim of occiput. The heel of the contact hand is placed upon the mastoid process, fingers pointing cephalad, wrist extended.

As soon as the contact is taken, long axis traction is provided with the indifferent hand while contact hand removes joint slack in

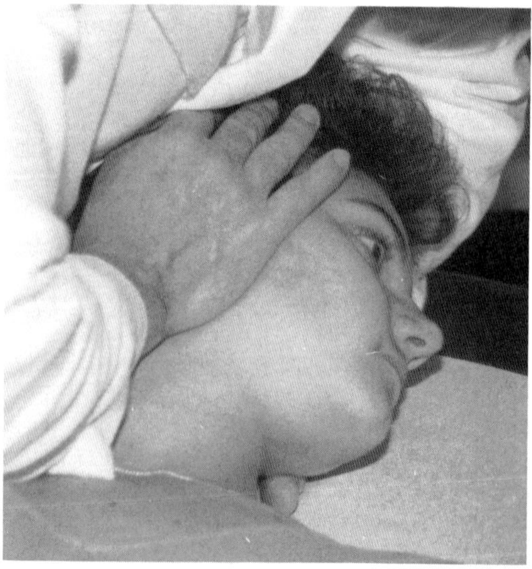

Figure 7.4. Correction of articular, lateral flexion fixation of occiput on atlas on the right side.

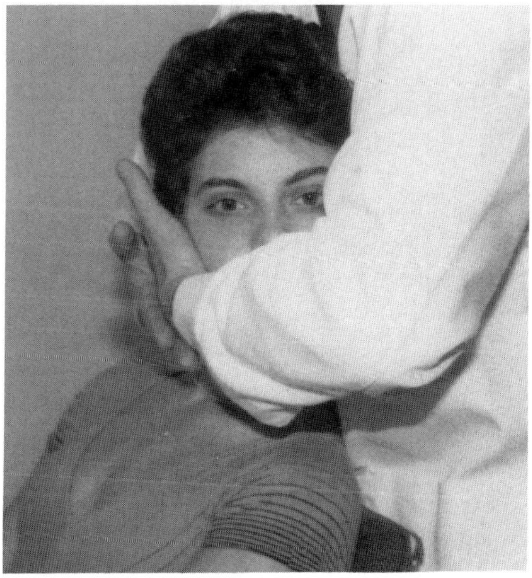

Figure 7.5. Sitting occipital lift technique for correction of a combined rotation and lateral flexion type lesion.

a lateral flexion direction. As the exact point of fixation is reached, the shoulder of the contact arm is lowered. The thrust is a single, shoulder drop, short amplitude impulse under traction, across the occipital condyles.

Motion Palpation Finding:

- Lack of anterior rotation and lateral flexion of occiput on atlas. (No separation of mandible and TVP of atlas on the right and no lateral shift of occiput to the left.)

Fixation. Rotation and lateral flexion on the same side.

Adjustive Procedure. This procedure involves the additional component of gravity during the adjustment (Fig. 7.5). The advantage of using a gravity-assisted technique has been shown to be more effective when postural muscles play a significant role in either the production or the maintenance of the spinal lesion.

The patient is instructed to sit in a slightly slumped position with both legs extended and arms folded in the lap. The selection of a Gonstead cervical chair is ideal when performing this adjustment. This specialized equipment provides the lean-back position for the patient, which will facilitate the downward traction that is necessary as a countertraction for this adjustment.

The doctor positions himself behind the patient so that the patient's head can be placed against the lower aspect of his chest. The patient's head is then rotated against the doctor's chest, with the fixation side to the outside (right side). The doctor's indifferent hand is then placed, with the hypothenar process against the right mastoid process of the patient. It is very important that the doctor's wrist is in a neutral position and that his forearm is not contacting the jaw of the patient. Once the contact Is made, it is reinforced by the palmar aspect of the doctor's other hand against the dorsum of his indifferent contact.

Remove joint slack by maintaining full rotation and guiding the occiput into lateral flexion. Cephalad traction is provided by straightening the doctor's legs and creating an increasing degree of lateral flexion with the reinforced contact hand.

A reinforced, double-hand, lift type of impulse is given as the force is centered in a combined rotation and lateral flexion plane at the occiput atlas condyle at the point of fixation.

If the muscles on the opposite side are involved in the lesion complex, the adjustment is directed so that the muscular components on the convex and the articular components on the concave side will be affected simultaneously. This is achieved by an additional lateral flexion component toward the concavity as necessary. This can be achieved by the doctor's body position.

Contraindications of this maneuver may include temporomandibular joint (TMJ) dysfunction and vertebral artery syndrome.

Motion Palpation Finding:

- Lack of anterior glide of occipital condyles indicated by no separation of TVP—mandible space during jaw-jutting test.

Fixation. Anterior glide bilaterally.

Adjustive Procedure—Supine Occipital Extension. The patient is lying supine on an elevated head piece (Fig. 7.6). The doctor stands at the head of the patient.

A two-handed contact is used. One hand contacts the chin by cupping it. The other hand is placed under the occiput, secured

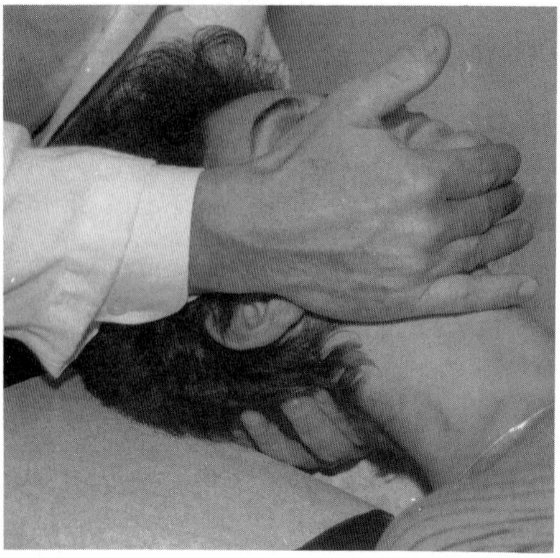

Figure 7.6. Mobilization procedure, when occipital extension is restricted bilaterally.

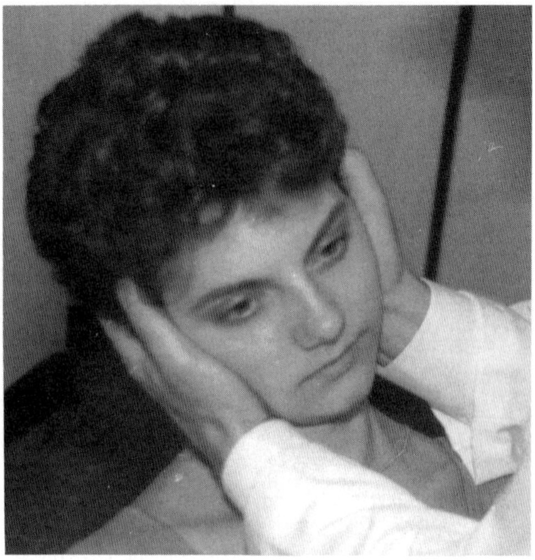

Figure 7.7. When posterior rotation of the occiput is restricted, the SCM muscle (left side of photograph) may be involved. Note the stretching the left SCM fibers.

against the rim by the web of the cupped hand. Both hand contacts should be firm, yet not stiff. Joint slack is taken up by first positioning the occiput into extension and then applying long axis traction cephalad. Traction should be applied progressively and through the doctor's body lean. It may be repeated three or four times. A moderate amplitude of impulse may be given at the height of traction.

Contraindications may include TMJ dysfunction.

Motion Palpation Finding:

- Restricted posterior rotation of occiput.
- Fullness and resistance against palpating fingers at the insertion of the sternocleidomastoideus (SCM) into the mastoid process.

Fixation. Posterior rotation of the occiput on atlas.

Muscular Involvement. Shortened or hypertonic SCM unilaterally.

Adjustive Technique. The patient is seated, leaning backward (Fig. 7.7). The doctor stands in a fencer stance at the side of the patient on the side of the involved musculature (left side lesion).

Double hand contact is used for the correction. The indifferent hand is placed against the contralateral temporal bone cupping the ear. The contact hand cups the ear on the side of the lesion with palmar contact against the mastoid process.

The patient's occiput is then positioned into maximal flexion and posterior rotation (on the side of involvement). This position should recreate the maximal point of restriction found during motion palpation. The doctor's contact forearm should be nearly parallel with the fibers of the involved musculature. Cephalad long axis traction is applied to the occiput with both hands to provide the appropriate amount of articular separation and muscular stretch to the involved SCM. A short amplitude thrust may be given in a superior and posterior direction.

Variation. This procedure may also be performed in a supine lying position. Contact, stance, line of drive, and thrust will be similar without the added advantage of gravitational counterstress.

Motion Palpation Finding:

- Lack of posterior glide bilaterally, indicated by restricted jaw retraction.

Fixation. Posterior glide flexion bilaterally; extended occiput due to posterior position and/or associated hyperlordotic cervical spine.

Adjustive Procedure—Supine Occipital

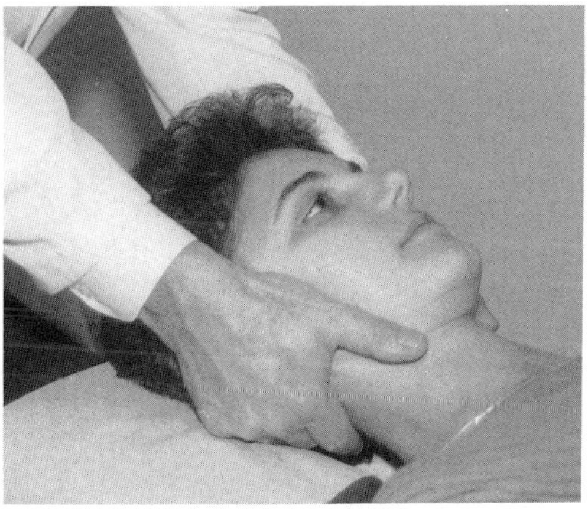

Figure 7.8. Long axis mobilization technique incorporating forced flexion to correct for restriction of bilateral occiput flexion on atlas.

Flexion. The patient is in a supine lying position with the doctor standing at the head of the patient (Fig. 7.8). The doctor may use body lean for traction.

Two-hand Contacts. This manipulation requires strong hands. The posterolateral aspect of the occiput is contacted with fingers secured at the rim of the occiput. *Cupped hand contact:* The thenar aspect of the hand is secured against the zygomatic ridge (zygomatic arch).

Traction is applied (with arms bent and elbows close to the doctor's body) in a cephalad direction. The thenar contacts force the occiput into flexion. Traction is applied progressively and released slowly. This may be repeated three to four times. A short amplitude impulse may be given by sudden ulnar deviation of both wrists at the height of traction.

Contraindications may include acute TMJ syndrome.

An alternative maneuver using a longer lever contact may be used (Fig. 7.9). In this position, one hand contacts the occiput with a webbed hand contact. The other hand is placed on the forehead of the patient with fingers extended. This contact should be firm yet not too stiff. Care should be taken of the patient's eyes and nose. The slack is taken up by cephalad pull of the occiput while leaning slightly backward to produce occiput flexion directed by the contact on the forehead.

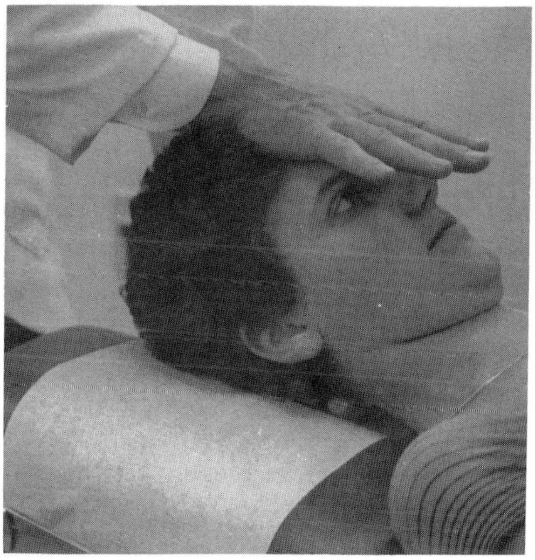

Figure 7.9. Alternative long axis, occiput flexion mobilization maneuver when strong flexion combined with a dynamic thrust is indicated.

A commonly used alternative is in the prone position (Fig. 7.10).

The contact used is a reinforced knife-edge contact. This contact should be firm yet not too stiff. The construction of the table will be the determining factor in this adjustment. If a terminal drop headpiece is available, this adjustment is greatly facilitated by the use of the terminal point headpiece. The patient's occiput is placed in the

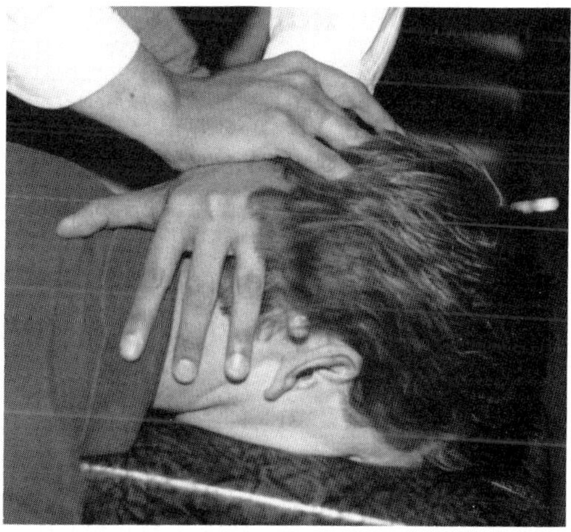

Figure 7.10. Commonly used prone flexion adjustment for the occiput. Terminal point headpiece mechanism facilitates the execution of the high velocity thrust.

maximal flexed position and then the headpiece is loaded, contact taken, and thrust executed using the terminal point mechanism.

Atlas-Axis Joint

Motion Palpation Finding:

- Restriction of anterior rotation of atlas on axis.
- Posterior malposition of atlas.

Fixation. Atlas on axis in rotation.

Muscular Involvement. Inferior and superior oblique on same side.

Adjustive Technique (Fig. 7.11). The patient is in a supine lying position with the doctor in a low squatting position at the head of the patient (Fig. 7.11).

Once the lesion is repalpated, an index contact is placed on the posterior arch of the atlas. The wrist of the contact hand should be straight; the thumb may be placed on the patient's cheek for added support and direction. As the contact is taken, the doctor steps to the side of contact but maintains squatting stance with equal weightbearing on both legs. The indifferent hand cups the patient's ear with fingers secured against rim of occiput.

Rotate the atlas and occiput anteriorly with both hands until the point of fixation of atlas-axis rotation is re-created. Provide slight occipital extension to lock the occiput atlas articulation, centering force to the atlas-axis joint complex. The line of drive is in a rotary direction with slight ulnar deviation of the wrist of the contact hand.

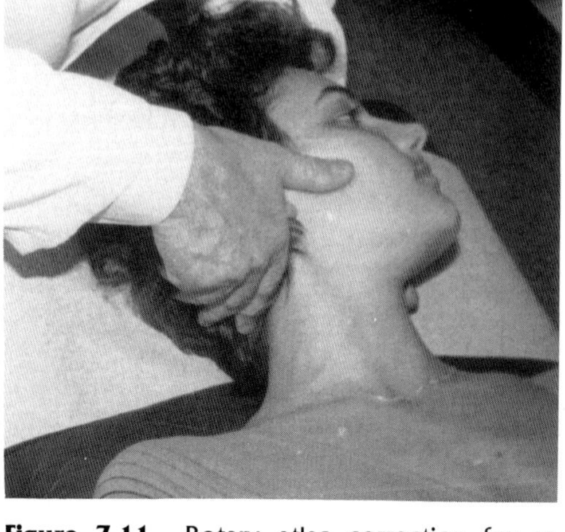

Figure 7.11. Rotary atlas correction for restriction on anterior rotation of atlas on axis.

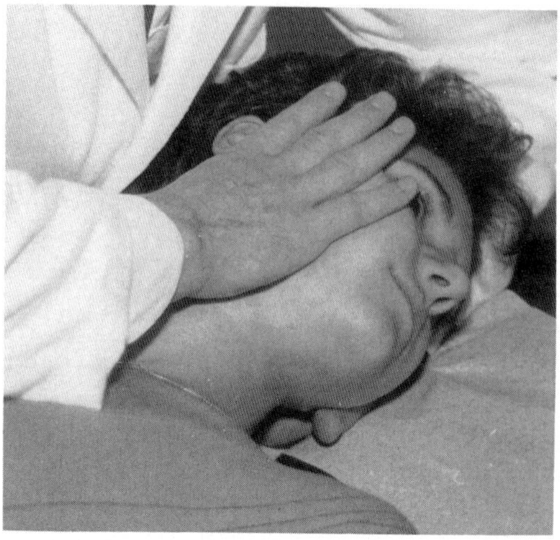

Figure 7.12. Doctor's thumb hooks the posterior arch of atlas on the right side, assisted by long axis cephalad traction. A useful alternative to correct anterior rotation fixation of atlas on axis.

The thrust is a single, short amplitude, high velocity impulse from posterior to anterior.

Caution. Extreme caution must be taken that the amount of rotation of the atlas-axis, occiput-atlas articulations re-create the exact point of fixation as found during the motion palpation. If excessive rotation is created and combined with excessive extension of the occiput on atlas, the vertebral artery complex may be compromised.

Alternative. To provide some long axis cephalad traction and to control the occiput extension, an alternative technique of thumb hook (Fig. 7.12) rotary atlas procedure provides a useful alternative. When this procedure is performed, the palmar aspect of the thumb is placed against the posterior arch of the atlas. The long axis traction is provided with both hands where the arms of the doctor are in line with the cervical spine. To perform the thumb hook rotary atlas procedure, the doctor must be in a much lower squatting stance, and the type of thrust used is a rotary thrust created by ulnar deviation of the contact hand.

Motion Palpation Finding:

- Lack of separation of atlas on axis beyond 25° of anterior rotation of atlas.
- Fullness and tenderness at spinous process of axis over the insertion of the inferior oblique muscle.
- Fullness and posterior malposition of atlas.

Muscular Involvement. Shortening and hypertonicity of the right inferior oblique muscle.

Fixation. Rotation-type lesion between atlas and axis.

Adjustive Procedure. The patient is in a supine lying position with the doctor in a low squatting stance at the head of the patient facing approximately 45° caudally (Fig. 7.13).

The indifferent hand is placed on the temporal bone cupping the ear of the patient. Contact is taken with a reinforced index fingertip against the spinous process of axis on the side of involvement. The patient's head is gently rotated *away* from the lesion until the contact finger senses axis rotation. Long axis cephalad traction is now applied while the contact hand prepares for a lateral to medial and superior to inferior thrust. The thrust is in a posterior direction and in line (parallel) with the direction of the fibers of the inferior oblique muscle.

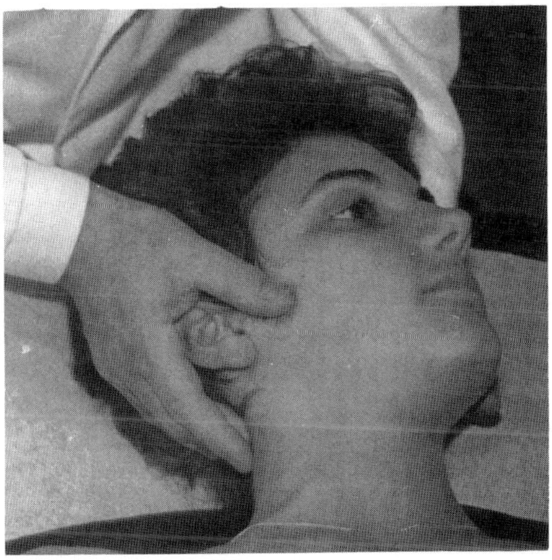

Figure 7.13. Correction for restriction of atlas rotation on axis when the right inferior oblique muscle is implicated.

Motion Palpation Finding:

- Lack of reciprocal motion between occiput-atlas and atlas on axis during right lateral flexion.
- Restricted range of left lateral flexion of occiput on atlas and atlas on axis restricted lateral and anterior rotation of atlas on axis on the right.
- Lack of lateral joint play between occiput-atlas and/or atlas-axis on the right to joint challenge.
- Static, right lateral malposition of atlas.

Muscular Involvement. Shortened or hypertonic right rectus capitis lateralis and right inferior oblique; shortened or hypertonic left obliquus capitis superior.

Fixation. Lateral flexion at occiput-atlas or atlas-axis combined with rotation fixation of atlas on axis.

Adjustive Technique. The patient is in a supine lying position with the doctor in a low squatting position at the head of the patient facing approximately 45° caudal on the side of the lesion (right) (Fig. 7.14).

Rotate the patient's head onto a cupped indifferent hand with fingers firmly secured against rim of occiput. Create sufficient lateral flexion away from the lesion side to allow easy identification of the atlas transverse process. The padded pisiform of the contact hand is placed on the posterolateral aspect of the atlas transverse process (right side). Provide cephalad, long axis traction with the indifferent hand while the

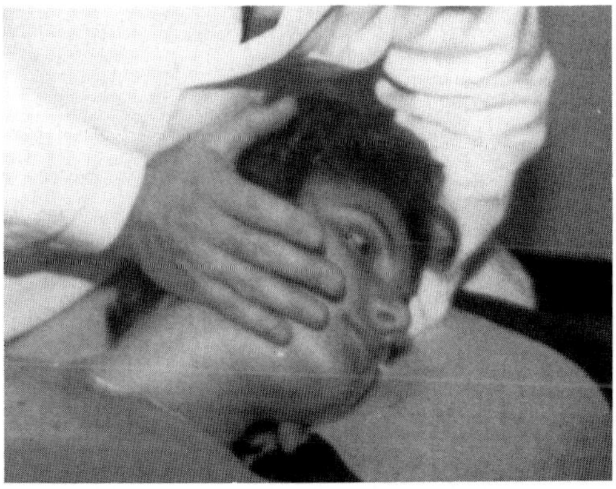

Figure 7.14. Correction for a combination of lateral flexion and rotation of the atlas on axis using a pisiform contact.

contact hand removes joint slack in a lateral flexion direction. The amount of rotation and lateral flexion movement should recreate the point of fixation found during motion palpation. The forearm of the contact hand should be close to the doctor's torso.

The line of drive is consistent with the facet facing of the occiput-atlas articulation and the direction of the fibers of the inferior oblique muscles, from lateral to medial and posterior to anterior. The thrust is a shoulder drop impulse under traction with very high velocity and short amplitude.

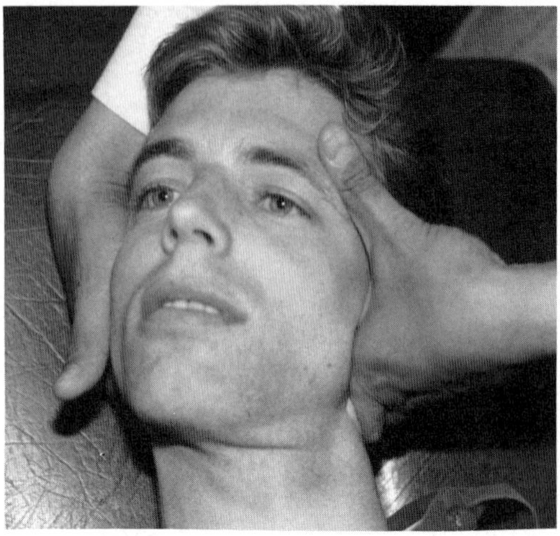

Figure 7.15. Lateral atlas correction, without rotary component, when the atlas is involved in a lateral flexion restriction.

Occiput-Atlas-Axis Joint

Motion Palpation Finding

- Lack of reciprocal motion between occiput and atlas and atlas-axis during right lateral flexion.
- Restricted range of left lateral flexion.
- Restricted lateral joint play between occiput-atlas-axis when the atlas is challenged from right to left.
- Static, right lateral malposition of atlas.

Muscular Involvement. Shortened or hypertonic left superior oblique and right acute capitis lateralis.

Fixation. Lateral flexion at occiput-atlas-axis.

Adjustive Procedure. The patient is in a supine lying position with the doctor in a squatting stance at the head of the patient facing approximately 45° caudal on the side of the lesion (Fig. 7.15). The indifferent hand is placed against the temporal bone with the patient's ear cupped and fingers secured against the rim of the occiput. Contact is made against the lateral aspects of the right transverse process of atlas with the index finger of the contact hand. Laterally deviate the patient's head without any rotation while joint slack is taken up from lateral to medial with the contact hand.

A sufficient amount of long axis traction is applied to provide articular separation at the occipital atlantal articulation. The amount of lateral flexion movement should re-create the point of fixation experienced during motion palpation. The thrust is a single, pectoral, very high velocity, short amplitude impulse from lateral to medial and from superior to inferior.

Caution. It is important that the amount of lateral movement is not excessive so that the articulations on the contact side (right side) are not compromised (i.e., jammed up).

UPPER CERVICAL RECOIL TECHNIQUE

No text such as this would be complete without addressing the group of techniques of diagnosis and treatment collectively known as "upper cervical techniques." While we cannot in this space convey the specifics and complexities of any of these techniques, a summary of this technique system is presented. We refer the reader directly to the primary texts, compilations, and articles written by authors in this field and the excellent review by Grice(23).

The notion of focusing exclusively on the upper cervical spine is universally credited to B. J. Palmer. Grice(23) notes that while B. J. Palmer initially advanced his father's tradition of a full spine approach to adjusting, "in the later years, [1934] . . . [he] went further by adopting the specific upper cervical technique . . . referred to as 'hole-in-one' (HIO)."

Since that time, many authors have written on the subject and developed techniques of diagnosis and/or treatment. These techniques generally have the following similarities, which form the foundation of upper cervical techniques:

(1) Adjustments are delivered primarily to atlas and, to a lesser degree, to axis;
(2) Adjustments are rendered in order to correct putative upper cervical misalignments (i.e., subluxations);
(3) Analysis of vertebral malposition is conducted in largest measure by static x-rays, which are taken from a number of views under precise stabilization techniques and are analyzed by marking systems that involve angles of various contiguous anatomical lines, localization of various anatomical landmarks for bilateral congruity and symmetry, and overall visual impressions of anatomical orientation;
(4) From the above analysis, a static "listing" is derived that, in codified form, describes the essentials of the spatial malposition that defines the individual patient's subluxation;
(5) Ancillary measurement techniques may be used including neurocalometer readings, nervoscope readings, blood pressure measurements, leg length checks, and the anatometer(24). It is not uncommon for upper cervical practitioners to regard all other clinical tests as "ancillary" in the sense that their findings are all potentially altered by the adjustment and are thus secondary to the atlas malposition.
(6) Adjustments are rendered to correct for the misaligned vertebra. Gregory states that correction involves "the establishment of a specific and accurate force vector, determined from x-ray findings, designed to restore to normal position the atlas vertebra"(24).
(7) Adjustive techniques are typically of the recoil variety, traditionally delivered by hand, but recently delivered by instrumentation as well (see the writings of Sweat and Fuhr). Grice has described the recoil adjustment in the following manner, which appears consistent with the methods as taught at the Palmer College(25): "The patient is placed in the side-lying position" (i.e., the laterality of the subluxation is placed on the 'up' side); the thrust is a dynamic adjustive thrust given in a specific direction with a specific depth, high velocity and low amplitude. A free-fall head piece or table cushion may be used with a set spring reset release to take up part of the force and allow for counter-resistance of the fixed vertebra." According to technique instructional material from Palmer College, "only the hands are used to deliver the toggle (adjustive thrust). The hands and arms are allowed to 'recoil' quickly, therefore assuring minimal discomfort to the patient."(25) (See Fig. 7.16).

Upper cervical recoil techniques are taught in many colleges. In some they form the mainstay of technique instruction; in others, they are relegated to an elective; and in a small minority of other colleges, they constitute the sole method taught.

The collective wisdom of the upper cervical techniques has contributed a great deal to the advancement of chiropractic clinical practice. Such insights as the importance of the upper cervical spine to the postural integrity of the patient, the impact of upper cervical dysfunction on the health

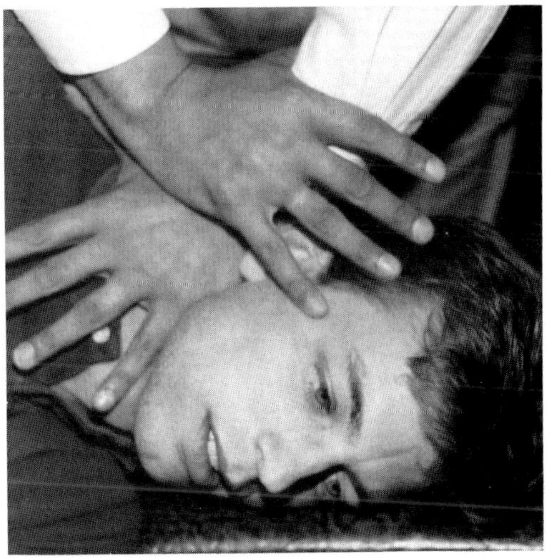

Figure 7.16. The toggle recoil adjustment. An alternative to the supine, lateral atlas, index correction, may be performed in the side posture position and may include torque in the delivery of the thrust.

of the "whole" patient (but particularly in local and cephalgic pain and dysfunction syndromes), the unique system of x-ray visualizations that have stood the test of time as the state-of-the-art in a thorough study of the area (see Chapter 2), and a unique form of adjustive technique that its practitioners generally perform to an extraordinarily high degree of precision have all contributed to a productive clinical tradition. It is unfortunate that in the minds of many modern chiropractors, the criticisms appear to outweigh these positive factors. These criticisms stem from the dogmatic presentation of these techniques, their rigidity to new and competing insights, their paradoxical attempt to expansively include everything clinical in the framework of a single structural problem, i.e., the chiropractic reductio ad absurdum, their reliance on a static paradigm derived from analytical measures far too imprecise for the methodological precision demanded by the practitioners, and a lack of coherence of their theory to accepted physiological reality provoking an excessive reliance on philosophical constructs to rationalize their own observations. Perhaps in this new era of chiropractic scientific clinical trials, the upper cervical techniques will be sorted out.

MOBILIZATIONS AND SOFT TISSUE TECHNIQUES

Lateral Mobilization (See Fig 7.17)

Indication

- Restricted lateral flexion in the cervical spine and/or upper cervical articulations.

The patient is in a supine position with the doctor standing or sitting at the head of the patient placing both hands under the patient's neck with fingers pointing caudal. The patient's head should be resting on the doctor's cupped hands. Starting from the lower cervical area, alternately, laterally mobilize cervical spine with fingertips of one hand pushing against spinous processes or articular processes while the other hand creates counterforce and appropriate long

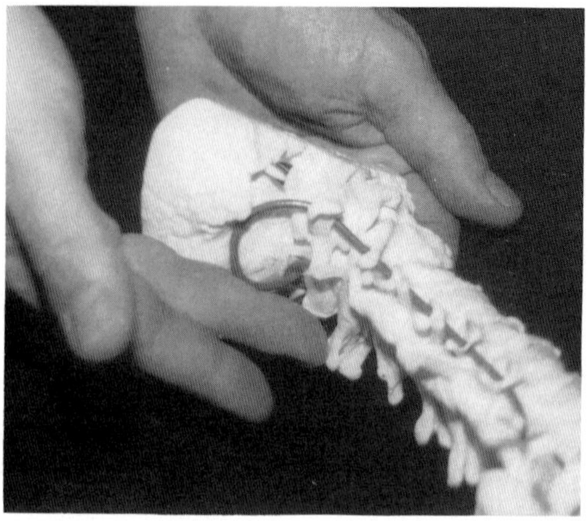

Figure 7.17. Finger positions on a skeletal model for lateral flexion mobilization in the upper cervical region.

axis traction. Smooth, rhythmical lateral mobilization in both directions can be achieved by alternating traction and fulcrum between the two hands. By changing contact and fulcrum, any segment can be mobilized.

Rotation Mobilization (See Fig. 7.18)

Indication

- Restricted movement in rotation of cervicals or upper cervical area.

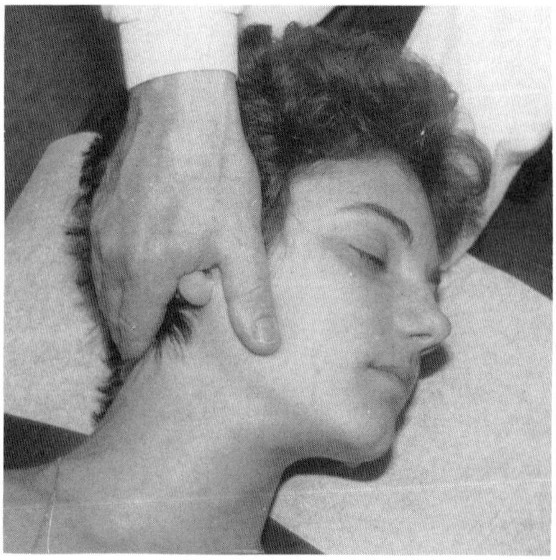

Figure 7.18. Anterior rotation mobilization of the upper cervical spine.

The patient is in a supine position with the doctor standing or sitting at the head, placing both hands under the patient's neck with fingers pointing caudal. The patient's head rests on the doctor's cupped hands. With fingertip contact against posterior articular processes, as one hand rotates vertebral segment, the other hand guides head and cervical rotation and provides appropriate cephalad traction. Rotation in the opposite direction is achieved by reversing the roles of the hands. This maneuver is repeated rhythmically several times, tending to increase the range of rotation each time. By changing contact, any segment can be mobilized.

Figure of Eight Mobilization (See Fig. 7.19)

Indication

- Restriction in both lateral flexion and rotation of any cervical or upper cervical articulations.

The patient is in a supine position with the doctor sitting or standing at the head, supporting the occiput in the palm of his hands with fingers pointing cephalad and medially. Providing the appropriate amount of long axis traction with both hands, the head and the neck are carried through a movement of elevation-rotation-side bending and extension in a figure eight pattern.

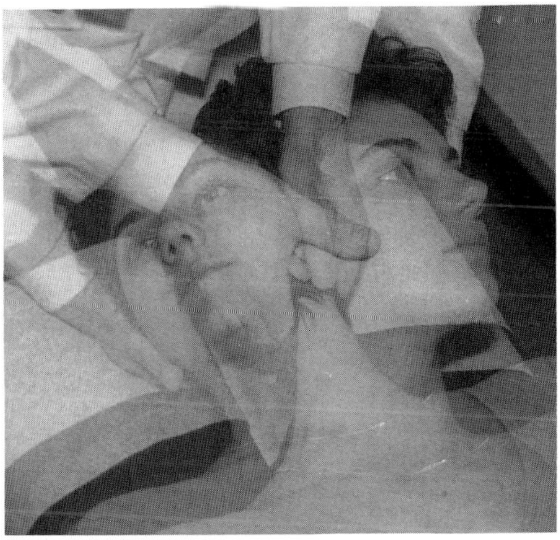

Figure 7.19. Double exposure demonstrating a figure of eight mobilization of the whole cervical spine including the upper cervical segment.

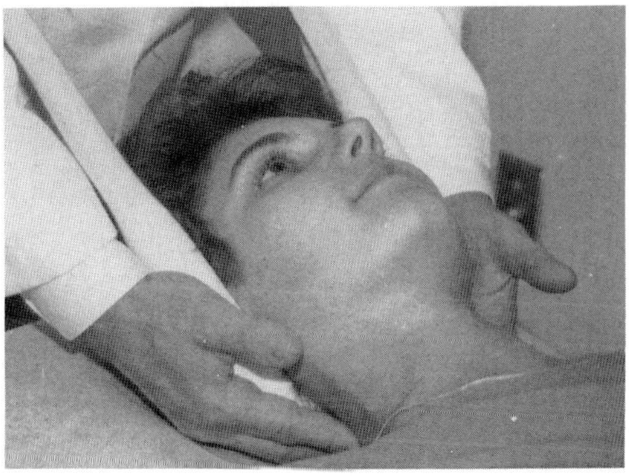

Figure 7.20. Long axis traction mobilization of the cervical spine with a padded tube of gauze as aid.

Long Axis Traction (See Fig. 7.20)

Indication

- General traction for any cervical articulation particularly effective in an acute lesion due to articular capsular effusion.

The patient is in a supine position with the pillow or headrest of the table elevated. The doctor sits or stands at the head, placing both hands under the patient's neck with fingers pointing caudal. Cephalad traction is achieved slowly and progressively and released slowly. To ensure maximal articular separation, the appropriate amount of cervical flexion is necessary.

Alternately, a towel or padded tube of gauze wrapped around the doctor's waist may be used. Long axis traction is achieved by the doctor leaning backward to an appropriate degree. This allows both hands of the doctor to be utilized for articular mobilization or adjustment under traction.

Paraspinal Muscle Kneading

Indication

- Contracted or hypertonic paraspinal musculature.

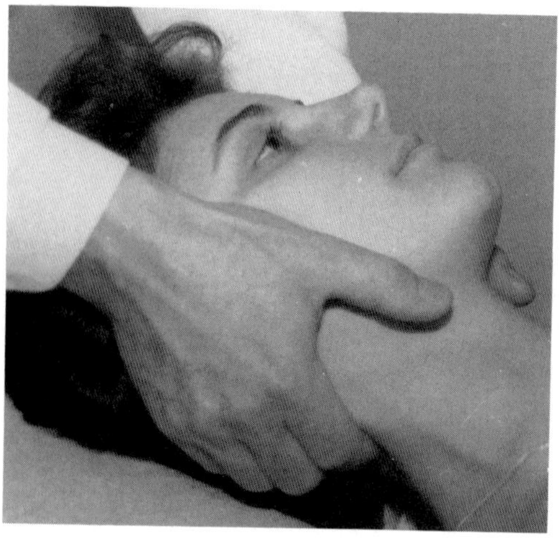

Figure 7.21. Soft tissue stretching technique of the cervical paraspinal musculature.

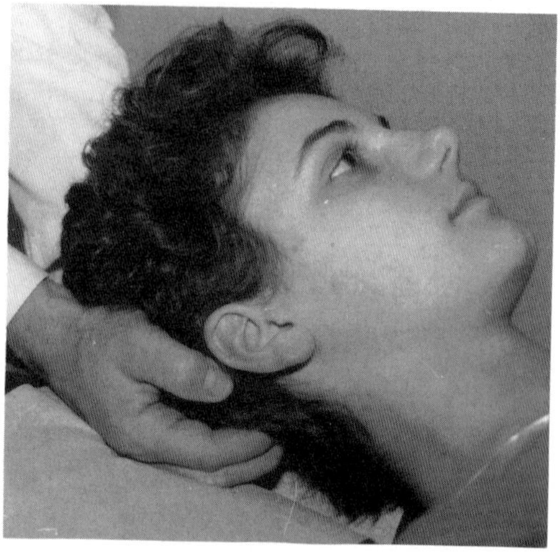

Figure 7.22. During transverse friction technique, the insertion of suboccipital muscles are deeply and gradually pressed against the bony rim of the occiput.

Procedure

The patient is in a supine position with the doctor sitting or standing at the head of the table (Fig. 7.21). The doctor places his hands, with fingers spread, on either side of the posterior cervical muscles. Starting from the spinous processes, gently pull anteriorly and laterally the paraspinal muscles in an alternate stretching and relaxing fashion. This procedure can be used locally or progressively to cover the entire posterior and lateral cervical musculature.

When indicated, this procedure may be combined with long axis cephalad traction for added ligamentous stretch.

Suboccipital Trigger Point Technique

Procedure

With the patient in a supine position, the doctor places occiput into his palm with fingers resting against the rim of the occiput (Fig. 7.22). Once the contracted, fibrotic trigger points are located, transverse friction massage can be applied. This procedure can be very painful and typically will reproduce frontal or temporal pain. If additional muscle stretching is required, the occiput and the cervical spine can be flexed progressively while friction massage is continued.

This procedure may be combined with occipital flexion manipulation when treating long occipital extensors semispinalis cervicis, semispinalis capitis musculature, or any postural muscles associated with postural occipital extension malposition. This combined procedure provides additional dynamic stretching to contracted suboccipital musculature (Fig. 7.23).

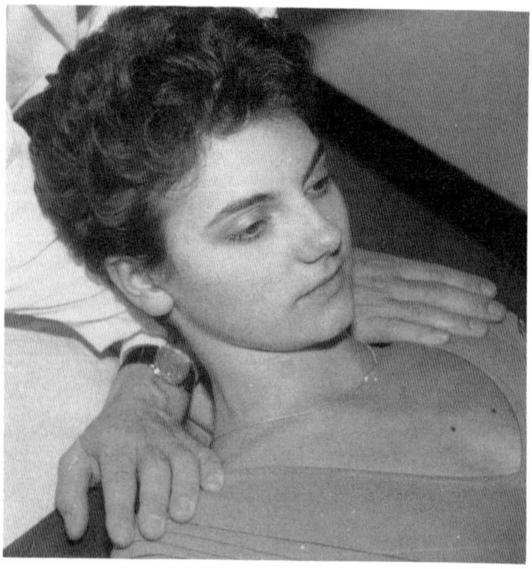

Figure 7.23. Progressive stretching technique of contracted suboccipital postural musculature. Caution must be exercised to prevent excessive muscle straining.

Table 7.1
Pathomechanical Approach to the Chiropractic Management of the Upper Cervical Spine

Fixation	Motion Palpation Findings	Static Palpation Findings	Muscular Involvement	Adjustment
Occipitoatlantal joint				
Rotation	Lack of anterior rotation of occiput over atlas	Posterior occiput with deep muscular fullness/tenderness on same side	Superior oblique	Rotary occiput
Lateral flexion	Lack of lateral shifting of occiput at end of lateral flexion range with lack of reciprocal atlas shifting	High mastoid process (high ear) on same side. Prominent atlas transverse on contralateral side. Deep muscular fullness/tenderness on contralateral side	Rectus capitis posterior major or minor on same side. Superior oblique on contralateral side	Lateral occiput
Rotation and lateral flexion on same side	Lack of anterior rotation and lateral flexion of occiput on same side	Posterior and lateral mastoid process. Muscular fullness and/or tenderness on same side	Rectus capitis posterior minor and splenius capitis on same side. Deep suboccipitals on contralateral side	Sitting occipital lift
Anterior glide bilaterally	Lack of anterior glide of occiput over atlas	Bilaterally posterior and superior mastoid process. Alordotic cervical spine. Retracted chin postural head carriage.	Longus capitis, rectus capitis, platisma	Supine occiput extension mobilization and/or adjustment
Posterior glide bilaterally	Lack of posterior glide of occiput over atlas	Postural occipital extension. Bilaterally deep mastoid processes. Deep muscular fullness and/or tenderness	Bilaterally rectus capitis posterior major and minor. Bilaterally semispinalis capitis	Supine, prone occiput flexion mobilization and/or adjustment. Soft tissue techniques
Posterior glide unilaterally	Lack of posterior glide of occiput over atlas	Anterior and inferior mastoid process. Tenderness at insertion of SCM muscle	Sternocleidomastoideus	Sitting occipital lift
Occiput on cervical spine				
Occiput flexion unilaterally or bilaterally	Lack of forward flexion of occiput on cervical spine	Fullness and resistance against palpating finger behind greater occipital protuberance. Superficial muscular fullness and/or tenderness under greater occipital protuberance	Semispinalis capitis, unilaterally or bilaterally	Supine semispinalis capitis
Occiput flexion and rotation unilaterally or bilaterally	Lack of forward flexion and rotation of occiput on cervical spine on same side	Fullness and superficial muscular tenderness behind mastoid process	Splenius capitis	Supine splenius capitis
Atlantoaxial joint				
Rotation	Lack of separation of atlas transverse beyond 25° of anterior rotation	Fullness/tenderness at spinous process of axis. Fullness and posterior malposition of atlas	Inferior oblique	Finger push on axis

Table 7.1 (*continued*)

Fixation	Motion Palpation Findings	Static Palpation Findings	Muscular Involvement	Adjustment
Rotation	Lack of anterior rotation of atlas	Posterior malposition of atlas	Inferior and superior oblique	Rotary cervical, alternative thumb hook cervical
Lateral flexion	Lack of lateral glide of atlas on axis during joing challenge from lateral to medial	Lateral and inferior malposition of atlas	Inferior oblique unilaterally	Lateral atlas with index or pisiform contact

Acknowledgments
The author wishes to express his gratitude to Drs. Grice, Fligg, and Vernon for their advice; Ellen Laine for her gracious pose during many hours of photo sessions; Dan McGinty for technical assistance; and Veronica Nass and Elaine Edwards for the many hours of typing and retyping of the manuscript.

References

1. Palmer BJ. The subluxation specific—the adjustment specific. Davenport, IA: Palmer School of Chiropractic, 1934.
2. Kfoury PW. Catalogue of chiropractic techniques. St. Louis: Logan College of Chiropractic, 1977.
3. Illi FWH. Highlights of 45 years of experience and 35 years research. Presented at European Chiropractic Union Convention, 1971.
4. De Jarnette MB. Sacro-occipital technique of spinal therapy. Nebraska City, NB: Self-published, 1940.
5. Pierce W, Stillwagon G. Pierce-Stillwagon Technique. In: Kfoury PW, ed. Catalog of chiropractic techniques. St. Louis: Logan College of Chiropractic, 1977.
6. Gregory R. The upper cervical monograph. Vol 2. Nos 4 and 5, 1978.
7. Grice AG. A biomechanical approach in cervical and dorsal adjusting. In: Haldeman S ed. Modern developments in the principles and practice of chiropractic. New York: Appleton-Century-Crofts, 1980.
8. Cole WV. The effects of the atlas lesion after 96 hours and after 6 weeks. J Am Osteopath Assoc 1948;48:7.
9. Buchmann J, Bulow B. Functional disturbances of the upper cervical spine in newborn. Manuelle Med 1983;21:59.
10. Frykholm R. Cervical migraine. In: Hirsch C ed. Cervical pain: proceedings of the symposium on cervical pain. Stockholm: Pergamon, 1971.
11. Johnston RJ. Vertebrongenic autonomic dysfunction—subjective symptoms: a prospective study. J Can Chiro Assoc 1981;25:51.
12. Hulse M. Dysequilibrium, caused by a functional disturbance of the upper cervical spine: clinical aspects and different diagnosis. Manual Med 1983;1:18.
13. Lewit K. The contribution of clinical observation to neurobiological mechanisms in manipulative therapy. In: Korr I ed. The neurobiologic mechanism in manipulative therapy. New York: Plenum, 1978.
14. Haldeman S. The clinical basis for discussion of mechanisms of manipulative therapy. In: Korr I ed. The neurobiologic mechanism in manipulative therapy. New York: Plenum, 1978.
15. Lomax E. Manipulative therapy, a historical perspective from ancient times to the modern era. In: Goldstein M ed. The research status of spinal manipulative therapy. Bethesda: Natl Inst Neurol Communicative Disorders Stroke Mono 15, 1975.
16. Sandoz R. Some physical mechanism and effects of spinal adjustments. Swiss Annals Vol VI, 1976.
17. Janse J. Principles and practice of chiropractic: an anthology. Lombard: National College of Chiropractic, 1946.
18. Wyke BD. Articular neurology and manipulative therapy. In: Dewhurst D ed. Aspects of manipulative therapy. Carlton: Lincoln Institute of Health Sciences, 1980.
19. Fassbender HG. Rheumatic pain (der rheumatische schmerz). Med Welt 1980;36:1263.
20. Dvorak J, Dvorak V. Manual medicine, diagnostian. New York: Thieme Stratton, 1984.
21. Travell J. Identification of myofacial trigger point syndrome: a case of atypical facial neuralgia. Arch Phys Med. 1981;62:100.
22. Good AB. Spinal joint blocking. J Manipulative Physial Ther 1985;8:1.
23. Grice AS. A biomechanical approach to cervical and dorsal adjusting. In:Haldeman S, ed. Modern developments in the principles and practice of chiropractic. New York: Appleton-Century-Crofts, 1980.
24. Gregory RR. The atlas subluxation complex and its correction. In Kfoury P, ed. Catalogue of chiropractic techniques. 1977.
25. Palmer upper cervical technique. In: Kfoury P, ed. Catalogue of chiropractic techniques. 1977.

3 Clinical Section

8 Differential Diagnosis of Headaches

L. M. Barbuto, D.C., F.C.C.S.(C)

The understanding of the pathogenesis of head-face pain is, to say the least, very primitive. Nonetheless, if a clinician has an appreciation of the mechanisms of head pain, he/she can proceed to reason a clinical diagnosis and institute the appropriate therapy. To start, the practitioner must take the time to get a reasonable understanding of the patient presenting with head pain.

Pain is a clinical nemisis; no subject in the entire health compendium involves such a wide variety of causes. To further complicate matters, pain is a subjective symptom that cannot be measured effectively. For our particular purposes, we will review pain as it pertains to the production of headache.

The term headache is conventionally used to describe any discomfort (usually pain) in the upper half of the head, from the forehead to the back of the neck excluding the face below the eyebrows. The area so defined is supplied by the second cervical sensory root and its extension, the greater occipital nerve, and by the first divisions of the trigeminal nerves. The sensory root of the first cervical nerve is inconspicuous and often believed to be absent. Gray(1), however, noted that it is absent in only 8% of cadavers, and Kerr(2) has stimulated it during posterior fossa surgery producing orbital, frontal, and vertex pain correlating with uppermost to lowermost root stimulation. Cameron goes so far as to hypothesize that it may be compressed by muscles in spasm(3).

Headache is a common problem, affecting approximately 70–75% of men and more than 80% of women in a one-year period(4, 5). At any given time, between 5 and 10% of the population are seeking intermittent headache relief in the United States(6). Headache and head pain are, needless to say, symptoms and not a disease in and of themselves. As a sole symptom, it is not diagnostic of any specific disorder.

Headache may indicate the presence of psychic overload such as anxiety or personal or life style difficulties or it may reflect the presence of organic disease. More recently, the role of the cervical spine in the production of head pain is attracting more attention(7, 8).

In spite of what is known about head pain, there still exists a large void in our understanding between organic pain and the variations of response to it. Patients' complaints of pain often do not correlate with degree of impairment or, on the other hand, with improvement noted in other aspects of their lives(9). Whereas pain may be related to nociceptive input, suffering is not.

Although the symptom of pain is the object of medical and social research measured in billions of dollars yearly(10), the precise relationship between pain patients and certain personality traits such as anxiety, depression, and hypochondriasis still remains unclear. Thus one appreciates that the resolution of the many difficulties that beset the evaluation of pain in the head depends a great deal upon the history and the communicative and observational interaction that takes place during the doctor-patient consultation(s).

Pain may be considered as an abnormal

emotional state that is called into being usually by the development of chemical and/or structural changes in various tissues of the body that give rise to activity in afferent systems within the neuraxis that normally are relatively quiescent. Its variation may be attributed to a complex combination of psychological, somatic, and visceral reflex responses and hormonal changes that are simultaneously evoked by such activity. Wyke(11) puts forth that it is not so much the nature or intensity of tissue disturbance that determines whether or not it will be painful, as the extent to which the afferent activity that it evokes is channeled into those central pathways whose cerebral connections are such that they evoke the experience of pain when appropriately activated.

Pain mechanisms as they pertain to headache have traditionally been delineated into general categories and include head pain of psychogenic origin, such as hysterical or conversion, neuralgia, direct pressure on pain-sensitive tissues, traction, inflammation, generalized dilation of intracranial vessels as in anoxia, fever, or toxic reaction to drugs, muscle contraction, and vasodilation. There are many causes of pain in the head but comparatively few ways in which it can be produced. A rational approach to the problem of head pain is to list and classify all of the known structures from which pain could arise and to clarify the neuroanatomic pathways (see Table 8.1).

Excluding the highly complex discussion associated with perception and interpretation, the physiological and structural considerations of pain may be summarized as follows: Fine unmyelinated nerve endings in head and neck tissues are excited by adequate stimuli. Some forms of stimulation of these nerve endings (receptors) may give rise to nonpainful sensations such as pressure. The more intense stimuli, especially chemicals released from damaged tissues, produce impulses that are interpreted as pain. These receptors are very numerous in the skin, less so in deeper tissues such as muscles and fascia, and relatively sparse in most of the viscera. Fibers involved in the transmission of pain sensation synapse in the posterior horn of gray matter in the spinal cord within a few segments of their entry into the cord, and the second-order neurones cross to the other side and then ascend in the lateral spinothalamic tract. The lateral spinothalamic tract is relayed by the nucleus ventralis posterolateralis (VPL) of the thalamus and is projected to the sensory cortex in the postcentral gyrus(12).

Table 8.1
Pain-sensitive Structures

Extracranial	Intracranial
Scalp and neck muscles	Arteries at base of brain, and their major branches
Blood vessels, especially arteries	Dural venous sinuses and adjacent dura
Mucosa of sinuses, nose	
Jaw and cervical spine joints	
Eyes	

The neuroanatomical source of head pain is based on a series of anatomic studies by Ray and Wolff(14), who delineated the pain-sensitive structures of the head. They found that all of the extracranial tissues are pain sensitive in varying degrees whereas the skull itself and most of its contents (brain, parenchyma, much of the dura and pia mater, ependyma lining ventricles, choroid plexus) will not produce pain(13). This presents as one of the great paradoxes of life in that the parenchyma of the master sensory organ of man is in itself insensitive. The other important pain-sensitive structures in the head are those cranial nerves that carry with them sensory fibers: cranial nerves V, VII, IX, X, and also the previously mentioned cervical nerves. The cervical and trigeminal afferents converge on common neurons in the trigeminocervical nucleus. Thus noxious stimuli from the neck travel along the cervical afferents and converge on neurons that also receive cervical afferents or trigmeninal afferents from the head. It is this later convergence that results in neck pain being misinterpreted as arising from the head.

CLASSIFICATION OF HEAD PAIN

Because of the multifaceted etiologies of head pain, a systematic classification may give clues to appropriate therapy and should

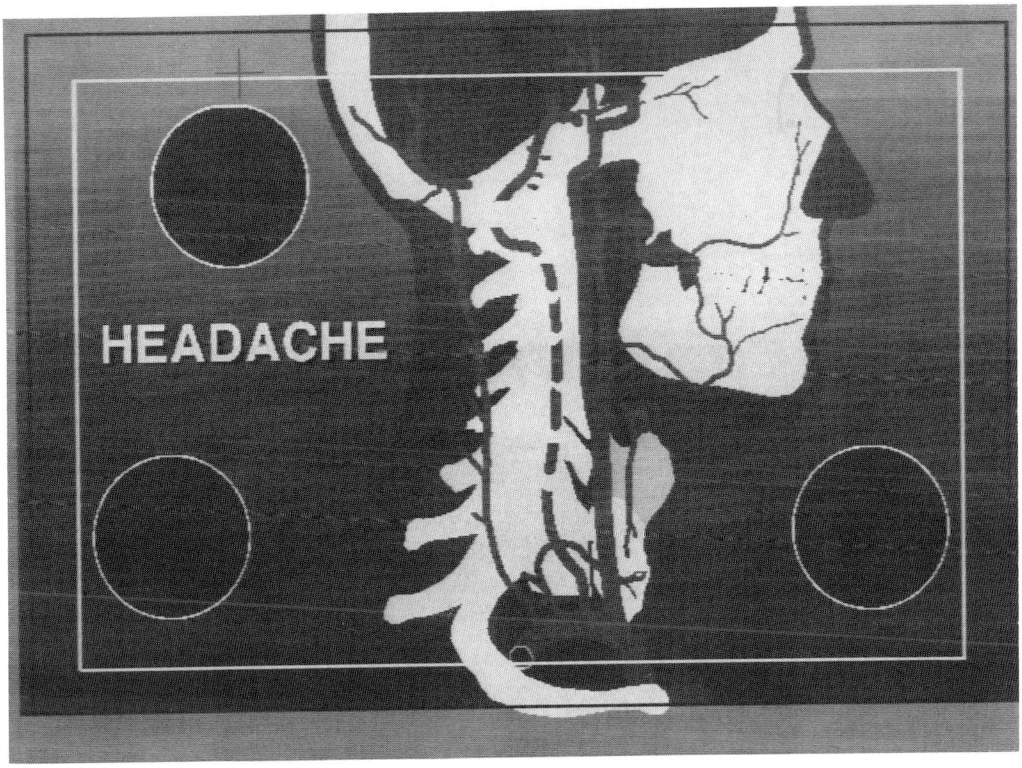

Figure 8.1.

obviously be used as a general reference and aid in establishing the appropriate diagnosis. Therefore, knowledge of an overall classification of head pain is without saying essential in dealing with the headache patient. There are a number of ways to classify headache. The definitive classification used by most researchers and headache specialists is that of Friedman et al(15). Suffice it to say conventional medicine has always emphasized the organic and vascular causes of head pain, almost to the exclusion of other types of headache, such as the somatic model(8). Accordingly, the classification presented here is more specific and takes into consideration the frequency of presentation. It must also be appreciated that most chronic headaches have an axis of interaction involving somatic, neurogenic, vascular, and autonomic components(6) (Fig. 8.1).

Cervicogenic Headache

As depicted in the classification of headaches in Fig. 8.2, the role of the cervical spine in producing head pain or the concept of cervicogenic cephalalgia is still very much in controversy. Head pain in cervical origin has usually been vaguely coined "tension" headaches, which indirectly implies that its etiology is of a psychogenic nature. While it goes without saying that certain psychological traits are present in headache sufferers, it would be remiss for us not to consider the important role that the cervical spine has in producing head pain(17–19). The vast functional disturbances that arise from chronic occupational overuse syndromes, i.e., static muscle load, trauma(20), degenerative and functional joint instability(21), myofascial hypertonicity(22), congenital abnormalities(23), rheu-

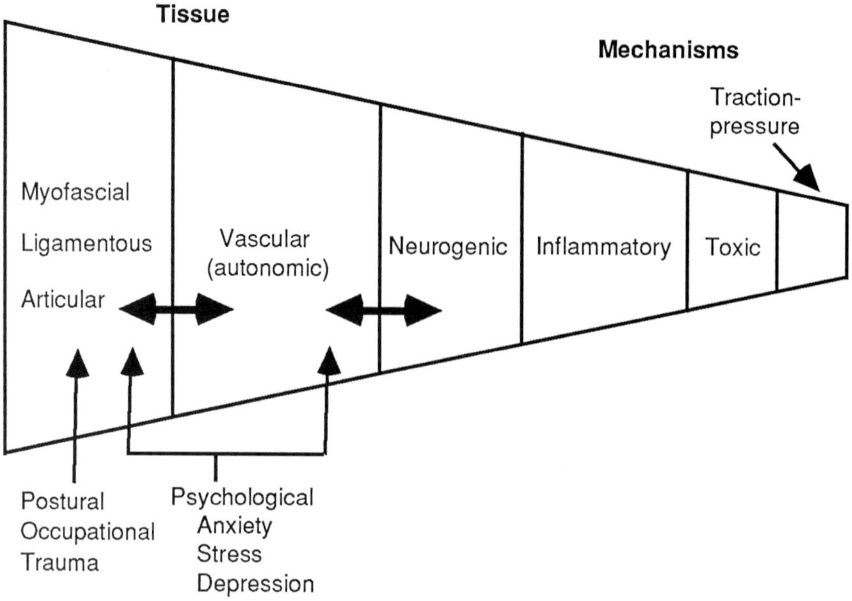

Figure 8.2. Classification of headaches.

matoid arthritis(24), and many more, must ultimately have a direct effect on neuromuscular reflexes and hence on the myofascial and articular components of the cervical spine. It is these functional pathologies that develop from the tissue overload that eventually require a more indepth look and reorganization.

Headache of cervical origin is elaborated upon in Chapter 9, however, a classical example is as follows: A 33-year-old female presented with chronic head pain of an intermittent nature. The onset was nontraumatic and insidious; initially it responded to mild analgesics. Her pain started in the suboccipital region and radiated into the temporal and frontal region. The pain was of a moderate dull nature and was described as "constrictive or band like." The headache was usually associated with sustained neck postures and posterior neck tension.

The postural and palpatory examination revealed an accentuated upper dorsal kyphosis, with associated fixations. Her cervical spine compensated with an anterior carriage to the neutral biomechanical stress line, with resultant hypermobility in the C4–5–6 region. The occiput-atlas-axis relationship demonstrated joint dysfunction, and there was unilateral suboccipital tenderness.

Ligamentous Headache

One of the many mechanisms causing vertebrogenic head pain is cervical ligamentous overload(25). Its most characteristic clinical feature is anteflexion headache(26). This type of headache is most frequently found in young functional hypermobile individuals, but other conditions causing ligament strain can also precipitate it in those with normal motion(27). The main causes of ligamentous head pain is trauma, followed by prolonged positional strain in which muscle activity is at a minimum. This is usually the case in prolonged sitting or standing where the head and neck are flexed forward.

The clinical presentation is as follows: A 23-year-old patient presented with posterior neck irritability and headaches. The neck irritability was usually brought on by prolonged neck flexion followed by headache. The patient described that the pain was worsened by any position in which the neck was held in a sustained flexion, such as reading, writing, and typing.

Exercises previously prescribed did not

help, however, lying down, massage, and moist heat sometimes did. A previous diagnosis of tension headaches had been made and analgesics had been prescribed.

The examination revealed that the most typical signs were found on forced and prolonged flexion, with palpable hypermobility of the cervical spine. The range of motion was full and on extension the examiner's finger appeared to disappear into the cervical lordosis. Unlike headache associated with articular and muscle dysfunction, there was not an abundance of muscular hypertonicity or myofascial trigger points.

Greater Occipital Neuralgia Headache

A review of the neuroanatomy shows that the second cervical nerve root of which the greater occipital nerve is a continuation emerges behind the lateral articular masses of the axis and atlas. The root, however, is not protected posteriorly by the pedicles and facets, which elsewhere in the vertebral column complete the root canal. Its respective ganglia, instead of occupying intervertebral foramina, lie on the vertebral arches of the axis. The nerve courses laterally and slightly upward and soon divides into a primary division. The anterior primary ramus passes between the arches of the axis and atlas.

The posterior primary ramus passes backwards through the posterior arches of axis and atlas gaining access to the cervical soft tissues(28). The posterior primary ramus of C2, which continues into the scalp as the greater occipital nerve, emerges between the bony surfaces and is capable of being traumatized by movement that would tend to approximate these two surfaces(29).

The clinical presentation is as follows: A 33-year-old female presented with a 6-month history of morning headaches of a nonprogressive nature. The headache had no associated prodrome and had a hemicranial distribution. The pain was usually constant, dull, and aching in character. It was usually unilateral and was possibly worsened by neck rotation and/or forward flexion. The frequency was variable as was the duration of the headache. On occasion she had noticed nonspecific ocular irritability on the ipsilateral side.

Exercise sometimes made it worse, and ergot preparations did not alleviate her pain. There was a possible associated history of trauma, such as a whiplash injury(30).

The examination revealed that there was generalized suboccipital tenderness associated with restricted joint mobility unilaterally. Sustained pressure over the occipital bony protuberance reproduced the pain in a more intense fashion and possibly referred pain following the course of the C2 nerve distribution.

Posttraumatic Headache

Headache following head trauma has been well documented in the literature(31–33) as a form of persistent pain varying in intensity and duration. In most cases it is an unreliable index of the severity of head injury when unaccompanied by neurological signs. It may be severe in concussion or slight in serious injuries. This paradigm requires that a careful history be taken and the mechanism for the head pain be ascertained. Posttraumatic headache of a chronic nature develops in approximately 40 to 60% of persons who experience head injury(34). Associated symptoms include vertigo, light headedness, insomnia, inability to concentrate, and irritability. While it is recognized that many headaches associated with head trauma are outside the scope of our discussion, a brief review of their mechanisms would likely assist in further readings.

Muscle Contraction

Reactive muscular contraction both in the head and neck as a result of head injury and pain may also involve dysfunction of regional blood vessels and nerves.

Cranial Dilation of Blood Vessels

This mechanism is predominately temporal. Increased pulsation of the dilated blood vessels and the action of the accumulated substances in the vascular walls and perivascular tissues apparently lower the threshold to pain.

Scar Formation

This condition is characterized by tenderness at the site of injury with a palable scar that is often visible. Pain is localized to the immediate site and is believed to be stimulating bulbous nerve endings in traumatized tissue. Although it might be expected that chronic changes within the skull, for example, meningeal adhesions, would play an important part in the production of headache after head injury, similar headaches are rare after surgery on the brain(35).

Intracranial Hemorrhage and Hematoma

These conditions are described under Intracranial Disorders Producing Headaches (p. 148).

Concussion

Concussion has been described as a condition of widespread paralysis of the functions of the brain following head injury and having a strong tendency to spontaneous recovery(36, 37). It is thought to be due to direct injury to nerve cells without any gross organic changes in the brain substance. After a slight head injury, the person may be merely dazed or unconscious for a few seconds, but his higher mental functions may be impaired for a period lasting up to several hours. Although a patient may recover rapidly from concussion, persistent disabling symptoms are extremely common. The three late manifestations are headache, giddiness, and mental disturbances.

The headache tends to be severe and to occur in paroxysms that may last for several hours, often against a background of constant pain. It may be brought on or exacerbated by physical exertion and excitement.

Vascular Headache

The vascular headaches over the years have been related to a series of changes or disturbance of vascular regulation in the cerebral circulation. This may involve the branches of the external carotid artery and possibly to a lesser extent the internal carotid artery. Summaries of migraine headache, its characteristics, symptomatology, and clinical presentation, have been well documented by Diamond et al(38) and Graham(39). The vascular theory asserts that the migraine attack is initiated by cerebrovascular spasm, or by concomitant reduction of cerebral blood flow, and that the headache phase is characterized by extracranial vasodilation. Vernon(8) suggests that six categories may serve to better explain the multicausative nature of this headache. These etiological classifications are:

1. Autonomic/vascular
2. Biochemical/platelets
3. Cellular/immunological/allergy
4. Psychophysiological
5. Neurogenic
6. Somatic

For our particular purposes we will review the cardinal features of vascular headaches as they pertain to migraine and their variations (see Table 8.2).

Migraines may be defined as recurrent attacks of headaches, widely varied in intensity, frequency, and duration. The attacks are commonly unilateral in onset and are usually associated with anorexia and sometimes nausea and vomiting. Some are preceded by or associated with conspicuous sensory, motor, and mood disturbances and are often familial(39). Other reported elements of migraine include pounding or throbbing pain, photophobia, and decreased urination.

The "classic migraine" usually begins suddenly as a vivid, stereotyped visual or neurologic prodrome without headache. This usually lasts 10 to 30 minutes, gradually receding as the headache begins. The headache itself is usually pulsatile, unilateral (often contralateral to the prodromal symptoms), and accompanied by nausea, vomiting, anorexia, and photophobia/phonophobia. The headache usually lasts for 1 to 6 hours, during which time the patient is often incapacitated by pain and the need to seek shelter in a quiet, dark environment. The combination of massage and pressure over the scalp vessels along with rest often provides some relief until the patient is able to sleep. The prodromal

Table 8.2
Vascular Headaches: Characteristics

Diagnosis	Classic	Common	Cluster	Opthalmoplegic	Complicated
Age	30	30	30–50	10	30
Onset	S*	I	S	I	I
Genetic	Yes	Yes	No	Yes	No
M:F ratio			6:1		
Site	U-B	U-B	U	U	B
Duration (hrs)	⅓–10	24–96	¼–2	24–240	Daily (wks/mos/yrs)
Prodrome	Succinct neurological	Euphoria, depression, irritability, vague	Burning, flush, pallor, tearing, prickling, sweating		
Timing	Anytime	On awakening	Day/night	Anytime	
Quality	Steady throbbing	Steady throbbing	Steady		
Intensity	1+ to 3+++	1+ to 3+++	4+		

*S, sudden; I, insidious; U, unilateral; B, bilateral.

symptoms are most often visual in character. These may include flashes of color, wavy lines, shimmering spots or stars, and all varieties of transient visual loss (rarely, total blindness). These visual symptoms are nonspecific with the exception of the fortification spectra phenomenon, which is virtually pathognomonic of migraine.

The neurologic prodomes experienced vary with the cerebrovascular anatomy involved by the vasospastic phenomenon of migraine. These usually occur contralateral to subsequent headache and include hemisensory paresthesias, hemiparesis, or dysphasia. Other symptoms such as vertigo, diplopia, dysarthria, and weakness are not rare. Absence of these prodromata with the typical unilateral throbbing headaches characterizes the "common migraine" syndrome.

Cluster Headache (Sphenoplatine Neuralgia)

Cluster headache is probably a vascular type headache, about one-tenth as common as migraine, whose diagnosis is usually apparent from the clinical history alone. The headache usually unilateral (frontotemporal or oculofrontal), extremely severe, and stereotyped. It begins suddenly, lasts for 30 to 60 minutes with gradually increasing intensity, is usually nonthrobbing, and is often associated with unilateral nose and eye symptom-tearing, running nose, and occasionally, Horner's syndrome. The headache itself may be confused with various other disorders—migraine, sinusitis, acute glaucoma, for example. It is the recurrent periodicity, the clustering of the headaches, that is often diagnostic. These clusters last an average of 1 to 3 months. During this time, headaches occur once or several times each day, often at the same time each day, frequently wakening the patient from sleep or other restful relaxation. The headache sufferer is almost always frantic, agitated, and in severe panic as a result of the pain. (This is different from the migraineur, who usually seeks hibernation during the headache.) Most sufferers of cluster headaches enter a period of remission during which they are totally free of headache for months or years until another cluster recurs. The family history is usually unimpressive, unlike that of migraine sufferers. Most patients with cluster headache are middle-aged males and not uncommonly, they have a characteristic facies that has been described as "alcoholic" or "acromegalic" (unexplained). Alcohol and other vasodilators often precipitate attacks(7).

The differential diagnosis of recurrent cluster headache is very limited. The periodicity and timing of the headache (episodic, 45-minute duration) may be mimicked by pheochromocytoma, but those patients usually have other symptoms and signs (sweating, tachycardia, hypertension, pallor) during their headache, which is itself usually generalized and more often throbbing (unlike cluster). The location, severity, and type of pain may be mimicked by temporal arteritis, but those patients usually have more of a persistent headache and an elevated erythrocyte sedimentation rate. Trigeminal neuralgia may superficially resemble cluster, especially when repetitive bursts of neuralgic pain add up to a 30- to 60-minute duration, but the timing and quality of trigeminal neuralgic pain are often distinctive.

Intracranial Disorders

The term intracranial disorders, though primarily applied to neoplasms, is extended more broadly to include other space-occupying lesions that produce a clinical picture of headache (see Table 8.3). Suffice it to say that brain functions are primarily dependent upon the maintenance of the circulation of blood and cerebrospinal fluid at their appropriate pressures. It follows that the intracranial contents react to a change in their volume or pressure when mechanical displacements of brain tissue occur as in tumors. The mode of onset of symptoms secondary to intracranial disorders then are extremely variable and largely dependent upon the nature and site of the disorder. Red light warnings of organic disease from the patient's history may include:

1. Episodic fainting in relation to headache
2. Abrupt onset of a severe headache for the first time
3. Neurological abnormalities associated with headache
4. Elevation in body temperature associated with headache
5. Onset of headache after age 50
6. Headache associated with an increase in pressure (coughing, bending, valsalva, coitus)
7. History of recent blood pressure elevation
8. Personality change
9. Headache following history of head trauma
10. Disturbance of pulse rate and respiration
11. Constant sensory disturbances
12. Onset of visual field defects

Table 8.3
Intracranial Disorders Producing Headache

Intracranial Hemorrhage	Neoplasms	Hematomas
Subarachnoid	Primary	Epidural
Cerebellar	Secondary	Subdural

Neoplasms

The headache associated with brain tumor may be mild, severe, or absent, depending upon its site of origin. Headache is one of the cardinal signs of brain tumor, particularly of rapidly expanding tumors, producing traction on the pain-sensitive structures of the head. This is especially the case of the ventricular system compromised by obstruction of absorption or flow of cerebrospinal fluid, causing hydrocephalus. Headache is sometimes a prominent finding with increased intracranial pressure. But with more slowly growing tumors, headache may be transitory, mild, or easily relieved by common analgesics, and the patient's description of his head pain in this situation may be pedestrian. The most severe head pains are not usually related to tumor but to vascular headaches or the major neuralgias. Some generalizations concerning headache as an aid to localization in patients with brain tumor are collected below.

- Although the headache of brain tumor may be referred from a distant intracranial source, it approximately overlies the tumor in about one-third of all patients.
- If the tumor is above the tentorium, the pain is frequently at the vertex or in the frontal regions.
- If the tumor is below the tentorium, the

pain is occipital and cervical muscle spasm may be present.

- Headache is almost always present with posterior fossa tumor.
- If the tumor is midline, it may be increased with cough or straining or sudden head movement. (This also occurs with migraine.)
- If the tumor is hemispheric, the pain is usually appreciated on the same side of the head.
- If the tumor is chiasmal, at the sella, the pain may be referred to the vertex.

THE QUALITY AND INTENSITY OF BRAIN TUMOR HEADACHE

This type of headache is usually a deep, aching, steady, dull pain. It is not rhythmic and is seldom throbbing. It is usually intermittent but in a minority of patients, it is continuous. The headache is sometimes severe, but rarely is it as intense as that of migraine or the headache associated with ruptured cerebral aneurysm, meningitis, certain febrile illnesses, or that induced by certain drugs. It is usually relieved by acetylsalicyclic acid or cold packs applied to the scalp, both indications of its moderate intensity. It rarely interferes with sleep. It is aggravated by coughing or straining at stool, and sometimes it is worse in the erect than in the recumbent position. It is also commonly aggravated by the onset of a minor infection. If there is any variation in intensity during the 24-hour cycle, it is usually worse in the early morning.

Even when the tumor directly compresses or extensively stretches the cranial nerves containing pain afferents, the pain is not equal in intensity to that of tic douloureux and indeed is often mild or absent.

Unless the pain is severe, nausea with tumor headache is usually slight. Vomiting occurs with displacement or compression of the medulla and is sometimes "projectile," perhaps because it is unexpected when accompanied by nausea. The headache, when occipital or suboccipital, is sometimes associated with "stiffness" or aching of the muscles of the neck and tilting of the head toward the side of the tumor.

Intracranial Hemorrhage

As a rule, the patient who suffers intracranial hemorrhage of any kind does not walk into the clinic simply complaining of headache. These events are usually catastrophic, resulting in obvious neurologic compromise. The two types of intracranial bleeding that deserve special emphasis are subarachnoid and cerebellar hemorrhage. These headaches present with a history of sudden acute head pain in individuals who may never have experienced headache and may occasionally present with subtle or no neurologic abnormalities. Let us first consider subarachnoid hemorrhage.

Subarachnoid hemorrhage produces sudden, severe headache, usually reaching peak intensity within a minute or two of onset. On occasion, strenuous physical exertion precipitates the event (by raising intracranial pressure) and the head pain is often associated with vomiting, transient loss of consciousness, or subsequent meningismus (with positive Kernig's sign, etc.). The headache may be mistaken for migraine unless a careful history is taken. In those patients who remain conscious, the headache will last for several days until a reduced level of awareness, nuchal rigidity, preretinal hemorrhage, and neurologic impairment become obvious. Approximately 20–30% of patients manifest no abnormal neurologic findings(1) and have a good prognosis if diagnosis is made early and the condition is managed correctly. Computed tomography (CT) scan will be diagnostic in more than half of patients and is the initial procedure of choice(2) followed by lumbar puncture and arteriography. Untreated subarachnoid hemorrhage is nearly always fatal.

Cerebellar hemorrhage is a life-threatening event that usually presents with sudden (often occipital) headache, vomiting, dizziness, and ataxia. While most patients are drowsy or comatose and exhibit cranial nerve dysfunction and ataxia on examination, some are fully alert and demonstrate neurologic findings that may be quite subtle. Most patients demonstrate appendicular ataxia, truncal ataxia, ipsilateral gaze palsy, and peripheral facial nerve paresis.

The patient usually has a history of hypertension, trauma, and/or use of anticoagulents. The mortality rate from cerebellar hemorrhage is high, even under ideal circumstances.

Epidural hematoma is a rare form of head pain but deserves some attention. The classical scenerio is that of brief loss of consciousness usually after some head trauma (fracture), thereafter followed by a lucid interval of minutes to days when the person appears to be normal. The sudden onset into coma with focal neurologic compromises such as hemiparesis, dilated pupils, etc. announces the seriousness of the problem. During this lucid phase, there may be vomiting, worsening headache, and neurologic deterioration. The head pain is best identified with CT scan following minor trauma, which may be the cause of intracranial bleeding, especially in the elderly, alcoholic, anticoagulated, or in those with advanced arteriosclerosis.

Subdural hematomas often present with no apparent neurologic deficits upon neurological examination. These patients may, however, present with history of minor head trauma with slowly worsening head pain. Subtle personality changes (inattention, intermittent drowsiness, slowed mentation) is best determined by family members or those closest to the patient. The CT scan is virtually always diagnostic.

Ocular Headaches

Pain around the orbit or headache associated with visual complaints should be investigated thoroughly with a careful history, examination of external orbit, pupil reactivity and size, ocular movements, visual acuity, and fundoscopic evaluation. Orbital or periorbital pain with a normal examination should suggest migraine, cluster headache, trigeminal or postherpetic neuralgia—here the history alone is often enough to make a diagnosis. Headache associated with photophobia is very common in migraine, systemic viral infections, and subarachnoid hemorrhage, yet in these conditions examination of them is often nonrevealing. On the other hand, when orbital pain is associated with visual loss, pupillary dilation or constriction, or cranial nerve palsies, many serious conditions must be considered. Headaches in the orbit or periorbital area should suggest several possibilities. Some of the more common causes of ocular headache and their salient features are as follows.

Acute Glaucoma. The patient is usually quite sick, often vomiting repeatedly. The globe is almost always tender or hard, the pupil is dilated, the cornea is unclear, and the conjectiva is injected. On occasion, using medication with anticholinergic properties or episodic pupillary dilation (moving into the dark) will precipitate intermittent brief eye pain. The symptoms may resolve completely and only the history is suggestive.

Optic Neuritis. Although not a very common cause of orbital pain, optic neuritis should be suspected when the patient presents with orbital-face-head pain with a decreased pupillary light reflex, blurring of the disc and hyperemia of the retina, or painful eye movement. The visual acuity is almost always diminished.

Iritis. Seen in some of the arthritides, iritis is also a cause of orbital pain, which is well localized and self-limiting. It is usually associated with pain, conjunctival injection, decreased visual acuity, and a unilateral small pupil often with extreme photophobia.

The common diagnosis of simple *eye strain* is a much overdiagnosed cause of headache. Since the pain is usually preceded by prolonged reading or close work, it is customary to assume that the mechanism for pain production was the eye. However, it is quite obvious that other mechanisms come into play, such as the concept of static muscle load while the head and neck are held in prolonged flexion, and the secondary effects on the ligaments and joints of the cervical spine. However, it would be fair to assume that those with presbyopia, strabismus, or astigmatism have a greater incidence of orbital pain following prolonged reading or eye use.

References

1. Goss CM, ed. Gray's anatomy. 29th American ed. Philadelphia: Lea & Febiger, 1973.
2. Kerr FWL. A mechanism to account for frontal

headache in cases of posterior fossa tumors. J Neurosurg 1961;18:605–609.
3. Cameron BM. Cervical spine sprain headache. Am J Orthop 1964;6:9.
4. Korczyn AD. Carel RS, Pereg I. Correlation of headache complaints with some physiological parameters in a healthy population. Headache 1980;20:196–198.
5. Newland CA, Illis LS, Robinson PK, Batchelor Bg. Waters WE. A survey of headaches in an English city. Res Clin Stud Headache 1978;5:1–20.
6. Appenzeller O. Headache. Clinical and pathogenetic aspects. Adv Pain Res Ther 1979;3:345–58.
7. Edmeads J. Headaches and head pains associated with diseases of the cervical spine. Med Clin North Am Vol 62. No 3, May 1978.
8. Vernon H. Vertebrogenic migraine. J Can Chiro Assoc 1985;29:20–24.
9. Sternbach R. Pain patients: traits and treatment. New York: Academic Press, 1974. 135 p.
10. Bonica J. General clinical considerations in recent advances on pain. Bonica J, Procacci P, eds, Chapt 11. Springfield, IL: Charles C Thomas, 1972.
11. Wyke BD. Neurological aspects of the diagnosis and treatment of facial pain. Scientific Foundation Of Dentistry. London: William Heinemann Books Ltd. 1976. 279 p.
12. Bowsher D. Termination of the central pathway in man: the conscious appreciation of pain. Brain 1957;89:723–746.
13. Dalessio DH. Mechanisms and biochemistry of headache. J Post Grad Med 1974;56(3):55–61.
14. Ray BS, Wolff HG. Experimental studies in headache: pain-sensitive structures of the head and their significance in headache. Arch Surg 1940;41:813–856.
15. Friedman AP, et al. Classification of headaches. Ad Hoc Committee. JAMA 1962;179:717–718.
16. Gitelman R, Fitz-Ritson D. Migraine headaches: chiropractic abstracts. J Chiro 1983;17:67–69.
17. Newill RGD. Headache and giddiness of cervical origin. J Roy Coll Gen Pract 1972;22:51–53.
18. Schlesinger EB. Treatment of headache and neck pain associated with disorders of the neck and cervical spine. Mod Treat 1964;1:1404–1411.
19. Sheldon KW. Headache patterns and cervical nerve root compression—a 15 year study of hospitalization for headache. Headache 1967;6:180–188.
20. Blumenthal LS. Injury to the cervical spine as a cause of headache. Postgrad Med 1974;56(3): 147–153.
21. Stoddard A. Cervical spondylosis and cervical osteoarthritis. Man Med 1970;8:31–33.
22. Graham JR. Treatment of muscle contraction headache. Mod Treat 1964;1:1399–1403.
23. McRae DL. The significance of abnormalities of the cervical spine. Am J Roentgenol 1960;84:3–25.
24. Bland JH. Rheumatoid arthritis of the cervical spine. Bull Rheum Dis 1967;18:471–476.
25. Hackett JS. Joint ligament relaxation treated by fibroosseous proliferation. Springfield, IL: Charles C Thomas, 1956.
26. Lewit K. Ligament pain and anteflexion headache. Eur Neurol 1971;5:365–378.
27. Penning L. Functional pathology of the cervical spine. Amsterdam: Excerpta Medica, 1968.
28. Cunningham DJ. Textbook of anatomy. 7th ed. New York: Oxford University Press, 1937, pp. 992–1008.
29. Hunter CR, Mayfield FH. Role of the upper cervical roots in the production of pain in the head. Am J Surg Nov 1949;743–749.
30. Seletz E. Whiplash injuries—neurophysiological basis for pain and methods used for rehabilitation. JAMA 1958;168(13):1750–1755.
31. Jones OW Jr. Brown HA. The treatment of post traumatic head pain. J Nerv Ment Dis 1944;99:668.
32. Friedman AP. Posttraumatic headache: its basic mechanisms and character. State J Med, 1961;61:1875.
33. Penfield W, Norcross NC. Subdural traction and posttraumatic headache, study of pathology and therapeusis. Arch Neurol Psychiat 1936;36:75.
34. Elkind AH. Friedman AP. A review of headache: 1955 to 1961. NY State J Med 1962;62:1220.
35. Adams H, Graham D. The pathology of blunt head injuries. Scientific Foundations of Neurology. London: Heinemann, 1972.
36. Gronwall D, Wrightson P. Cumulative effects of concussion. Lancet 1975;2:995.
37. Ommaya AK, Gennarelll TA. Cerebral concussion and traumatic unconsciousness. Brain 1974;97:663.
38. Diamond S, Falk J, DeVeno T. Biofeedback in the treatment of vascular headache. Biofeedback Self-Regul 1978;3(4):385–408.
39. Graham JR. Migraine headache: diagnosis and management. Headache 1979;19(3):133–141

9 Vertebrogenic Headache

Howard Vernon, D.C., F.C.C.S.

"In my experience, cervical migraine is the type of headache most frequently seen in general practice and also the type most frequently misinterpreted. It is usually erroneously diagnosed as classical migraine, tension headache, vascular headache, hypertensive encephalopathy or post-traumatic encephalopathy. Such patients have usually received an inadequate treatment and have often become neurotic and drug-dependent."

Frykholm (1971)

Headache is one of the most ubiquitous and frequent complaints in our society(1). Headache is the most frequent reason for patients attending their general physician. Medications for headache constitute one of the largest groups of prescribed and self-administered drugs(2). While there are many varieties and categories of headaches, muscular contraction and migraine-type headaches constitute the vast majority of headaches, especially of those seen by primary care practitioners(3).

Chiropractic interest in headaches dates back to the inception of the profession. As early as 1928, Loban(4) gathered anecdotal statistics on the results of chiropractic treatment of migraine. Since that time, a host of chiropractic writers (and other practitioners of manual therapeutics) have addressed the topic. The clinical literature is composed of a variety of studies—from single case studies, multiple case reports, to retrospective, open and controlled clinical trials. While this literature will be reviewed in depth in this chapter, the consensus of these studies, as well as of numerous theoretical treatises on the mechanisms of benign headache, is that the cervical spine plays a very important but largely undervalued role in the etiology of such headaches and that chiropractic treatment can be efficacious in the management of this broad category of headaches.

Despite this consensus of opinion and data, the role of the cervical (especially the upper cervical) spine is poorly understood (and almost wholly unaccepted) by most orthodox practitioners and their patients. According to the data of Kellner, Hall, and Coulter(5), headache constitutes only 9% of the chief complaints seen by Canadian chiropractors. The diagnosis of occipital headache occurred in only 3% of cases in a recently reported survey conducted by a respected Swiss chiropractor in his clinic(6). In all eight editions of the Swiss Annals from 1960 to 1986, there exist only three articles on headaches(6–8). A review of the typical medical literature on headache reveals very little attention to the role of the cervical spine. In the last three years, the journal HEADACHE has published only six articles on headache and the cervical spine. Three of these dealt with the effects of biofeedback treatment, focusing solely on the large regional musculature(9–11). Three of these do, in fact, deal with the cervical spine as a wholistic entity comprised of bone, joint, muscle, and nerve structures, each component being capable of involvement in headache(12–14).

The current medical paradigms of psychosomatic and vascular etiologies of the vast majority of headaches are, therefore, firmly entrenched (see Figs. 9.1 and 9.2). This is so much so that even when a vertebrogenic origin attributed to the cervical

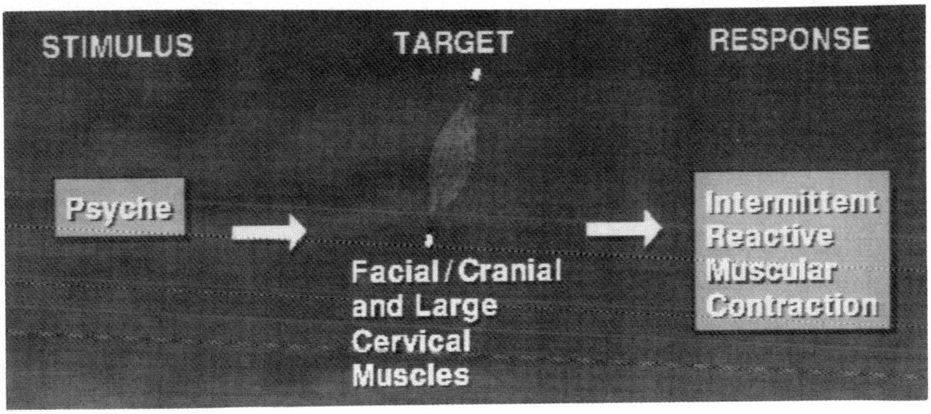

Figure 9.1. Current medical model of muscle contraction headache.

spine is considered by the orthodox literature, it is typically viewed as a minor variant form which does not reflect on or refute the major paradigmmatic categories.

The proposition and elucidation of a vertebrogenic model of headache is, therefore, a daunting task. This chapter will carefully review and substantiate such a model. Much of the supportive literature will be reviewed, and, to avoid repetition, representative studies will be reviewed in depth while the remaining studies will be listed and referred to in general. The literature generally assumes two forms: (1) the clinical and theoretical review paper, which generally reviews the mechanisms of headache attributable to the cervical spine and describes its diagnostic features; and (2) the research report, which either compiles data on a specific sample of headache sufferers or in the rarer cases, actually reports on a clinical experiment involving manipulation therapy and/or chiropractic treatment. Since the majority of authors have treated headaches attributable to the cervical spine as a single category within which the typical forms of migraine and nonmigraine types are viewed as derivations of the major mechanism of vertebrogenic headache, then this chapter will, as well, review the general category of vertebrogenic headache first, and then consider the manipulative management of muscle contraction and migraine headaches separately, as subcategories.

REVIEW OF THE LITERATURE: THEORETICAL AND DESCRIPTIVE MODELS OF CLINICAL MECHANISMS

Barré(15) and Lieou(16) were among the first to implicate the cervical spine in the

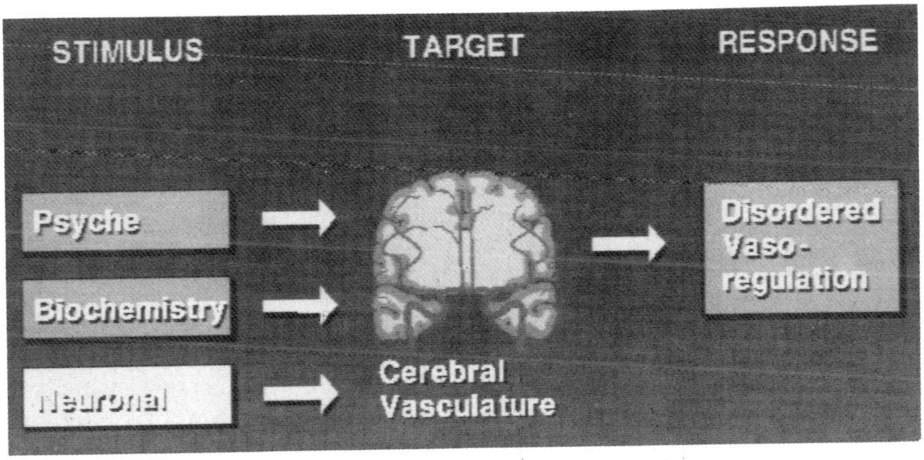

Figure 9.2. Current medical model of migraine.

Table 9.1
Literature Review of Articles Written on Vertebrogenic or "Cervical" Headache

Barré (1925)	Shultz (1977)
Bartschi-Rochaix (1948)	Gelb (1977)
Beckwith (1949, 1952)	Gutmann (1977)
Hunter (1949)	Mountjoy (1977)
Geiger (1952)	Edmeads (1978)
Gayral and Neuwirth (1954)	Henderson (1979)
Skillern (1955)	Hoyt et al (1979)
Kovacs (1955)	Schoenholtz (1979)
Jackson (1958)	Kramer (1981)
Seletz (1958)	Edeling (1982)
Grillo (1961)	Ward (1982)
Brain (1963)	Bogduk (1979, 1981, 1985)
Trevor-Jones (1964)	Freitag (1983)
Figar and Jansky (1965)	Schmidt (1983)
Travell (1967)	Bouquet et al (1983)
Chocret (1967)	Sjasstad et al (1983, 1987)
Robertson (1968)	Gallagher (1985)
Dutton and Riley (1969)	Graham (in Aronoff) (1985)
Lewit (1971, 1977)	Vernon (1985)
Ghavamian (1971)	Graff-Radford, et al (1987)
Boake (1972)	Turk and Ratkolb (1987)
Frykholm (1972)	
Hargrave-Wilson (1972)	
Webber (1973)	
Pozniak-Patewicz (1975)	

genesis of a wide array of neurological symptoms, foremost among which were headache and vertigo (see Table 9.1). In their writings, they linked irritation of the cervical sympathetic system to circulation disturbances, primarily as a disturbance of vasomotor tone, in the distributions of the vertebral artery or the internal auditory artery.

In 1948, Bartschi-Rochaix(17) coined the term "migraine cervicale" to describe a type of headache, potentially very severe in character, which was caused by disturbances of the cervical spine. The impact of these mechanical disturbances was thought to be mediated through the autonomic nervous system. At this stage of its development, the vertebrogenic theory focused largely on changes in the vertebral artery and the resultant symptomatology arising from transient ischemia of the posterior cranial structures.

Following Bartschi-Rochaix, Beckwith(18, 19), Hunter and Mayfield(20), Geiger(21), Gayral and Neuwirth(22), Skillern(23), and others(133) addressed the topic. Kovacs(24) summarized the emergent model in his article entitled "Subluxation and deformation of the cervical apophyseal joints: a contribution to the etiology of headaches." He bridged the gap between theories focusing largely on the arterial system as it was affected by the neck structures and those whose focus expanded to include the nervous system more directly as a source of mediation between the spine and pain or disturbances about the head. Kovacs recognized that subluxation or backward displacement of contiguous articular surfaces of the cervical apophyseal joints could constrict the vertebral artery directly or it could provide a source of mechanical irritation to the vertebral sympathetic plexus. The result would be the same—intermittent constriction or even spasm of the vertebral artery and/or those arteries in the posterior cerebral distribution. Kovacs proposed that subluxation of the cervical apophyseal joints would produce both direct encroachment of the vertebral artery by the facet processes and by osteophytic proliferation from the uncovertebral joints in the lower and upper portions of the cervical spine. In the latter region, laterally displaced osteophytes from C1–C2 or C2–C3 might encroach the vertebral artery with or without subluxation.

However, Kovacs went further than these structural considerations. He emphasized the role of functional changes in intervertebral joint behavior. He proposed a sequence of events that lead to joint derangement: restriction and disturbance of joint motion would lead to reflex muscle spasm, which would alter the curve of the cervical spine and accelerate degenerative changes, which would then compromise the vertebral artery and nerves. This shift to a functional perspective is pivotal in the development of the modern vertebrogenic model and would be reiterated and expanded by numerous successive authors.

Kovacs culminates his important work by citing his anecdotal experience with manipulation for headache of cervical origin. His report is a very favorable, albeit nonquantified one.

The landmark work of Dr. Ruth Jackson appeared in 1958(25). Headache and a variety of neuro-otological symptoms were found to be attributable to direct mechanical irritation of the ascending posterior cervical sympathetic system, especially (and perhaps too exclusively) in the typical trauma of the cervical spine, namely the whiplash injury.

Another important work appearing in 1958 focused more exclusively on headache arising from the neck in nontraumatic circumstances. Seletz's "Headache of extra-cranial origin"(26) both summarized the existing model of vertebrogenic effects on the arterial supply to the cranium and proposed what we might call a neurogenic model arising from vertebral derangements. In this neurogenic model, Seletz emphasized the following:

(1) The uncovertebral joints may directly irritate the cervical nerve roots and thus cause pain and muscular dysfunction.
(2) Noxious stimulations from the cervical joints and muscles might produce reflex irritation of the spinal accessory nerve (XI) and thus produce spasm of the sternocleidomastoid and trapezius muscles inducing a local occipital headache syndrome.
(3) Such spasms of the trapezius muscle may produce entrapment (see Fig. 9.3) and give rise to unilateral occipital neuralgic headache.
(4) However, the most important contribution to this neurogenic model arose from Seletz's discussion of a mechanism that had been discussed three years earlier by Skillern(23) involving the connections in the spinal cord between the sensory pathways of C1 and C2 and the second order neurons of the spinal tract of the trigeminal nerve (V). It is the convergence of this peripheral sensory pathway from the joints of the upper cervical spine with the trigeminal nerve that creates the most fertile mechanism for head pains to arise from the structures of the neck. This mechanism is so important that it will be amplified in the separate section on mechanisms of vertebrogenic headache (vide infera).

One of the first important chiropractic contributions to the vertebrogenic model is provided by Grillo(7). Writing in the Swiss

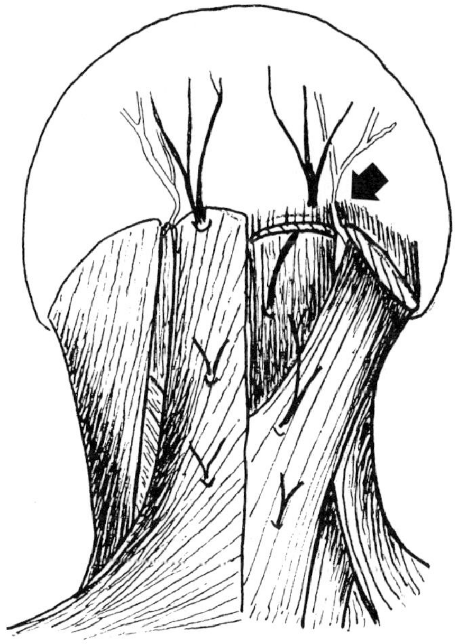

Figure 9.3. Entrapment of the greater occipital nerve in the production of occipital neuralgia.

Annals II on the "Differential diagnosis of therapy and headache," he presented a complete review of the knowledge of the day on migraine and what he termed "vertebragenous headaches." He described these latter as a syndrome of neck-cranial-facial pains, presenting unilaterally with tenderness in the suboccipital region and with associated "neurovegetative symptoms." He proposed that the major cause of this syndrome was mechanical irritation of the nerve roots, particularly in the foraminal environs. This, of course, was consistent with the prevailing paradigm in chiropractic thinking at that time.

Grillo proposed three etiological categories of "vertebragenous headache":

(1) *Somatic root-irritation type.* This is the true foraminal encroachment envisioned in the then current, chiropractic paradigm. Grillo noted, however, that since there were no true intervertebral foramina between C0–C1 and C1–C2, the upper cervical nerve roots would be spared any significant mechanical irritation. This is a point with which this author does not agree. However, this opinion lead Grillo to place greater

emphasis on the other two categories, namely:

(2) *"Anterior sympathetic syndrome."* This syndrome would involve the ascending sympathetic ganglionated chain with special emphasis on the superior cervical ganglion, irritation of which would produce autonomic and vasomotor disturbances in the cranium leading to head pain; and

(3) *"Posterior sympathetic syndrome."* This involves the mechanism previously elaborated by Barré, Bartschi-Rochaix, and Jackson, i.e., the vertebral artery, vertebral nerve, and the accompanying sympathetic plexus.

Grillo refers to the therapeutic success of chiropractic in the treatment of vertebrogenic headache but not in the treatment of migraine. This follows from the fact that he viewed these as separate and distinct entities.

In the decade from 1961 to 1971, numerous authors contributed articles toward the development of this model(27–35, 138, 139). However, Boake's article in 1972 stands out as a landmark effort. Boake(36) provided a thorough description of the "cervical headache" as being unilateral, of chronic duration, with maximal pain in the fronto-orbital distribution while occipital pain is always present, associated with neck stiffness, tenderness, and spasm over the facet joints of C2 and C3 and with "trigger radiations" possibly present. He proposed that this sort of headache was responsible for 70% of all headaches seen by medical doctors (see Table 9.2).

Table 9.2
Boake's Description of the Cervicogenic Headache*

Symptoms	Unilateral Long duration Maximal pain is fronto-orbital Occipital pain is always present Neck stiffness Tenderness over facets of C2 and C3 with muscle spasm and trigger radiations 70% of all headaches
Mechanisms	(1) Major cause: trauma to apophyseal joints leading to fixation; muscle spasm is secondary (2) Emphasizes convergence of afferents from C1 and C2 with spinal tract of V. (3) Cervical afferents (especially C1) found in facial region (4) Irritation of Postganglionic fibers especially from SCG

*Adapted from Boake HK. Cervical headache. Can Fam Phys 1972; 18:75–78.

Boake proposed a number of mechanisms to explain the etiology of cervical headache. It is interesting to note how his proposals amalgamated those of the previous vascular model and extended the neurogenic model. He proposed, as the major cause of cervical headache, trauma to the apophyseal joints of the upper cervical spine leading to joint fixation or blockage of motion. In his view, muscle spasms associated with the craniocervical region and which were typically associated with headache of the "tension" type were secondary to these joint disturbances. Boake further emphasized the convergence of sensory input from C1 and C2 with the spinal tract of the V, as well as the role of the postganglionic sympathetic fibers from the superior cervical ganglion (SCG). He included a description of the fiber projections from the SCG as they "ascend in a plexus around the internal carotid artery and branch off to the opthalmic division of the fifth cranial nerve and via the nasociliary nerve to the dilator pupillae and levator palpebrae superioris." He noted that, given these projections, mechanical stimulation of the SCG might be capable of producing changes in the iris as well as "clear rhinnorhea, lacrimation, and puffiness of the eyelid." Interestingly, although he did not state so, these last mechanisms describe the symptomatology of cluster headaches to a very large degree.

Boake also mentioned that work current to his time had demonstrated that afferent fibers from C1 appeared to arise from some parts of the facial region (vide infera).

Again, I would like to bypass important work through the decade of the 1970s(37–43, 140) and examine, in more detail, the more recent work of Edmeads(69). Edmeads' description of the cervical headache is illustrated in Table 9.3. Edmeads organized his presentation around an ana-

Table 9.3
Cervicogenic Headache according to Edmeads*

(1)	Persistant occipital or suboccipital pain
(2)	Reproduction with neck movements
(3)	Abnormal postures
(4)	Occipital, suboccipital or nuchal tenderness plus trigger phenomenon
(5)	Limitation of neck movements
(6)	Abnormal mobility of cervical joints
(7)	Sensory abnormalities attributable to the upper cervical nerve roots

*Adapted from Edmeads J. Headaches and head pains associated with diseases of the cervical spine. Med Clin North Am 1978; 62(3):533–541.

tomical model. He delineated the different and distinct tissues and structures that comprise the cervical spine and then described their particular contribution to the entity of "headaches associated with diseases of the cervical spine." His perspective was decidedly "somatic" in nature. He first described the role of the cervical joints, emphasizing their capacity to produce local and radiating pains that would mimic headache. According to Edmeads, the primary mechanism of joint involvement is via degenerative changes although he does admit to irritations of the spinal joint ligaments that would be more characteristic of "predegenerative" dysfunction.

The role of the musculature of the cervical spine is ascribed to two categories—direct or primary involvement of the muscular structures in myofascial pain processes and secondary involvement due to reflex muscle spasm caused by the underlying joint disturbances.

Edmeads then considered the cervical nerve structures. He noted that the C2 nerve root is particularly susceptible to mechanical irritation and thus capable of initiating local or referred pain and muscle spasm. He provided an amplification of Boake's mention of C1 afferents in the facial area by citing Kerr's work(44) in which three divisions of the C1 nerve root were located and selectively stimulated giving rise to the following findings:

Stimulation of the

upper rootlet	gave rise to	orbital pain;
middle rootlet	gave rise to	frontal pain;
lower rootlet	gave rise to	vertex pain.

Included in the section on nerve structures was the vertebral nerve, irritation of which was acknowledged to mediate pain and reflex vasospasm of the vertebral artery. Regarding this structure itself, compression and/or occlusion of the vertebral artery was noted as a possible cause of occipital headache. However, Edmeads did not share the opinion of previous writers that disturbances of the vertebral artery could contribute to migraine or migraine-like headache.

Despite this diversity of structures in the cervical spine capable of initiating or contributing to a headache syndrome, Edmeads summarized these into three major mechanisms of pain propagation from the cervical spine to the head:

(1) Referred pain in the C1 and C2 distributions. These distributions include both the classical dermatomal areas in the posterior cranial region and the less distinct frontofacial distributions of C1 afferents as described by Kerr(44).
(2) Referred pain in the trigeminal distribution via the spinal tract of V. This pain projection is typically in the ophthalmic division of V, giving rise to temporal and frontal pain.
(3) Autonomic irritation of the postganglionic sympathetic fibers.

Edmeads concurs with North American writers in contending that this autonomic disturbance arises largely in the "postconcussion syndrome"(45, 132). He contrasted this with the European tradition in orthopedic and manual medicine, which views the autonomic component as a more fundamental consequence of functional disorders of the intervertebral joints.

While Edmeads provided the most thorough review of the mechanisms involved in the "cervical headache," his central thesis is that this symptom complex arises out of "diseases" of the cervical spine. As such, he places greatest emphasis on degenerative diseases of the cervical spine as well as frank trauma (i.e., whiplash or postconcussion syndrome). Minor emphases are placed on congenital anomalies and on pathologies that typically affect the region, i.e., rheumatoid arthritis, neoplasm and ankylosing spondylitis.

Unfortunately, far less emphasis is placed on functional derangements of the vertebral column. Cervical headache is, in the final analysis, viewed by Edmeads as a variant type of headache usually associated with degenerative joint disease or trauma. There is no sense given of an integration of the somatic model so thoroughly reviewed by him and the medical muscle contraction and migraine models. In these latter categories, the psychosomatic and vascular paradigms, respectively, appear uncontestable, and the cervical headache is then portrayed as a distinct but far less important headache type. This belies the fact that the literature supports the contention that cervicogenic headache may be found in individuals far younger and with far less frank trauma then would be necessary to fulfill Edmeads' model of headache arising from diseases of the cervical spine.

While there have been numerous studies in recent years(46–51, 55, 56, 58–60, 80, 134, 141–145, 149), I would like to focus on the work of Nikolai Bogduk(52) and Ottor Sjaastad(61). Bogduk's contribution to the vertebrogenic model of headache consists of several articles on the neurology of the upper cervical region(53, 54) as well as the clinical manifestations of disturbances of this region of the spine, culiminating in a short report on "Headaches and cervical manipulation"(52) in which he reviews the previous literature and responds to the criticism generated by a major clinical trial in which chiropractic treatment of migraine was investigated(75) (vide infera). It is this response which forms the basis of his position on the vertebrogenic model of headache. Bogduk initially debunks the concept of a "cervical migraine" citing the (at the time) obvious biochemical and autonomic mechanisms for which he fails to find any justified correlation with the cervical spine. This is in spite of the fact that he provides an excellent review of the mechanisms previously proposed to explain the "cervical migraine" phenomenon—i.e., he cites Bartschi-Rochaix's work, noting that mechanical irritation of the vertebral artery, vertebral nerve, and the ascending sympathetic chain can initiate an "autonomic barrage" sufficient to create cerebral vasospasm. In addition, he accepts Kovac's contention that subluxation of the cervical apophyseal joints may compromise these structures. However, he reserves his most enthusiastic support for the role of the apophyseal joints in nonmigrainous headache. He asserts a direct, causative role for mechanical derangements of the cervical apophyseal and most importantly, craniocervical, synovial joints in the production of headache. This mechanical derangement is characterized as a "chronic hypomobility"—commonly referred to by chiropractors as a fixation(62). While we will amplify this mechanism in the latter section of this review, suffice it to say that support for this mechanism is fundamental to the chiropractic model of vertebrogenic headache. This mechanism allows us to explain the role of the cervical spine in headache in a much younger population, contrary to the limitations of the "degenerative disease" model proposed by Edmeads.

Bogduk does, in fact, include osteoarthritic afflications of the apophyseal joints in the group of mechanisms of headache production attributable to the cervical spine. He also includes derangements arising from meniscoid entrapments, but this is seen as a secondary mechanism of joint hypomobility.

Sjaastad's contribution consists of a series of studies published primarily in Cephalalgia from 1983 to 1987(61) on what he has termed "cervicogenic headache." This is described as a variant of the chronic paroxysmal headache. The cervicogenic headache is almost always unilateral, accompanied by autonomic symptoms, and provocable by movements of the head, primarily forward flexion. This description, purported to be quite recent in its discovery, is remarkably reminiscent of that of Grillo's description of vertebragenous headache in 1961. Sjaastad has proposed that this headache may be due to entrapment of the occipital nerve, or to a C2–C3 rhizopathy. He also feels that this diagnosis may be very underreported and that confusion has probably existed between it and common migraine, a point that this author will amplify below.

Table 9.4
Experimental and Case Studies in Manipulative and/or Chiropractic Treatment of Benign Headache

Muscle Contraction	Case Studies
Lewit (1971)	Mannen (1983)
Ng (1980)	Miller et al (1984)
Vernon (1982)	
Schimek and Mohr (1984)	
Jirout (1985)	
Droz (1985)	
Graff-Radford et al (1987)	
Turk and Ratkolb (1987)	
Migraine	
Figar and Jansky (1964)	
Wight (1978)	
Parker et al (1978)	
Parker et al (1980)	
Sachse et al (1982)	

Research Studies in Vertebrogenic Headache

As discussed earlier, the research study differs from the clinical or theoretical descriptive study in that the models proposed assume the form of an hypothesis (or set of hypotheses) that is then tested with data gathered directly from a clinical population. These studies include single case studies, descriptive surveys or "open trials," and randomized controlled studies. These studies have also been categorized as exploratory, in which a broad view of clinical experience and patient management is taken, or explanatory, in which a more precise "experimental" approach is taken with the objective of delineating the mechanisms whereby a particular treatment intervention exerts its effects. I will discuss this literature in chronological order for muscle contraction and migraine headaches separately. Table 9.4 presents what is, to my knowledge, a complete list of these studies as of 1987.

Muscle Contraction Headache

Lewit, in 1971(33), studied 41 late adolescents (21 females and 20 males) who had sustained anteflexion injuries in gymnastic activities and who were presenting with headache. Of these subjects, 71% were found to have fixation of the craniocervical joints and 53% were found to have hypermobility. Manipulation was reported to be the single most effective treatment from a number of physical modalities.

Lewit also reported on a series of 93 adults who had sustained head/neck traumas. Of these subjects 96% demonstrated movement restriction in the upper cervical spine. Manipulation was reported to be very successful in treating the headache associated with these injuries.

Ng, in 1980(63), investigated the association between static vertebral misalignment as viewed on plain film x-rays and the incidence of occipital headache. Thirty-eight subjects suffering exclusively from occipital (i.e., muscle contraction) headache were studied (10 males, 28 females). These subjects were compared to an age- and sex-matched control group. Lateral inclinations of C1, C2, and C3 were measured using a standardized x-ray marking technique. Lateral curvature of the entire cervical spine was also measured. Statistically significant differences were found between headache sufferers and controls in the incidence and degree of lateral tilting at C1 and C3, while a tendency toward a similar distortion existed at C2. No differences were found in the lateral spinal curve in the two groups. Ng concluded that abnormal static mechanics of the upper cervical spine may be associated with occipital headaches.

Mannen, in 1980(64), reported a single-case study in which headache was relieved by a course of chiropractic treatment.

Vernon, in 1983(65), in a descriptive survey, studied two groups of headache sufferers presenting at a chiropractic college outpatient clinic. One group (15) was studied retrospectively by mail survey, while the other group (18) was studied prospectively within the clinic. Headache sufferers were asked to rate the level of headache frequency, duration, and severity, as well as the presence of four "neurovegetative" symptoms—nausea, dizziness, tinnitus, aura. These ratings were made for the condition before and after treatment. In the prospective group, a fixed number of treatments (9) was used. Subjects were also asked to rate the level of subjective improvement by rating their response to three questions:

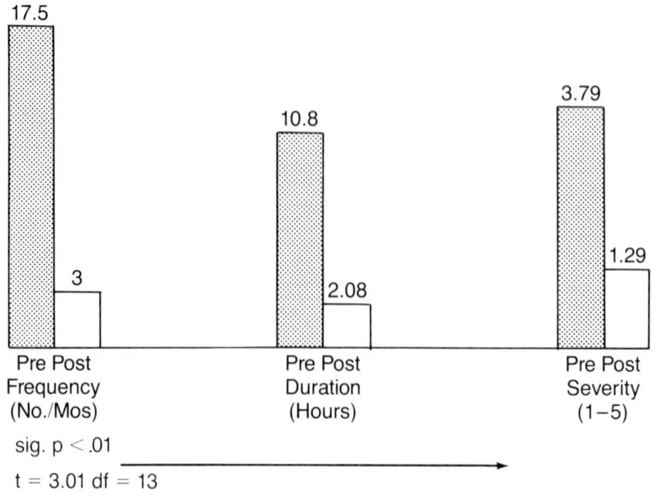

Table 9.5. Retrospective study group comparison of the mean values of the dependent variables before and after treatment. The average subject in this study suffered frequent, long, and intense headaches prior to treatment. Significant improvement was demonstrated following chiropractic manipulative therapy.

(1) How much improvement did they obtain?
(2) How satisfied were they with chiropractic treatment?
(3) Would they return for similar chiropractic treatments?

These ratings formed a satisfaction index (scored out of 15).

The results of the study in both the retrospective and prospective groups are displayed in Tables 9.5 to 9.9. The levels of statistical significance are very high on all of the indices. The satisfaction index scores range from 12.2 to 12.7 of 15 or 90%. Of seven subjects who reported nausea present prior to treatment, 100% were relieved of that symptom. Similarly, 9 of 9 or 94% of subjects reporting dizziness reported complete relief.

In 1984, Schimek and Mohr(66) conducted a descriptive survey of 78 patients with chronic headache. It is assumed that these subjects were suffering from benign headaches of the muscle contraction, migraine or mixed types. The approach taken in this study was to determine the characteristics of these patients at presentation to a manual therapy clinic as opposed to the outcome of manipulative treatment. The clinical protocol is very similar to that used included a determination of the presence of active and latent trigger points, the presence and degree of "vertebral blockage" patterns of referred pain, and patterns of x-ray findings in the cervical spine. This clinical protocol is very similar to that used by many chiropractors in the examination of chronic headache sufferers.

These authors conclude their study with the following statements: ". . . pathological nociceptive impulses from a blocked joint increase, reflexly, muscle tension in certain neck muscles. Referred pain develops which may be co-related with a certain

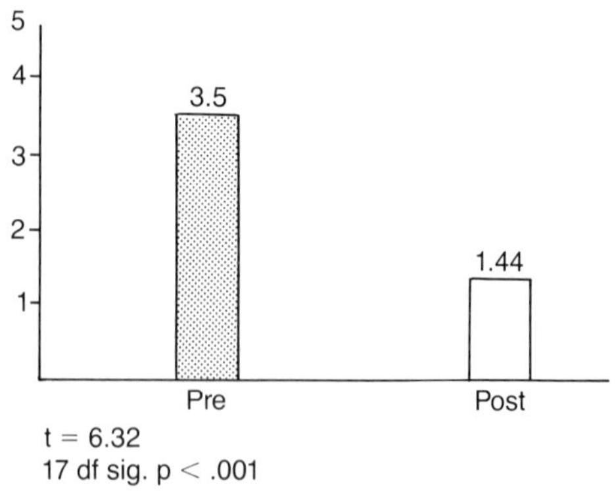

Table 9.6. Comparison of mean scores of headache frequency (no/mos).

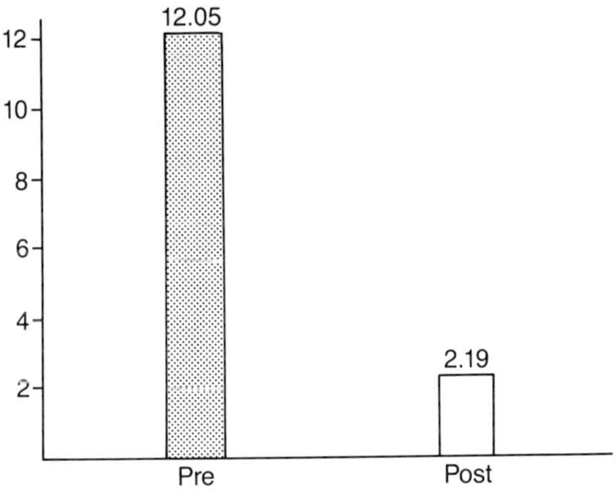

Table 9.7. Comparison of mean scores of headache duration (hours).

area of the head. . . . Vertebral dysfunction is of primary importance in the development of chronic headache and is considered to be its generator. . . ."

Miller, Maxwell, and De Boer, in 1984(67), reported on a single case study of "longstanding, uncomplicated tension headache." According to the authors, 13 adjustive treatments were rendered, resulting in a reduction in headache frequency from 2.6/day to 1.0/day within one week. Use of analgesic medication similarly decreased.

In 1985, Jirout(68) reported on 200 patients who had previously been involved in a roentgenological study of motion blockage at the C2–C3 segment. Of subjects

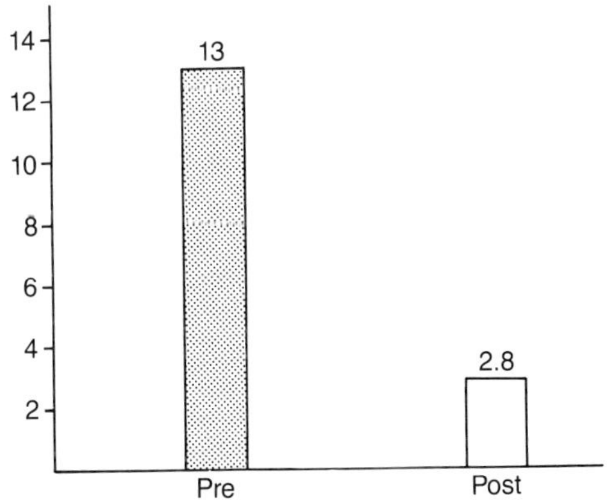

Table 9.8. Comparison of mean values of headache severity (1–5).

Table 9.9
Response of Autonomic Symptomatology to Chiropractic Manipulative Therapy in the Prospective Group

	Number of Subjects (Pre)	Number of Subjects Relieved (Post)[a]
Nausea	7	7 (100%)
Dizziness	9	8 (88.9%)
Tinnitus	2	1 (50%)
Aura	4	2 (50%)
Total	22	18

[a] 3 df $X^2 = 11.34$ $p < .01$.

with this vertebral dysfunction 90% reported the presence of headaches. Manipulation produced complete relief in approximately 80% of this sample.

Droz and Crot reported in the 1985 Swiss Annals VIII on "Occipital Headaches"(6). A retrospective survey was conducted of clinic files from 1962 to 1963 and from 1973 to 1983. Of approximately 10,000 patient files surveyed, 332 (approximately 3%) were found to suffer from "occipital headaches" (taken here to mean a variant of muscle contraction headache). Average values of number of treatments and case outcome were compiled. The average number of treatments was nine. Treatment outcome was rated as very good (90% relief), good (75%), slightly better (50%), same, or worse. Of the sample, 80% had a very good result, while 10% had a good and 3% had a slightly better outcome. As such, 93% had a positive treatment outcome, while 7% had no improvement. Droz noted that the vast majority of successful cases had no more than 10–15 treatments, so that treatment success can be achieved quickly, but in cases in which the number of treatments exceeds 15, a poorer prognosis is to be expected.

Most recently, Turk and Rotkolb (150) have reported on 100 cases of cervicogenic headache treated by manipulation. Nine manipulative treatments produced significant reduction of headaches in 75% of subjects. At six-month follow-up, 65% still had significant improvement while 35% had recurrence of symptoms. A significant reduction of analgesic usage was noted.

The research literature then includes five descriptive surveys (two in the paper by

Lewit) of treatment outcome and three studies describing the characteristics of vertebrogenic dysfunction in chronic benign headache sufferers. Included in these three are one study noting an association between findings of segmental misalignment on static x-ray studies of the upper cervical spine and two studies noting the association of upper cervical vertebral motion dysfunction with chronic headaches.

Migraine Headache

In 1964, Figar and Jansky(29) studied vascular reflexes of subjects who suffered from "vertebrogenic migraine." This is a diagnostic entity fully accepted by the authors. Vascular reflexes were studied by photoplethysmography of the superficial temporal artery. Both the resting state levels and those evoked as a response to external stressors were studied. Subjects were stimulated by acoustically loud noise, psychological-mental arithmetic, and nociceptive stresses. Nine migraine patients were compared to nine age-matched control subjects. Subjects were studied in between their headaches.

In the normal controls, the vasomotor response of the superficial temporal artery was uniformly and bilaterally vasodilatory. In the patients, 23% showed parallel vasoconstriction, while numerous others showed asymmetric reactions. The authors concluded that vertebrogenic migraine is associated with abnormal cerebrovascular tone and regulation.

A landmark descriptive survey of a chiropractor's clinical experience in the treatment of migraine was reported by Wight in 1983(70). In this study, 87 patients (57 female and 30 male) were included, 34 with common migraine and 53 with classical migraine. The results of typical chiropractic treatment regimes were as follows: In the common migraine group, 85% of the females and 50% of the males were greatly improved; in the classical migraine group, 78% of the female and 75% of the male patients were greatly improved. The overall success rate for both migraine categories for both sexes was 74.7%. In those not reporting a greatly improved status after treatment, a reduction of severe attacks was achieved for 81.5% of female and 45.8% of the male patients in the common migraine group, and 43.2% and 34.5%, respectively, of the classical migraine group.

Wight also cites the improvement rates reported in three other chiropractic surveys by Loban(4), International Chiropractic Association, and Rose(72). These are shown in Table 9.10.

The most important study and indeed the only randomized clinical trial on chiropractic manipulation and migraine was conducted by Parker, Tupling, and Pryor in 1978(73). In this study, 85 subjects (33 male, 52 female) with a mean age of 41 years and a mean headache duration of 19 years were randomly allocated to three treatment groups. Of these subjects, 70% suffered common migraine while 30% suffered classical migraine. The subjects received a baseline assessment consisting of psychological tests (especially regarding attitudes toward manipulative therapy), x-ray analysis of the cervical spine, and a migraine diary wherein daily data on headache duration, intensity, and frequency were

Table 9.10
Chiropractic Surveys of Migraine Patients as Reported by Wight[a]

		Improvement (%)				
Cities	Number	Complete		Marked	None	Worse
Loban (1928)	89	58	90	32	10	0
ICA survey (1953)[b]	76	40	87	47	11	2
Rose (1973)	17	27	72	45	27.5	0

[a]Adapted from Wight JS. Migraine: a statistical analysis of chiropractic treatment. Am Chiro Assoc J Chiro 1978; 12:363–367.
[b]ICA, International Chiropractic Association.

gathered. Medical and neurological tests were conducted to ensure that no organic cause existed for the headache condition. After the baseline examination, subjects were randomly allocated to one of three treatment groups—chiropractic manipulation, medical manipulation, a control/mobilization performed by physiotherapists. Subjects underwent a two-month pretreatment stage, a two-month treatment stage, and a further two-month follow-up period.

This study tested a number of hypotheses which essentially compared the treated and nontreated groups as a whole, compared to each other and separately on the response to headache frequency, severity, and duration. These hypotheses were tested with statistical tests using a probability level of .01.

An average of seven treatments were performed in the treatment phase. The mean improvement level for all three groups was 28%. Only one hypothesis achieved an acceptable level of statistical significance (.01), that being that headache severity (i.e., pain intensity) was reduced in the chiropractic manipulation group. Measures of treatment expectation of the subjects and the treators indicated a higher degree of expectation of treatment response by the patients and the chiropractors in the chiropractic manipulation group. The authors concluded that such high expectations had a direct effect on pain ratings and, as such, the finding that a single significant hypothesis did attribute treatment success to chiropractors was probably due to a placebo-type response.

This study was the subject of much criticism and independent review. An independant statistical consultant was commissioned by the New Zealand Commission on Chiropractic(74) and asked to revise the statistical tests in order to more properly analyze the available data. Several problems were delineated, which, in the opinion of that consultant, contributed to the negative findings of the clinical trial.

First, the control group did in fact receive a form of treatment, i.e., mobilization, so that a true treatment—no treatment comparison could not be conducted. Second, the alpha level of .01 was very stringent—even higher than that of many medical clinical trials. Third, some of the statistical tests were inappropriate. A revision of the statistical analysis was performed that did not produce an aceptable level of statistical significance in any of the hypotheses, even at a lowered (.05) alpha level. However, the consultant noted that subjects in the chiropractic manipulation group consistently scored higher in every rating than did the other two groups. Given that a relatively low number of treatments was performed on average (7), and that the chiropractic manipulation group was favored in all of the statistical tests, the consultant concluded that the study had a low power. This meant that it was not designed effectively enough to detect a difference between treatment groups when such a difference might, in fact, have been present.

A follow-up study was published in 1980 by Parker and his colleagues that was very much a response to his critics(75). It was noted that at a 20-month follow-up period, a further 19% of subjects had achieved an improved rating. This constituted a 47% success rate for manual therapy in the treatment of migraine. An interesting aspect of the data that did not receive statistical analysis was that 14 of the subjects in the study achieved a complete recovery. Of these, 8 were in the chiropractic manipulation, 1 in the medical manipulation, and 5 in control/mobilization groups.

The follow-up study attempted to correlate certain psychosocial variables with treatment success. Only one—sex (.01)—achieved the appropriate level of statistical significance to be accepted as a correlate of therapeutic success. In this regard, female patients responded better than male patients to the forms of manual therapy studied by Parker et al.

It should be evident from the preceding discussion that the "Parker clinical trial" raised more questions than it provided answers for. It appears to have been a study with very worthwhile intentions, but which fell heir to an important but often overlooked error known as Type B error. This is the statistical error in which a clinical trial fails to demonstrate significant differences when they do in fact exist. In other words, this appeared to have been a false negative trial. Upon reflection, a 47% total success rate, with the chiropractic group producing a significantly larger number of complete recoveries, is an impressive set of findings which should encourage further study.

Sachse, Eckhardkt, Lieb, and Sachse(76), in 1982, presented a report on 22 migraine patients in which a structural assessment very similar to a chiropractic clinical examination was conducted. They found the most frequent segmental fixations to be at C0–C1 and C7–T1 as well as in the first costovertebral joint (first rib restriction). They found the most severe tenderness to palpation present in the shoulder (scapular) region and over the posterior arch of atlas. The most severe muscle hypertonicity was found in the trapezius and levator scapula muscles.

The author is currently engaged in a prospective controlled clinical trial of chiropractic manipulation compared to placebo ultrasound therapy in the treatment of adult migraine headaches. The headache history, headache diary, and headache examination form are shown in Figures 9.4–9.6, respectively. Together, these forms comprise a complete chiropractic headache protocol suitable for office use. Other outcome measures that will be utilized in this clinical trial include static and dynamic x-ray studies of the cervical spine, photoplethysmography of the digital blood supply, and psychological assessments (Self-Efficacy Index, Lifestyle Stress Index, State Anxiety Index). Profiles of one treated subject in a pilot study conducted in 1985 at the Canadian Memorial Chiropractic College are shown in Figures 9.7 and 9.8.

Summary

What is the consensus from the experimental literature on the efficacy of manipulative treatments in the management of benign headache? At present, there appears to be evidence for, if not agreement about, the following:

(1) Subjects with muscle contraction headache often have signs of upper cervical joint dysfunction.

Ng demonstrated that muscle contraction headaches were associated with x-ray evidence of static misalignment of the upper cervical vertebrae, while Jirout, Lewit, and Shimek and Mohr have all noted the presence of motion dysfunction in the upper cervical motion segments in headache sufferers. Sachse et al found typical motion restrictions and typical myofascial dysfunction in migraineurs.

(2) Spinal manipulation appears to produce a very favorable response in those who receive it, although no true comparison to a control group exists.

The consensus of the treatment studies including those by Lewit(33), Vernon(65), Jirout(68), Mannen(64), Miller, Maxwell, and De Boer(67), Droz(6), and Wight(70) is that manipulation produces from 75 to 90% relief in a typical treatment regime averaging 9–10 treatments. Parker, Tupling, and Pryor(73) found the success rate for manual therapy in migraines to be 47% after 20 months.

(3) Cervical joint dysfunction appears to be related to both the pain and the vascular disorder of migraine headaches.

Figar and Jansky's work substantiates the role of cervical spine dysfunction in the creation of abnormal vasoregulation in the superficial temporal artery(126, 127). Their findings are similar to those of Feuerstein et al(77) who showed abnormal vasoregulation in between headaches in migraineurs who eventually underwent biofeedback therapy.

(4) No prognostic criteria have yet emerged that could predict a favorable response to manipulative treatment. This is largely due to the relatively small number of studies and the small aggregate number of subjects in these studies.

Parker, Tupling, and Pryor found that treatment expectation might play a role in treatment response to manual therapy, however, this could certainly be said for a variety of conservative management techniques(78). In addition, they found that sex appeared to correlate with outcome, however, since more female patients, suffer from migraine, it is reasonable to see more female patients responding to the treatment offered in that study.

Patient Name ____________________ Date ________

1. Age ________

2. M F

3. Occupation ______________________________

4. Onset ______ Total Duration ______ Hours ______
   ± ________ Weeks

5. Initial Precipitating Event

	No	Yes
1. Trauma	____	____
2. Menses	____	____
3. 1° Work stress	____	____
4. Childhood	____	____
5. Illness	____	____
6. Other	____	____
____________	____	____

Typical Headache

6. Frequency
   Daily ________
   ________/Week
   ________/Month
   ± ________/Month

7. Duration
   ± ________/Hours

8. Severity

   ____
   0 none — 10 worst
   ± ________

9. Location

	No	Yes*
1. Occipital	____	____
2. Temporoparietal	____	____
3. Frontal	____	____
4. Facial	____	____
5. Orbital	____	____
6. Vertex	____	____
7. Mandibular	____	____

10.

	No	Yes*
1. Neck pain	____	____
2. Upper back pain	____	____

11.

	No	Yes*
1. Unilateral		
Right	____	____
Left	____	____
2. Bilateral	____	____

12.

	No	Yes*
1. Focal	____	____
2. Diffuse	____	____
3. Radiating	____	____

13. Character

	No	Yes*
1. Pressure	____	____
2. Steady ache	____	____
3. Throbbing	____	____
4. Stabbing	____	____

14. Associated Symptoms

	No	Yes*
1. Nausea	____	____
2. Vomiting	____	____
3. Dizziness	____	____
4. Aura	____	____
4.1 Visual	____	____
4.2 Smell	____	____
4.3 Kinesthetic	____	____
4.4 Other	____	____
____________		
5. Visual disturbance	____	____
6. Abdominal pain	____	____
7. Photophobia	____	____
8. Phonophobia	____	____
9. Jaw pain	____	____

15. Diurnal

	No	Yes*
1. Awakes at night	____	____
2. Morning	____	____
3. Afternoon	____	____
4. Evening	____	____
5. All day	____	____
6. Variable	____	____

16. Precipitation

	No	Yes*
1. Hunger	____	____
2. Tension/stress	____	____
3. Fatigue	____	____
4. Weather changes	____	____
5. Movements of head/neck	____	____
6. Certain foods	____	____

____
____

17. Aggravation

	No	Yes
1. Menstruation	____	____
2. Sneeze/cough	____	____
3. Exertion	____	____
4. Head/neck movements	____	____
5. Motion	____	____
6. Noise	____	____
7. Light	____	____

18. Medications

	No	Yes
1. None	____	____
Analgesic		
2. Aspirin	____	____
3. Tylenol	____	____
4. Fiorinal	____	____
5. Ibuprofen	____	____
6. Other	____	____
Abortive		
7. Ergot	____	____
8. Cafergot	____	____
9. Other	____	____
Preventative		
10. Inderal	____	____
11. Isoptin	____	____
12. Methysergide	____	____
13. Other	____	____
14. Hormonal/BCP	____	____

19. Self-Help

1. Lying down	____	____
2. Massage	____	____
3. Heat	____	____
4. Cold	____	____
5. Food	____	____
6. Other	____	____

____
____

Figure 9.4. Canadian Memorial Chiropractic College Migraine Trial Headache History.

Past Treatment

20. Previous diagnosis? ________

21. Past diagnosis?
Specialist No ____ Yes ____

	No	Yes
1. CT scan	____	____
2. EEG	____	____
3. Other	____	____

____
____

22. Past Treatments

	No	Yes	Helpful? No	Yes
1. G.P.	____	____	____	____
2. Biofeedback	____	____	____	____
3. Acupuncture	____	____	____	____
4. Chiropractor	____	____	____	____
5. Dentist	____	____	____	____
6. Other	____	____	____	____

____
____

General Health

23. Do you have any separate pain in

	No	Yes
1. Neck	____	____
2. Upper back	____	____
3. Lower back	____	____

24. Are you taking any other medication?

	No	Yes
1. Anticoagulant	____	____
2. Valium	____	____
3. Antidepressant	____	____
4. Antihistamine	____	____
5. Other	____	____

____
____

25. Have you had any recent illnesses or operations?

No	Yes
____	____

26. Do you have

	No	Yes
1. High blood pressure	____	____
2. Vascular disease	____	____
3. Neurological disease	____	____
4. Other diseases	____	____

Lifestyle

	No	Yes
27. 1. Are you married?	____	____
2. Do you have children?	____	____
Boys #____ Girls #____		
28. Are you a smoker?	____	____
How much? ________		
29. Family History of Headache		
1. Mother	____	____
2. Father	____	____
3. Grandparent	____	____
4. Sibling	____	____
5. Children	____	____
30. How would you rate your job stress		
1. Low	____	____
2. Medium	____	____
3. High	____	____

Patient Summary

Migraine		Tension/Muscle Contraction/Cervical*
11.1 ____		5.1 ____*
13.3 ____		9.1 ____*
14.1 ____		10.1 ____*
14.2 ____		12.2 ____
14.4 ____	16.4 ____	13.2 ____
14.7 ____	17.6 ____	16.2 ____
14.8 ____	29.1 ____	16.5 ____*

Diagnosis ________
____
____

Vertebrogenic Pattern ________
____

Prognosis for Manipulation/Contraindications ____
____
____

Treatment Plan ________
____
____
____
____

Figure 9.4 (*continued*)

MECHANISMS OF VERTEBROGENIC HEADACHE

At this point, I will attempt to synthesize all of the information in the clinical, theoretical, and experimental literature into an integrated and coherent model. This model will be organized along two major lines—anatomical and physiological.

Anatomical Model

Table 9.11 displays the components of a generic vertebrogenic model organized along anatomical lines. The major categories of structures include:

(1) Extrasegmental—largely involves the large regional musculature and their fascial structures;

Patient #__________

Month Day Year	DAY 1	DAY 2	DAY 3	DAY 4	DAY 5	DAY 6	DAY 7	DAY 8	DAY 9	DAY 10	DAY 11	DAY 12	DAY 13	DAY 14	Office Use
1. Did you have a headache today? Answer YES or NO															
2. If YES, how long did it last? (in hours)															
3. How severe was it? (0–10) None .... = 0 Mild .... = 2 Moderate .... = 4 Heavy .... = 6 Severe .... = 8 Horrible .... = 10															
4. Rate your activity today. Normal .... = 0 Minimal Effect on Activity .... = 1 Interference with work/leisure .... = 2 Absent from work/school .... = 3															
5. Medication taken: (a) How much each time? ________ ________ ________															
(b) How often? ________ ________ ________															

Figure 9.5. Canadian Memorial Chiropractic College Migraine Trial Headache Diary.

Table 9.11
An Anatomical Model of Vertebrogenic Mechanisms

Extrasegmental	Intersegmental	Infrasegmental	Intrasegmental
Regional muscles	Joint dysfunction Ligaments Capsules Deep/short muscles	"Foraminal" area Nerve root Dorsal root ganglia	Reflex disturbances
Fascial attachments	Intervertebral disc		
"Postural" or configuration causes			

PATIENT NAME ______________________ AGE ______ M/F ______ (1/2)

Number of Headaches: ____/mo Headache Duration: ____hr Headache Severity: 1 2 3 4 5 6 7 8 9 10

STRUCTURAL EXAM:

1) Ranges of Motion (Full = 0, partial = 1, moderate = 2, severe = 3)

FLEX	____
EXT	____
RROT	____
LROT	____
RLB	____
LLB	____

2) Myofascial Triggers (Good = 0, Present = 2, Not Done = X)

	R (1)	L (2)
Frontalis	____	____
Temporalis	____	____
Occipitalis	____	____
Sub-occip	____	____
Mid-cerv	____	____
Lower-cerv	____	____
Traps	____	____
Scal	____	____
Rhomb	____	____
Pec Ma	____	____

3. Fixations (Score 2 for each fix or hyper, X = Not Done, 0 = Normal)

Lateral Bend L(2)		Lateral Bend R(1)	Rotation L(2)		Rotation R(1)	Anteroposterior Block L(2)		Anteroposterior Block R(1)
____	C0	____	____	C0	____	____	C0	____
____	C1	____	____	C1	____	____	C1	____
____	C2	____	____	C2	____	____	C2	____
____	C3	____	____	C3	____	____	C3	____
____	C4	____	____	C4	____	____	C4	____
____	C5	____	____	C5	____	____	C5	____
____	C6	____	____	C6	____	____	C6	____
____	C7	____	____	C7	____	____	C7	____
____	T1	____	____	T1	____	____	T1	____
____	T2	____	____	T2	____	____	T2	____
____	T3	____	____	T3	____	____	T3	____

Figure 9.6. Canadian Memorial Chiropractic College Migraine Trial Cervical Spine Examination Form.

(2) Intersegmental—involves the holding elements of the motion segment: anterior and posterior joint structures as well as the deep, short intersegmental muscles;

(3) Infrasegmental—involves structures in the intervertebral foramen or, in the case of the upper cervical vertebrae that lack true foramina, the bony environs of the nerve roots. Specifically, these structures include the ventral and dorsal nerve roots, the mixed spinal nerve, the dorsal root ganglion, the autonomic fibers, the recurrent meningeal nerve, and the vascular structures of the intervertebral foramina;

(4) Intrasegmental—applies to the spinal cord, in particular, the ascending pain pathways, the anterior horn cells, and those of the sympathetic nervous system. These spinal neuronal pools are involved in reflex connections that govern pain behavior, muscle tone and coordination, and autonomic tone (specifically vasomotor tone), respectively.

An anatomical model of vertebrogenic headache applies these categories to the

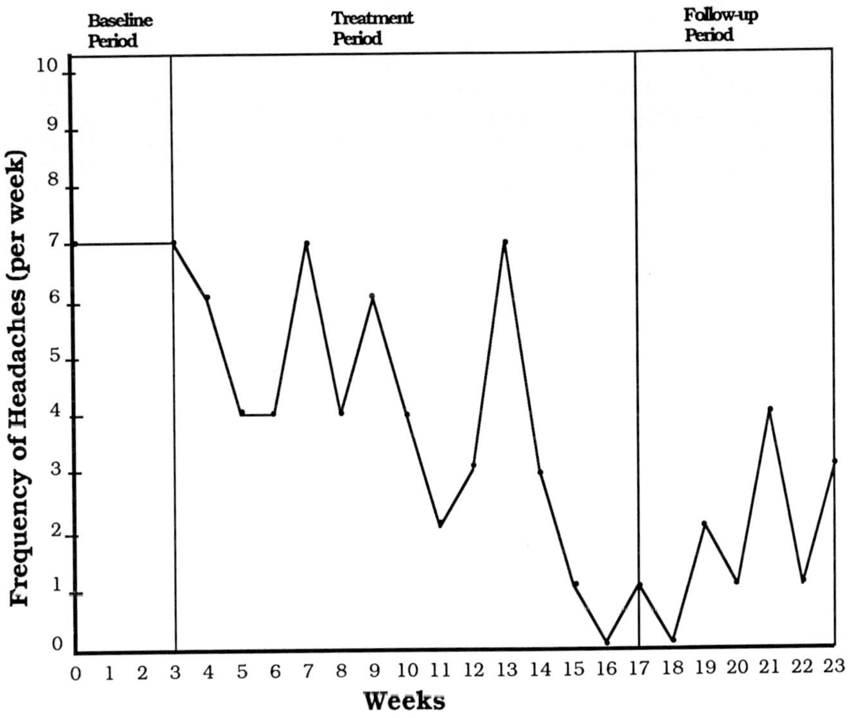

Figure 9.7. Data from a single case study of a migraine subject in the manipulated group. Headache frequency.

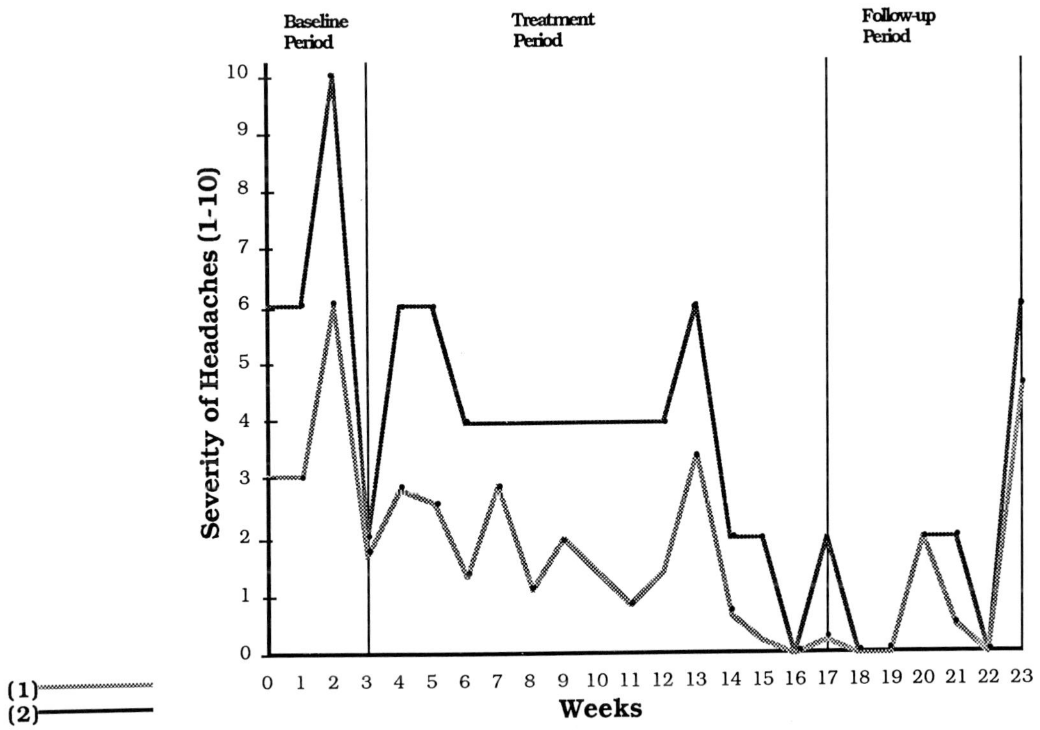

Figure 9.8. Data from a single case study of a migraine subject in the manipulated group. Headache severity.

craniocervical anatomy in order to rationalize mechanisms that could be productive of the kind of head pain and dysfunction clinically associated with benign headaches, i.e., muscle contraction, migraine (common and classic), and mixed types. This model will be applied presently to each of these headache categories separately.

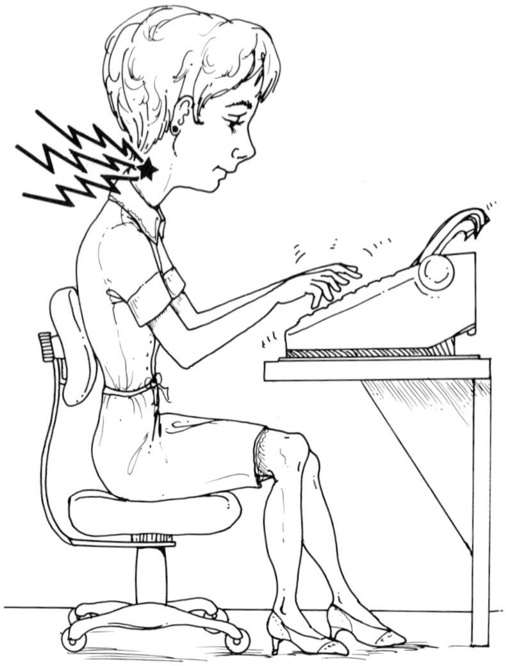

Figure 9.9. Line drawing of the typical postural maladaptation in the upper cervical spine (see text).

Vertebrogenic Muscle Contraction Headache

Mechanisms

Extrasegmental. The structures involved in this category are the large regional cervicothoracic and cervicocranial muscles, specifically, trapezius, sternocleidomastoid, levator scapula, splenius, and semispinalis capitus, and the occipitofrontalis muscle. In addition, one would include the fascial investments surrounding and interconnecting these large muscles that, as a group (excluding occipitofrontalis), we would define as "regional craniocervical extensors."

These muscular structures are susceptible to a variety of chronic low-level but accumulative stresses that alter their function and prepare the way for primary or secondary pain states. These stresses arise from postural strain as well as occupational strain and are aggravated when individuals assume slumped postures with cervical hyperlordosis and occipital extension (see Fig. 9.9) as well as seated postures that, involve forward tilt of the head and neck (especially with superimposed rotation) and constant upright support of the active arms. These postures are adopted daily by millions of workers in offices around the world (see Fig. 9.10). These muscles may suffer direct trauma as in anteflexion strains or in hyperextension-hyperflexion injuries of the whiplash type. Cervical joint derangement (see below) may also produce muscular dysfunction by inducing secondary arthrogenic contractions(79).

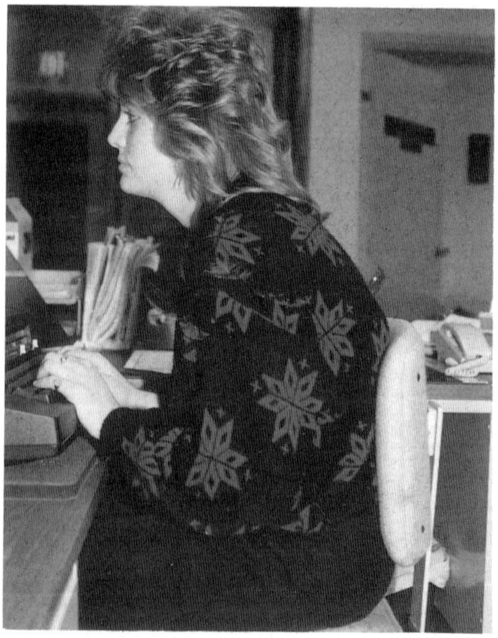

Figure 9.10. Typical upper cervical decompensated posture in modern desk workers.

How do these myofascial dysfunctions produce headache? The most direct mechanism involves irritation of the tendoperiosteal junctions producing low-level chronic foci of tenderness and pain. This produces local occipital or nuchal and suboccipital pain. Lewit(34) has remarked on "pain over the posterior arch of atlas" and others(38, 84, 85) have noted the presence of tenderness over the insertions of the large regional muscles to the posterior occiput and to the vertebral arches.

The second mechanism involves a chronic myofasciitis of the muscle structure as a whole, which is typically expressed as a low-level hypertonicity with a focal zone of pain and tenderness. This may or may not be accompanied by radiation zones of pain, typically in a cephalad direction into various predictable cranial locations. This phenomenon is referred to by various names but is most commonly known as the "trigger point" phenomenon of Travell(82–84). The trigger point phenomenon may be an actual focal lesion within the muscle structure, typically located in the vicinity of the motor point with local histopathological changes(84), or it may be a zone of referred pain and hypersensitivity resulting from proximal peripheral neuropathy as described by Gunn(81). Regardless of its origin, this myofascial dysfunction produces muscle-specific zones of radiating head pain that may completely mimic the pain of cranial muscular contraction. Some of these typical referral zones, adapted from Travell(147), are displayed in Figures 9.11–9.19.

Muscular hypertonicity or contracture as found in chronic postural dysfunction may also produce a secondary entrapment of accompanying neurovascular structures. There are two such conditions that are associated with headache: entrapment of the greater occipital nerve and the thoracic outlet syndrome. Skillern(23) and Arnold(86) described a syndrome resulting from entrapment of the greater occipital

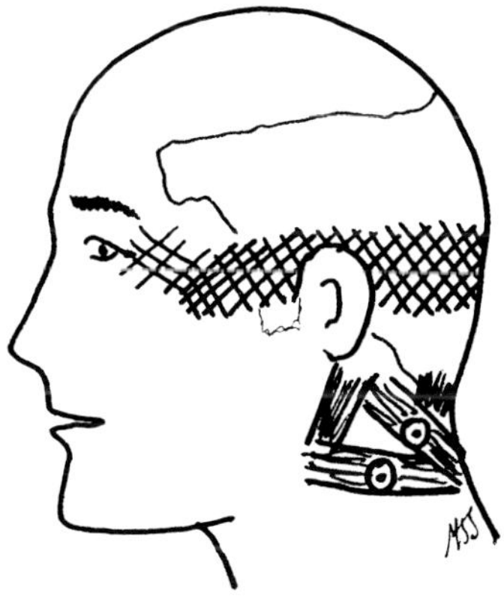

Figure 9.11. Trigger points and pain referral zone for the suboccipital muscles (after Travell and Simons (147)).

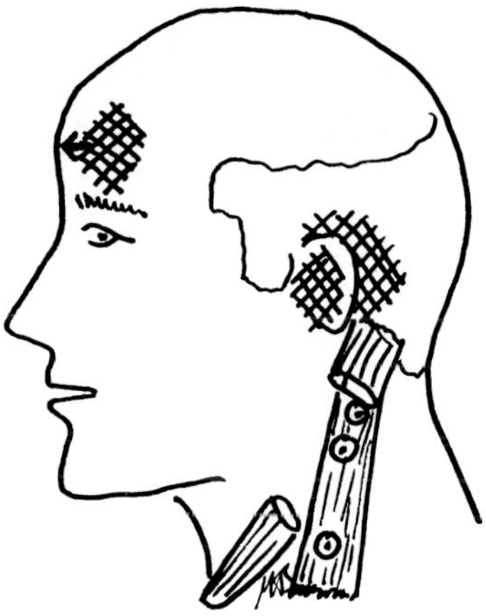

Figure 9.12. Trigger points and pain referral zone for the clavicular division of the sternocleidomastoid muscle. After Travell JG, Simons DG. Myofascial pain and dysfunction. The trigger point manual. Baltimore: Williams & Wilkins, 1983.

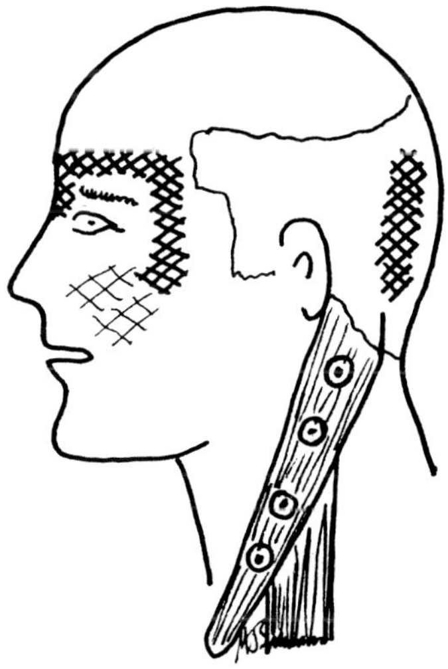

Figure 9.13. Trigger points and pain referral zone for the sternol division of the sternocleidomastoid muscle. After Travell JG, Simons DG. Myofascial pain and dysfunction. The trigger point manual. Baltimore: Williams & Wilkins, 1983.

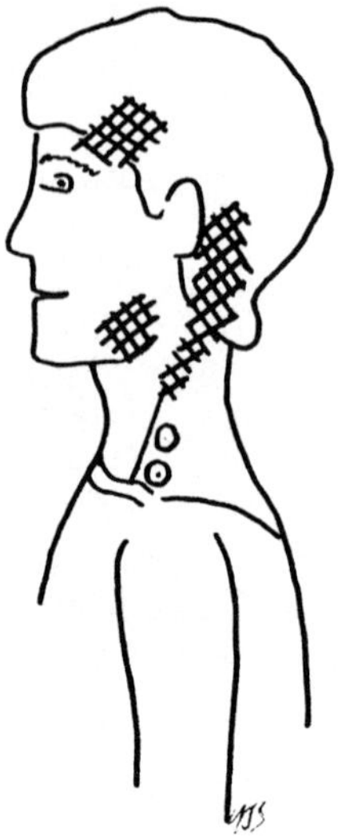

Figure 9.14. Trigger points and pain referral zone for the upper trapezius muscle. After Travell JG, Simons DG. Myofascial pain and dysfunction. The trigger point manual. Baltimore: Williams & Wilkins, 1983.

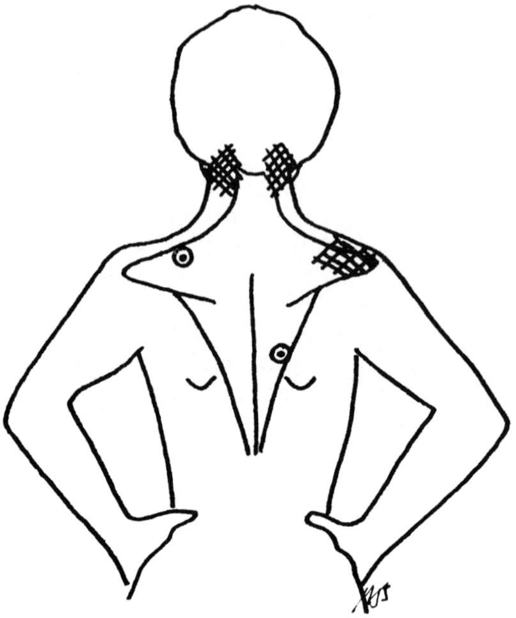

Figure 9.16. Trigger points and pain referral zone for the upper and middle trapezius muscles. After Travell JG, Simons DG. Myofascial pain and dysfunction. The trigger point manual. Baltimore: Williams & Wilkins, 1983.

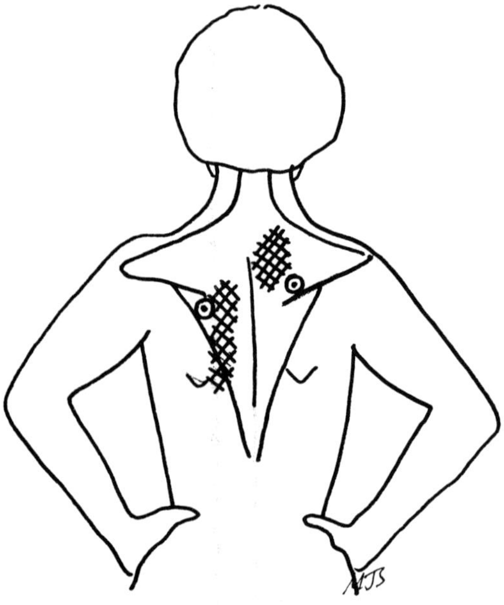

Figure 9.15. Trigger points and pain referral zone for the middle and lower trapezius muscles. After Travell JG, Simons DG. Myofascial pain and dysfunction. The trigger point manual. Baltimore: Williams & Wilkins, 1983.

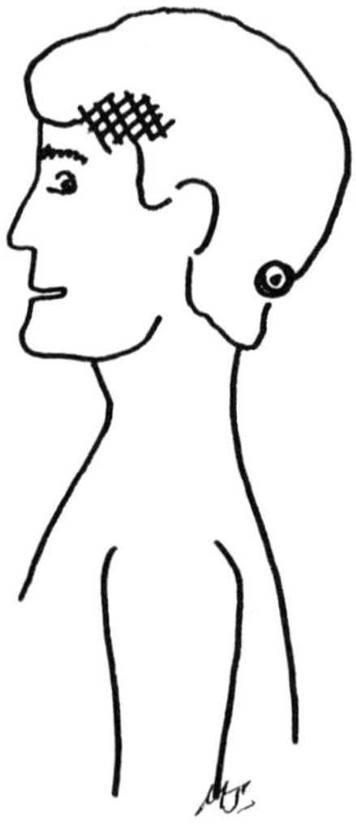

Figure 9.17. Trigger points and pain referral zone for the semispinalis capitus muscle. After Travell JG, Simons DG. Myofascial pain and dysfunction. The trigger point manual. Baltimore: Williams & Wilkins, 1983.

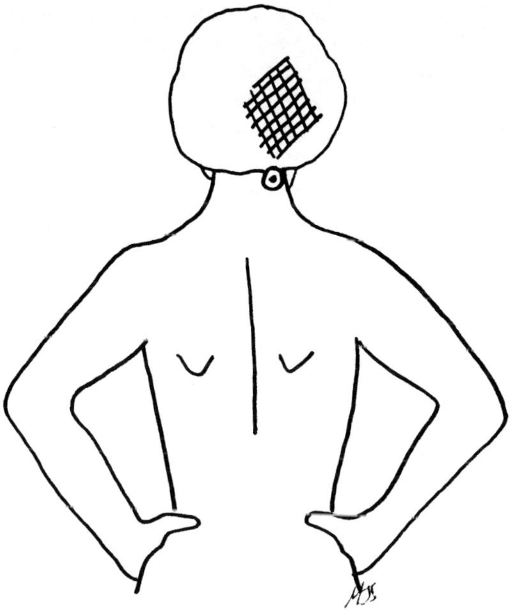

Figure 9.18. Trigger points and pain referral zone for the semispinalis cervicis muscle. After Travell JG, Simons DG. Myofascial pain and dysfunction. The trigger point manual. Baltimore: Williams & Wilkins, 1983.

nerve as it pierced the cephalad portion of the trapezius muscle. Bogduk(53) has refined our appreciation of the anatomical basis of this "occipital neuralgia." Entrapment appears to occur where the nerve courses between the insertions of the trapezius and the splenius capitus. Focal tenderness is uniformly present on the occiput unilaterally with sharp, more intense pain radiating forward over the cranium, very often to the frontal region. Conservative therapy(87), myofascial release(85), injection therapy, and occasionally removal of the C2 dorsal root have been proposed in the treatment of this type of headache(86).

According to Raskin et al(12), headache is the leading symptom of thoracic outlet syndrome. They proposed that muscular hypertonicity produced a nonspecific trigger to the existing headache mechanisms, that is, to vascular dysfunction or to cranial muscle tension.

In summary, the large occipital extensors may undergo stresses leading to greater and more persistent degrees of contraction, which then may irritate tendinous in-

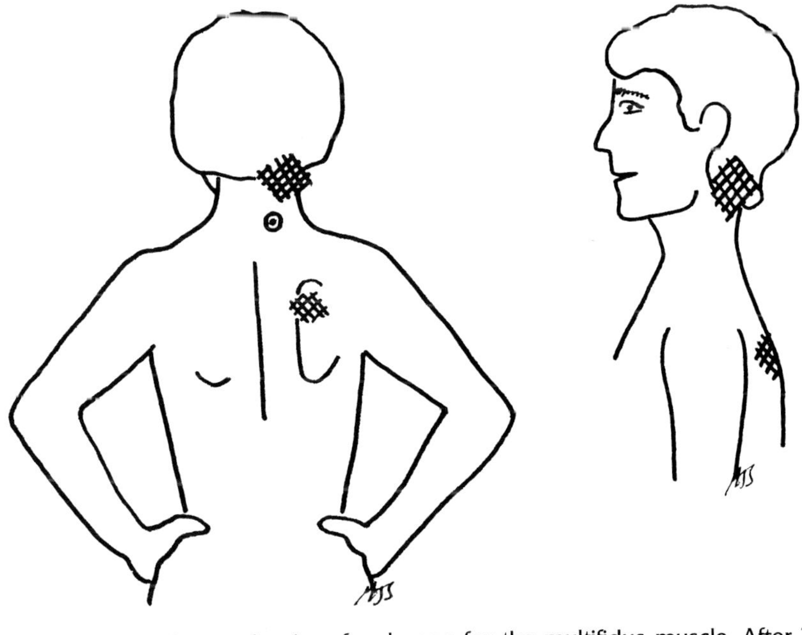

Figure 9.19. Trigger points and pain referral zone for the multifidus muscle. After Travell JG, Simons DG. Myofascial pain and dysfunction. The trigger point manual. Baltimore: Williams & Wilkins, 1983.

sertions, create focal trigger points with myotomal radiations, and entrap neural structures so that primary and/or referred head pain might arise.

Intersegmental. This category refers to the joint structures of the motion segment-posterior ligament complex, apophyseal joints, intervertebral disc, and uncovertebral joints, as well as the deeper short segmental muscles that have been labeled suboccipital muscles in the craniocervical region. Considering first the posterior motion segment, attention focuses on articular and ligamentous nociceptors (Type IV receptors of Wyke)(79) and the intraarticular nociceptors that appear to accompany intra-articular inclusions such as joint meniscoids(88). These nociceptors, when irritated by mechanical or chemical stimuli, transmit local joint pain that may then initiate arthrogenic muscle spasms especially of the segmental musculature(79). In addition, referred pain may arise as a consequence of activation of convergent neurones(89).

This referred pain has been described as a "sclerotogenous" type of referral. Feinstein et al(90) and Kellgren(91) have experimentally irritated facet joints and mapped the corresponding zones of pain. Representative depictions from Feinsten's work of pain referrals from upper cervical joints are shown in Figure 9.20.

Involvement of the cervical and craniocervical joints in headache takes two general forms: first, joint dysfunction and second, osteoarthritis. Joint dysfunction describes a spectrum of mechanical derangements affecting the static and dynamic capacities of a synovial joint. These have been alluded to by manipulative practitioners in all of their writings and have been described as "subluxations" (chiropractic)(146), "fixation" (chiropractic), osteopathic lesion, and joint blockage (medical manipulators). This dysfunction involves a static misalignment, a hypomobility, a paradoxical mobility, or an excess of mobility below the threshold of frank instability. The role of joint dysfunction in headaches was alluded to by numerous authors, some of whom were mentioned in the preceding literature review (see also Ref. 46). Certainly, Schimek and Mohr's(66) description of joint dysfunction as the "generator" of muscle spasm and pain about the head, Boake's(36) description of upper cervical joint dysfunction being responsible for 70% of all headaches, Jirout's(68) finding of headaches in 90% of individuals with C2–C3 dysfunction, and Bogduk's(52) mention of upper cervical hypomobility as the major cause of headaches previously termed "muscle contraction-type" all point to a consensus in the literature on the primary role of joint dysfunction in the production of headache.

Joint derangements of C0–C1, C1–C2, and C2–C3 may initiate direct sclerotogenous referral of cranial pain. The finding of C1 afferents in the facial region(44) gives rise to the possibility of a wide distribution of referred pain from the occiput-atlas segment. Joint derangements cause arthrogenic spasm of the suboccipital muscles, which may then lead to muscular pain syndromes in a manner similar to that described above for the regional musculature.

Pain arising from the upper cervical joints may converge with and facilitate the sec-

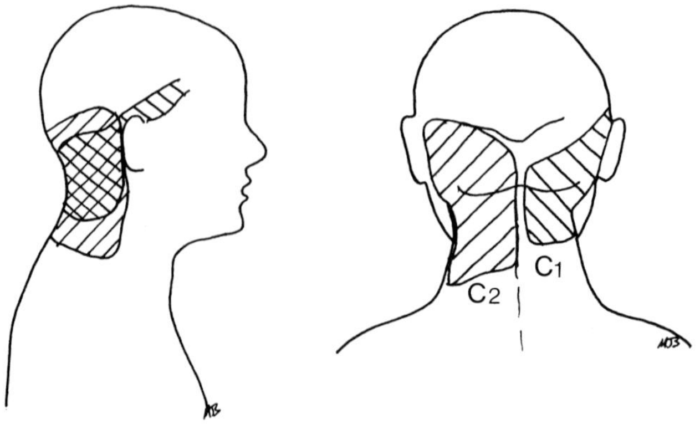

Figure 9.20. Zones of pain referral from the interspinous tissues of C1 and C2. After Feinstein B, et al. Experiments on pain referred from deep somatic tissues. J Bone Joint Surg 1954;36A:981–997.

ond order neurons in the spinal tract of the trigeminal nerve. Pain from upper cervical joint dysfunction may then appear to radiate to the frontotemporal region, an area distinct from the typical "dermatomal" distributions of the C1 and C2 nerve roots.

The second category of joint afflictions involved in headaches is osteoarthrotic changes. Edmeads' review(69) of this aspect of cervicogenic head pain is exhaustive. Suffice it to say that joint pain and stiffness that accompany the degenerative joint process often give rise to headaches.

At least one author(148) has implicated intervertebral disc lesions in disturbances of the spinal tract of the trigeminal nerve. These would likely occur at C2–C3 or C3–C4 as it is doubtful that the spinal tract of V descends any lower in the cervical cord(128). An important feature of osteoarthrosis is the degenerative changes that occur in the uncovertebral joints or the lateral atlantoaxial joints. Osteophytic outgrowths from these joints may affect the C2 nerve root (at C1–C2), the vertebral artery (at C1–C6), and the posterior sympathetic chain that ascends with the vertebral artery. Encroachments on these structures may initiate reflex spasm or occlusion of the vertebral artery or other neurogenic disturbances (see Neck-Tongue Syndrome in Chapter 12).

Infrasegmental. This mechanism involves disturbances of the nerve roots, dorsal root ganglia, and preganglionic sympathetic fibers in the environs of the intervertebral foramina or, as in the case of the C1 and C2 nerve roots, in the osseoligamentous environs of the posterior arches of the atlas and axis. Hunter and Mayfield(20) were the first to report on the significance and vulnerability of the C2 nerve root in the genesis of head and facial pains. The earlier chiropractic conception of a "pinched nerve" has given way to the concept of progressive, low-level compressive neuropathy created by a spectrum of predegenerate(81) and degenerative changes in the boney environs of the nerve root. Gunn(81) and Luttges and Triano(92, 93) have summarized these progressive alterations in nerve function. Gunn uses the term "denervation hypersensitivity" to describe the functional changes that arise from such a neuropathy. The nerve root is far more vulnerable to lower levels of compression than is the peripheral nerve(93). Luttges and Triano report significant reduction of conduction velocity at 10 times less compression of the nerve root than the peripheral nerve. Gunn's description of these changes is depicted in Table 9.12. The important consideration for our discussion on vertebrogenic headaches is the vulnerability of the C1 and C2 nerve roots, which are not protected by an intervertebral foramen or a nerve root canal. Inflammatory reactions around the synovial

Table 9.12
Effects of Denervation Supersensitivity and Chronic Nerve Root Irritation according to Gunn and Luttges and Gerren

Accord to Gunn[a]	According to Luttges and Gerren[b]
(1) Increased sensitivity at motor end plate to circulating neurotransmitters—especially to acetylcholine.	(1) Modification of receptor sensitivity.
(2) Spontaneous (ectopic) discharge or fibrillation.	(2) Altered fiber projection into cord.
(3) Increased ability to receive synaptic contacts.	(3) Altered sensory input into cord with subsequent changes in cord cells.
(4) Disturbed afference.	(4) Altered function of Schwann and other supporting cells.
(5) Denervated primary afferent fibers may reduce endorphin and enkephalin stores in laminae I, II, and III.	(5) Sprouting.
	(6) Abnormal reinervation.
	(7) Ventral root afferentation.
	(8) Altered temporal pattern of input.
	(9) Ephaptic transmission (sensory activation by sympathetics).

[a]Adapted from Gunn CC. "Prespondylosis" and some pain syndromes following denervation supersensitivity. Spine 1980; 5(2):185–192.
[b]Adapted from Luttges MW, Gerren RA. Nerve compression: nerves and roots. In: Haldeman S, ed. Modern developments in the principles and practice of chiropractic. New York: Appleton-Century-Crofts, 1979.

joints between C0 and C3, hypermobility especially at C1–C2, combined hyperextension/torsional impingement of the C2 dorsal root ganglion (see Chapter 1), and osteophytic encroachments from the posterolateral margins of C1–C2 and C2–C3 joints are all potential sources of nerve root irritation. According to the model of Gunn, these low-level chronic stresses, so much a part of the consequences of the typical pathogenesis of spinal degenerative joint disease, produce referred pains in the cranium, myalgic tender zones, sustained hypertonicity of the craniocervical muscles subserved by these nerve roots, and disturbed afference into the spinal cord resulting in a lowering of the "pain gate"(94) and facilitation of the motor pools. As such, the pain of "muscle contraction headache" may have a decidedly more neurogenic cause than is presently considered.

Included in this infrasegmental set of mechanisms is irritation of the ascending sympathetic chain structures. As Grillo pointed out(7), the autonomic structures are divided into posterior and anterior compartments. The posterior sympathetic structures ascend with the vertebral artery. They are loosely referred to as the vertebral nerve. Compression or rotational irritation can be exerted from the posterior facet joints in the manner described by Kovacs that was presented earlier.

The anterior chain is composed of the preganglionic fibers melding into three cervical ganglia: inferior, middle, and superior. Postganglionic fibers ascend from the superior cervical ganglion into the cranium. A discussion of sympathetic mechanisms in vertebrogenic headache will be presented below in the section on vertebrogenic migraine.

Intrasegmental. Normal reflex function and the consequent control of normal physiological responses depend in large part on the nature of sensory input into the spinal cord. Melzack and Wall(94) first proposed that particular patterns and intensities of sensory input might exert a modulating effect on the ultimate transmission of pain in the central nervous system. Korr and his colleagues(95–97, 98) proposed that somatic stimulation could have profound effects on the spinal motor and autonomic pools by creating what was called a state of central facititation or the "central excitatory state." In this state, more or less constant excitatory postsynaptic potentials combined with a release of inhibitory or suppressive mechanisms serve to increase the "gain" on output behavior of the effector pools or the second-order sensory pathways, thus producing persistent and inappropriate motor and autonomic discharge. This is expressed as sustained muscular contraction, sustained vasoconstriction, and hypersudation, as well as persistent transmission of pain(98).

When these disturbances of central or spinal reflex behavior are considered in the area of the upper cervical spine, attention must focus on the local motor pools and the spinal tract of the trigeminal nerve. The first-order sensory neurons of the trigeminus descend into the spinal cord and terminate on second-order neurons in the C1–C2 and possibly C3 neuromeres (see Figure 9.21). These second-order neurons also receive terminations from the C1 and C2 nerve roots. Boake refers to this situation as an "anastomosis" of nerve endings"(36). The practical considerations, for our purposes, are that disturbed or nociceptive impulses from the C1 and C2 nerve roots (via any of the sources of somatic irritation discussed above) will converge on and facilitate—by spatial and temporal

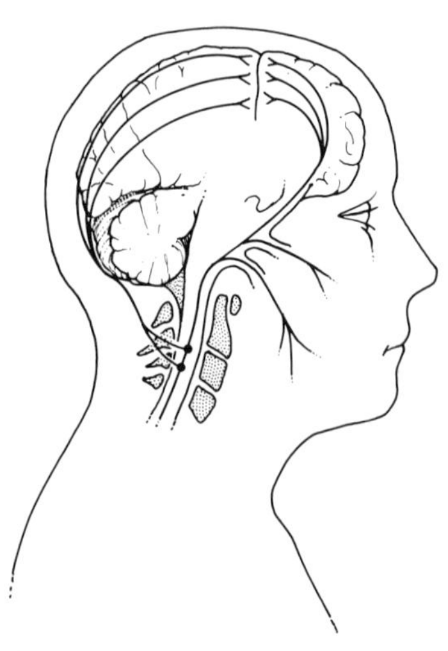

Figure 9.21. Synapse of C2 and C3 afferents with the spinal tract of the fifth cranial nerve in the nucleus subcaudalis.

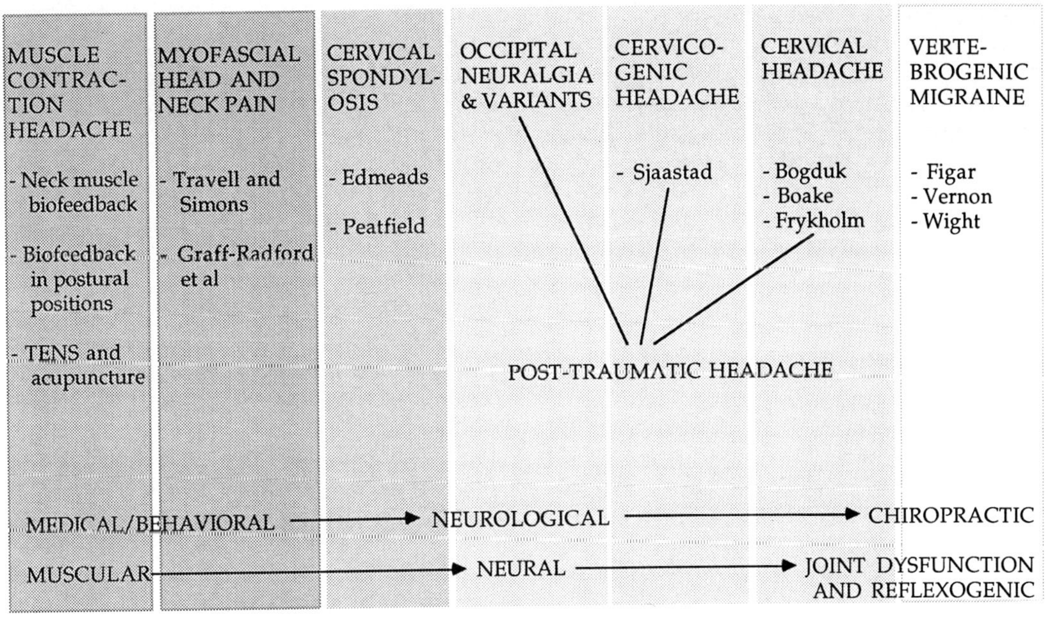

Table 9.13. Current status of vertebrogenic headache

summation—the second-order neurons of the spinal tract of the V. In the discussion below on vertebrogenic migraine, further central terminations from the locus ceruleus will be discussed. Thus, referred pain in the trigeminal sensory distribution can arise from upper cervical joint dysfunction. Facilitation of the motor pools would create sustained muscular hypertonicity in the craniocervical region consistent with the model of the arthrogenic reflex of Wyke(79).

In summary, central facilitation of the upper cervical cord by somatic input from joint dysfunction would create pain and muscle contraction in the cranial region again, pointing to a neurogenic etiology of muscle contraction headache pain contrasted with the psychogenic etiology of primary muscle contractions in the craniocervical muscles as proposed in the current medical model.

Vertebrogenic Migraine

There are several mechanisms that are of particular interest to a vertebrogenic model of migraine.

Mechanisms

Intersegmental. Osteophytic or facet joint encroachment on the vertebral artery, vertebral nerve, or sympathetic plexus has been implicated by numerous authors including Bartschi-Rochaix(17), Kovacs(24), Frykholm(37), and Edmeads(69) in the production of migraine-like prodromata and pain.

Infrasegmental. Irritation of the postganglionic fibers in the lowest cervical intervertebral foramina has been implicated in the production of cerebral vasoconstriction. Ghavamian(35) reported on relief of migraine symptoms in individuals undergoing surgical decompression of the lower cervical nerve roots. Direct irritation of the superior cervical ganglion(108) would produce vasoconstriction of the internal cerebral vasculature along with a host of other "vegetative symptoms" that have as their basis reflex reduction of blood supply to various cranial structures(71). This direct irritation can occur in posttraumatic states or possibly as a result of mechanical derangement (torsional hypermobility) of the atlantoaxial joint(99).

Intrasegmental. The vertebrogenic model of migraine proposes that disturbed somatoautonomic reflexes can be responsible for disordered cerebrovascular tone—specifically for the vasoconstrictive phase of the migraine cascade. Clinical and anecdotal observations support the existence of symptoms arising from the cervical spine, which are mediated by excessive discharge from the cervical sympathetic system (see Chapter 10).

Basic Scientific Evidence

It has been known for over 25 years that the arterial vessels on the surface and inside the brain are innervated by sympathetic nerve fibers that arise from the superior cervical ganglion (see Figure 9.22). Rosenblum(100) and Krog(101) provided early experimental evidence for the effect of neuronal influences on cerebral circulation. Several studies in the early 1970s(102–106) convincingly demonstrated the presence of adrenergic receptors on the pial vessels. The functional role of this innervation has been the subject of much study and debate. As reviewed by Wei et al, some of the early studies showed that pial vessels were responsive to chemical or electrical stimulation of the adrenergic fibers that terminated in their vessel walls(107), while other studies could not demonstrate such a response. Kobayashi, Waltz, and Rhoton(108) found that stimulation of the cervical sympathetic trunk produced ipsilateral reduction of cerebral blood flow in cats as well as arteriolar constriction. Inappropriate or dissociated responses of cerebral blood flow and arteriolar caliber also occurred leading them to propose "that vessels smaller than 50 microns are largely responsible for the regulation of cerebral blood flow (CBF), are innervated by sympathetic fibers, and may react to sympathetic stimulation differently than do larger arterioles. Impairment of vascular reactivity by stimulation may be an acute phenomenon induced by repetitive vasoconstriction" (Ref. 108 p 302). Wei et al on the other hand found that only arterioles larger than 100 microns were responsive to stimulation and manifested a narrowing of the vessel caliber (i.e., vasoconstriction). They found that physiological levels of experimental stimulation produced an average of 7% reduction in vessel caliber with a maximum of 18% under potentiated conditions. They concluded that such vasoconstriction could account for a "modest reduction in cerebral blood flow" (Ref. 107 p 654).

As reported by Rubin et al(109), a study

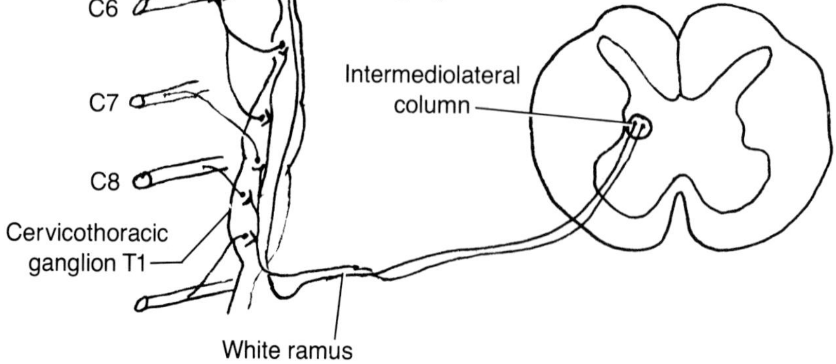

Figure 9.22. Sympathetic nerve supply in the cervical spine.

by Meyer et al(110) demonstrated a 30% decrease in the arterial flow in the internal carotid artery in the monkey upon stimulation of the cervical sympathetic trunk, while Edvinsson et al(102) found that regional cerebral blood flow is reduced in response to electrical stimulation of the cervical sympathetic nerves and that the magnitude of this response was related to the amount of local perivascular innervation. It is agreed that numerous factors determine the arterial response to sympathetic stimulation including vessel size(107) and the number of vasodilatory mechanisms and local circulating metabolites(106) (also see: 123–127, 129).

This brief review of the neurophysiological mechanisms of cerebrovascular regulation prompts us to ask about Its clinical relevance or application. It is obvious that if the vascular model of migraine is to be accepted, then these experiments support the contention that there is a role for the autonomic nervous system in the etiology of migraine. Rubin et al have written an important work that both reviews the implications of the "autonomic theory" of migraine and provides evidence in support of this theory. This theory is described as follows: "The neurological symptoms of the prodromal phase of classic migraine result from vasoconstriction due to the neurally released noradrenaline acting on alpha and beta adrenoreceptors. The vessels ultimately dilate possibly assisted by the presence of vasodilator metabolites accumulated during the constrictor phase or perhaps by a reflex inhibition of the constrictor drive" (Ref. 109 P 40). This theory is markedly in contrast to the biochemical model that asserts the role of serotonin as derived from altered platelet membranes in the vasoconstriction of cerebral arterioles(111). Rubin et al measured pupillary function and psychological measures of neuroticism, anxiety, and depression. They found a sympathetic dysfunction consisting of a hypofunction of the sympathetic nervous system under stress in common migraineurs. This hypofunctional disturbance of autonomic tone was correlated with higher states of personality dysfunction, i.e., higher neurotic and depressive tendencies. They assert that since the autonomic nervous system is the mediating system of emotional behavior in the physiological milieu of the body, emotional disturbances might manifest themselves as a disturbance of autonomic regulatory tone sufficient to produce the episodic and acute disruptions in cerebrovascular circulation characteristic of migraine.

The vertebrogenic model of migraine accepts the "autonomic theory" but asserts a somatic/neurogenic source of disturbed autonomic regulatory function. Is there experimental support for this contention?

Bouquet et al(57) have studied somatic and vegetative parameters thought to be associated in the etiology of migraine. They studied trapezius muscle tone (by eletromyography) and peripheral autonomic tone (by blood pressure, heart rate, and electrical skin resistance) in 12 migraneurs and 12 subjects with postconcussional vertigo. They found that trapezius muscle tone always increased on the side of increases in sympathetic tone that appeared in the period antecedent to a migraine or vertigo crisis. Trapezius muscle hypertonicity was always ipsilateral to the side of pain in the migraineurs. The muscle tone increases were correlated with increases in vegetative tone. Bouquet et al proposed the following model to explain the interaction of somatic structures and the autonomic system in the genesis of the migraine cascade: somatic dysfunction in the craniocervical region (consisting of muscular hypertonicity and joint/muscle nociception(66) creates disturbed afference (noxious irritation), which leads to activation of the spinoreticular tract that produces central facilitation of the autonomic system. From a behavioral point of view, this is experienced as tachycardia, increased aggressivity, hypersudation, peripheral vasoconstriction, and increase in postural muscle tonus (i.e., the state of "sympathicotonia" of Korr)(95), (also see below). This produces an overall state of vascular dysregulation, an increase in postsynaptic excitation potentials that in the somatic motor pools, creates excess muscular activity and, most surprisingly, a destabilization of the central aminergic system with increased aminergic discharges. This would lead to deactivation of the central pain inhibiting pathways and a vicious cycle of escalating dysfunction. Under potentiated conditions, this would lead to cerebral vasoconstriction via discharges from facilitated preganglionic cells.

These experimental findings are predicted by the "facilitation theory" of Korr(96), which states that nociceptive somatic input will facilitate the segmental effector pools (motor, autonomic, pain pathways) leading to abnormal input/output relationships. Hinoki and Niki(112) have found that excessive sympathetic discharge is a cause of muscular hypertonicity by causing overexcitation of β-receptors in injured neck muscles of subjects suffering from postwhiplash cervicogenic vertigo. These findings probably parallel those of Bouquet et al and allow us to conceptualize a vicious cycle of increased sympathetic and motor tone leading to transient cerebral vasoconstriction and cervicogenic vertigo. When this information is integrated with that describing the excitation of the peripheral sympathetic trunks in the cervical region (especially the superior cervical ganglion and the "third neuronal sympathetic pathway," according to Vijayan(45), then a very plausible mechanism emerges, which causally links somatic dysfunction to the autonomic disturbance that is responsible for the migraine phenomenon.

This somatoautonomic model can also be integrated with the emerging neuronal model arising from the work of Lance et al(113), Bates et al(114) and De La Torre et al(115) among others(135).

This work involves the experimental delineation of a neuronal center—the locus ceruleus—as the source of neural control of the migraine cascade. Their work on cats and monkeys has shown that low-frequency stimulation of the locus ceruleus produces vasconstriction of the internal cerebral vasculature; and increasing frequencies of stimulation produce vasodilation of the external carotid artery and its branches. These changes are predominantly ipsilateral. The vasoconstriction was presumed to be effected by noradrenaline since "the locus ceruleus is known to project to the cerebral cortex via noradrenergic fibers"(113). The vasodilation was found to be mediated by the facial and greater superficial petrosal nerves "employing a noncholinergic transmitter agent." This work also highlights the importance of the trigeminal nerve in the production of vasodilation of the external carotid circulation and in the modulation and transmission of pain in the frontotemporal region, which is so typical a location for the migraine headache. The trigeminal sensory system interacts with the second-order neurons found in the first to third cervical neuromeres via the spinal tract of the trigeminus. These same second-order neurons receive pain afferents from the first to third cervical roots.

The locus ceruleus projects a noradrenergic pathway to the upper cervical spinal cord that inhibits pain transmission. Lance et al hypothesize that "an exhaustion phase" might occur in the locus ceruleus output via the descending inhibitory pathways, which would then allow the trigeminal system to override vascular control and pain transmission systems thus effecting the migraine cascade. Lance et al conclude that "since the locus ceruleus is a central analogue of the sympathetic ganglia(113), any of the accepted migraine triggers could influence locus ceruleus activity."

In summary, two operational descriptions consistent with the clinical and experimental literature can be proposed:

(1) Somatic dysfunction of the C7–T4 vertebral levels causes joint pain and joint fixation. This leads to local segmental facilitation and consequently, to sustained discharges from the sympathetic chain. This leads to transient cerebral ischemia, which under potentiated conditions, might reach a threshold level sufficient to create cerebral ischemia that then activates the migraine cascade. Increased catecholamine levels would result from the subthreshold central excitation and would have direct effects on platelet membranes.

(2) Somatic dysfunction in the upper cervical spine-C0–C2 produces local pain and fixation. The upper cervical neuromeres become facilitated reducing the inhibitory effect of the descending pain pathways (at least one of which arises from the locus ceruleus) and increasing the facilitation of the second-order neurons in the spinal tract of the

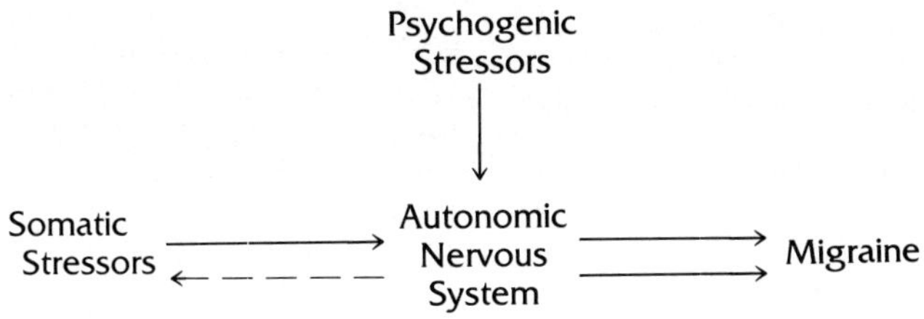

Figure 9.23. Somatoautonomic model of migraine etiology. *Dotted line,* somatosympathetic positive feedback cycle.

trigeminus. This leads to transient stimulation of the locus ceruleus, which, upon reaching threshold levels, results in focal and spreading vasoconstriction in the intracerebral circulation, which then leads to a secondary vasodilation of the extracarotid circulation with cranial pain being mediated by the ipsilateral trigeminal nerve.

Since, as Rubin et al have stated, emotional or psychogenic factors are also extremely important correlates of autonomic dysfunction and migraine(109), it is most appropriate to propose that the somatic and psychogenic components discussed above act in an integrated fashion, one potentiating the other in the manner described in Figure 9.23.

The Vertebrogenic Model: An Integrated Model?

While the Ad Hoc Committee on Headache definitions for muscle contraction, common and classical migraine, and mixed headache are undoubtedly distinct and, excepting the latter, nonoverlapping(116 and 136), there is a spectrum of thought on the etiology of benign headache types that ranges from a set of totally distinct etiological theories for each type to an integrated model that proposes a single underlying etiology or etiological complex for these various headache types. Exemplifying the former is the work of Oleson and his colleagues and Rose(117, 118, 119) in which it is proposed that even common and classical migraine are distinct both symptomatically and etiologically. At the other end of the spectrum, Featherstone(120) has asked whether muscle contraction headache and migraine are separate entities. He has proposed a "severity model" for which he supplies supportive data in the finding that various clusters of different headache symptoms do not correlate well with specific diagnoses such as muscle contraction headache or migraine, but that severity of a large pool of common symptoms does distinguish the groups. Muscle contraction headache sufferers experience the same type of symptoms as do migraineurs, however, the symptoms are far less severe, and in some cases, insignificantly so, than those of migraine sufferers. Muscle contraction and common and classical migraine are then linked to one another on a severity spectrum from low to high (see Figure 9.24 and Refs. 130, 131, 137).

Ramirez(121) has recently reviewed the biofeedback literature and draws attention to the tenuous nature of the assumption that muscle contraction headache results from increased tonicity of the craniocervical musculature. He cites differential and contradictory results from the therapeutic literature, as well as evidence of a lack of correspondence between high-tension states and head pain and low-tension states and lack of head pain(122). His conclusion is consistent with that of this author, that "increments in muscle tension are an *effect* of headache pain rather than the cause" (Ref. 122 p 339). While he does not propose an alternative mechanism for the production of headache pain, and while he ultimately favors psychosocial interventions in the treatment of headache, his articulation of an emerging hypothesis debunking the traditional model of muscle contraction headache is supportive of the etiological mechanisms proposed by the vertebrogenic model, i.e., that headache pain is

Severity	Low	————	High
Autonomic involvement	None	————	Substantial
Diagnosis			
Muscle contraction		Common migraine	Classical migraine
Mechanism(?)			
Somatic exclusive		Somatic/ autonomic, low	Somatic/ autonomic, high

Figure 9.24. Headache severity model. Adapted from Featherstone HJ. Migraine and muscle contraction headaches: a continuum. Headache 1985;25:194–198.

derived from noncranial sources of somatic pain, particularly from the upper cervical spine, which are referred to the cranial area.

Can the vertebrogenic model be interfaced with the severity model? And if so, would this increase the validity of the model itself? It is my proposal that a mechanism can be proposed that fulfills the requirements of the severity model, which are that a lower order activation of this mechanism would find, as its expression, muscle contraction headache and a higher order activation of the same mechanism would produce a set of consequences whose increasing severity would express itself as the migraine phenomenon. Simply put, this mechanism would have to produce, at one end of the spectrum, somatic head pain, and at the other end, somatic head pain plus vascular dysregulation. Figures 9.25 and 9.26 depict a model that conceptually links somatic dysfunction with facilitation of the central nervous system, which in a progressive fashion, would produce the necessary spectrum of events.

This model also allows us to propose that the somatic dysfunction-facilitation complex may act as a potentiator of other etiological processes. The effect of psychogenic stressors on the craniocervical muscles would be potentiated by coexisting somatic dysfunction. This would apply equally to the responsiveness of the sympathetic system to a variety of stressors that have been causally linked to migraine.

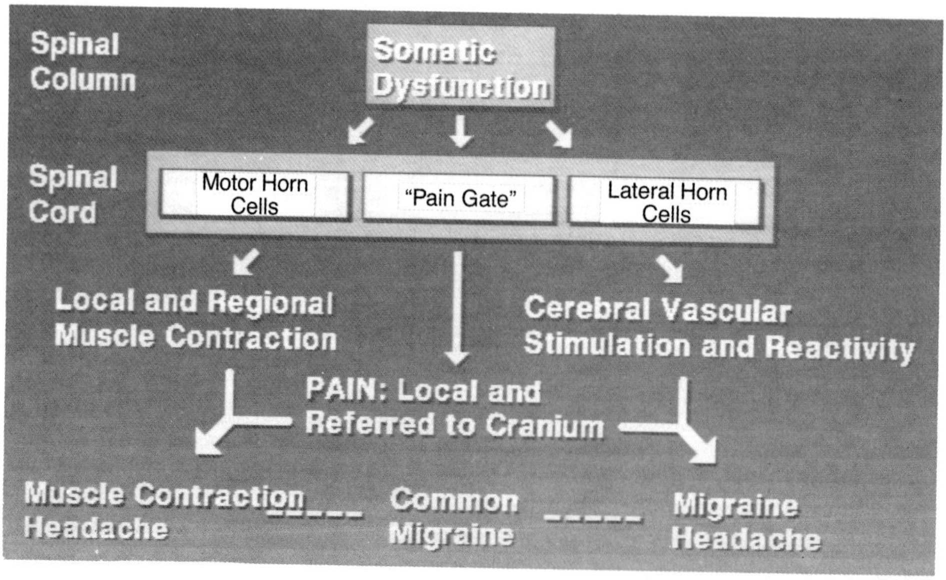

Figure 9.25. Facilitation theory of somatic dysfunction applied to a chiropractic model of benign headaches.

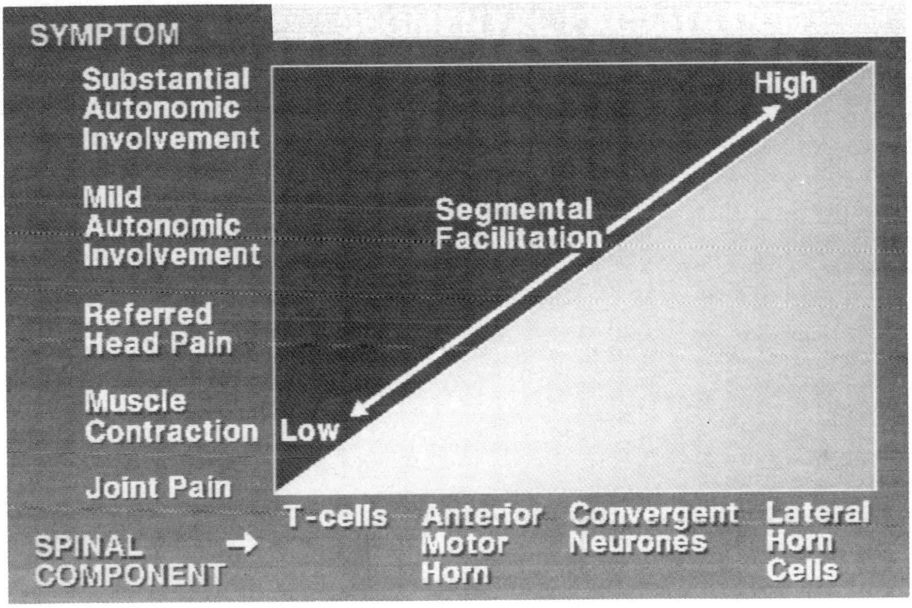

Figure 9.26. Model of progressive facilitation applied to headache.

CONCLUSION

It is the conclusion of this paper that the head pains of "muscle contraction headache sufferers" may in fact be the pain referred to the cranium by somatic structures in the craniocervical region, (Fig. 9.27) and somatic dysfunctions in this same region may be responsible for the autonomic dysfunction of migraine. (Fig. 9.28).

This allows us to propose three categories of headache sufferers:

(1) Those in whom the vertebrogenic component is etiological. This group ideally will derive primary benefit from spinal manipulative therapy;

(2) Those in whom the vertebrogenic component is secondary but synergistic. This group ideally could benefit from

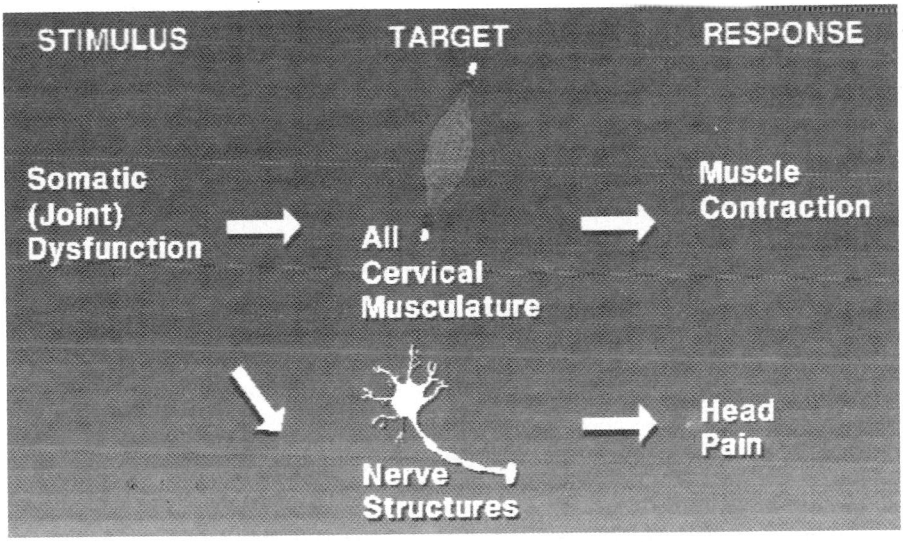

Figure 9.27. Chiropractic model of muscle and contraction headache.

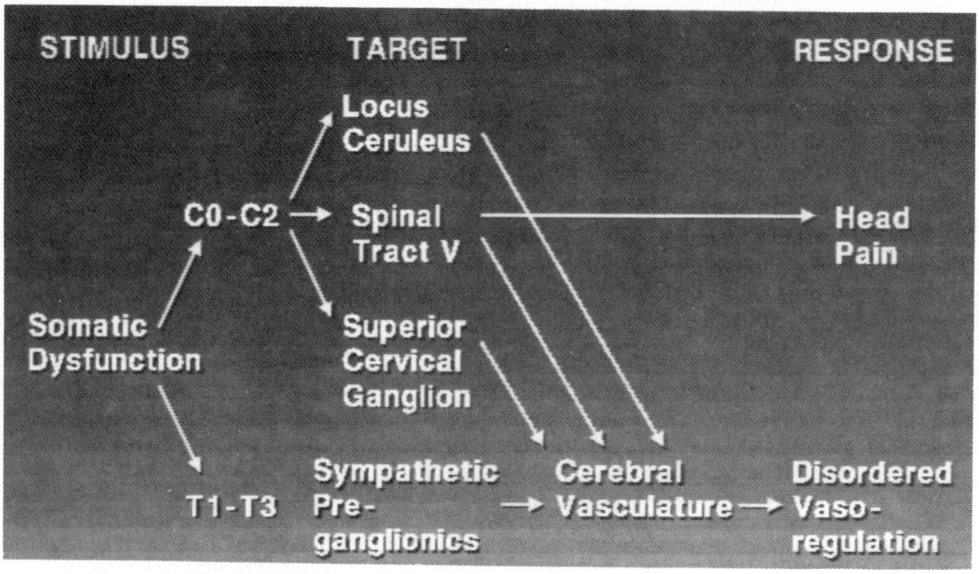

Figure 9.28. Chiropractic model of migraine headache.

spinal manipulative therapy in conjunction with other therapeutic meaures;

(3) Those in whom there was a negligible vertebrogenic component and for whom manipulation would provide no benefit.

The challenge of the future is to design effective research strategies with the following objectives:

(1) To determine the clinical ramifications of the vertebrogenic model and to demonstrate to what extent chiropractic manipulative therapeutics might be efficacious in the treatment of benign headaches;

(2) To further *explain* the mechanisms whereby vertebral dysfunction might promote headache and spinal manipulation might relieve it. As this is accomplished, the ultimate objective of integrating chiropractic management with orthodox therapies in the treatment of benign headache will be accomplished.

Refrences

1. Diamond S, Dalessio DJ. The practicing physician's approach to headache. Muscle contaction headache. Baltimore: Williams & Wilkins, 1978, pp 94–103.
2. Edmeads J. Headache. Sandoz Monograph, 1980.
3. Graham JR. Seven common headache profiles. Neurology 1963;13(2):16–23.
4. Loban JM. Technic and practice of chiropractic. 4th ed. Denver: Bunn-Loban, 1928.
5. Kelner M, Hall O, Coulter ID. Chiropractors—do they help? Toronto: Fitzhenry and Whiteside, 1980.
6. Droz JM, Crot F. Occipital headaches: statistical results in the treatment of vertebragenous headache. Swiss Annals VIII 1985, pp 127–136.
7. Grillo F. The differential diagnosis and therapy of headache. Swiss Annals 11, 1961, pp 121–166.
8. Valentini E. The occipito-cervical region. Ann Swiss Chiro Assoc IV, 1969, 225–232.
9. Hudzinski LG. Neck musculature and EMG biofeedback in the tratment of muscle contraction headache. Headache 1983;23:86–90.
10. Ahles TA, King A, Martin JE. EMG biofeedback during dynamic movement as a treatment for tension headache. Headache 1984;24:41–44.
11. Sturgis ET, Schaefer CA, Ahles TA, Sikora TL. The effect of movement and position in the evaluation of tension headache and non-headache control subjects. Headache 1984;24:88–93.
12. Raskin NH, Howard MW, Ehrenfeld WK. Headache as the leading symptom of the thoracic outlet syndrome. Headache 1985;25:208–210.
13. Solomon S, Guglielmo KM. The treatment of headache by transcutaneous nerve stimulation. Headache 1985;25(1):12–14.
14. Fortin JF, Biller J. Neck tongue syndrome. Headache 1985;25:255–258.
15. Barré J. Sur un syndrome sympathetique cervical posterieure et sa cause frequente: l'arthrite cervicale. Rev Neurol 1926;45:1246. Cit. by Sand-

strom J. Cervical syndrome with vestibular symptoms. Acta Otolaryngol 1961;54:207.
16. Lieou YC, Syndrome sympathetique cervical posterieur et arthrite chronique. These de Strasbourg 1928. Cit. by Sandstrom J. Cervical syndrome with vestibular symptoms. Acta Otolaryngol 1961;54:207.
17. Bartschi-Rochaix W. Headaches of cervical origin. In: Vinkin PJ, Bruyn GN, eds. Handbook of clinical neurology. Vol. 5. Amsterdam: North Holland Pub Co, 1968 pp. 192–201.
18. Beckwith C. Headache. J Am Osteopath Assoc 1949;48:385–387.
19. Beckwith C. Migraine pathophysiology and manipulative treatment. Yearbook Am Assoc Osteo path 1953, pp, 5–8.
20. Hunter CR, Mayfield FH. The role of the upper cervical roots in the production of pain in the head. Am J Surg 1949;78:743–51.
21. Geiger W. "Zur Zevicalen Migraine." Deutsch Med 1952; 7:198.
22. Gayral L, Neuwlrth E. Oto-neuropthalmologic manifestations of cervical origin. NY State J Med 1954;54:1920–26.
23. Skillern PG. Great occupital-trigeminus syndrome as revealed by induction block. Arch Neurol Psychiatry 1954;72:335–40.
24. Kovacs A. Subluxation and deformation of the cervical apophyseal joints: a contribution to the etiology of headache. Acta Radiol 1955;43:1–16.
25. Jackson R. The cervical syndrome. Springfield, IL. 3rd ed. Charles C Thomas, 1966.
26. Seletz E. Headache of extracranial origin. Calif Med 1958;89:314–319.
27. Brain L. Some unsolved problems of cervical spondylosis. Br Med J 1963;1:771–777.
28. Trevor-Jones R. Osteoarthritis of the paravertebral joints of the second and third cervical vertebrae as a cause of occipital headache. S Afr Med J 1964;38:392–395.
29. Figar S, Jansky M. Studies of vascular reflexes in cases of vertebrogenic migraine. Acta Univ. Carolina Supl 21:1964;76–79.
30. Travell J. Mechanical headache. Headache 1967;7:27–29.
31. Robertson AM. Manipulation in cervical syndromes. Practitioner 1968;200:396–402.
32. Dutton CB, Riley LH Jr. Cervical migraine: not merely a pain in the neck. Am J Med 1969;47:141–148.
33. Lewit K. Ligament pain and anteflexion headache. Eur Neurol 1971;5:365–378.
34. Lewit K. Pain arising from the posterior arch of the atlas. Eur Neurol 1977;16:263–269.
35. Ghavamian T. Cervical discopathy and a new concept in the sympathetics of the cervical spine and head. J Bone Joint Surg 1971;53A:1233.
36. Boake HK. Cervical headache. Can Fam Phys May 1972;18:75–78.
37. Frykholm R. Cervical migraine: the clinical picture. In: Hirsch C, Zotterman Y, eds. Cervical pain. Oxford England: Pergammon Press, 1972, pp 13–16.
38. Hargrave-Wilson W. The cervical syndrome. Am J Physiother 1972;18(4):144–147.
39. Webber TD. Diagnosis and modification of headache and shoulder-arm-hand syndrome. J Am Osteop Assoc 1973;76:697–710.
40. Pozniak-Patewicz E. "Cephalgic" spasm of head and neck musculature. Headache 1976;15:261–265.
41. Schultz DR. Occipital neuralgia. J Am Osteop Assoc 1977;76:335–343.
42. Gutman G. Kofelenke und Kopfshmerz. Man Med 1977; Heft 1:1–16.
43. Mountjoy G. Migraine mitigated by manipulation. Clin Trends Osteopath Med 1977;4:1–7.
44. Kerr F. Structural relation of the trigeminal spinal tract to the upper cervical roots and the solitary nucleus of the cat. Exp Neurol 1961;4:134–137.
45. Vijayan N. A new post-traumatic headache syndrome; clinical and therapeutic observations. Headache 1977;17:19–22.
46. Henderson DJ. Significance of vertebral dyskinesia in relation to the cervical syndrome. J Manipulative Physiol Ther 1979;2(1):3–15.
47. Hoyt W, et al. Osteopathic manipulation in the treatment of muscle-contracted headache. J Am Osteopath Assoc 1979;78:322–325.
48. Schoenholtz F. Conservative management of cervical tension cephalagia. J Chirop 1979;16(6):S-49-S-52.
49. Kramer J. Intervertebral disc diseases. Chicago: Yearbook Medical Publishers, 1981, pp 77.
50. Edeling J. The true cervical headache. S Abr Med 1982;62:531–534.
51. Ward RC. Headache: an osteopathic perspective. J Am Osteop Assoc 1982;81(7):458–66.
52. Bogduk N. Headaches and cervical manipulation. Med J Aust 1979;66(2):65–66.
53. Bogduk N. The anatomy of occipital neuralgia. Clin Exp Neurol 1981;17:167–184.
54. Bogduk N. A neurological approach to neck pain. In: Aspects of manipulative therapy. Glasgow EF, Twomey LT, Scall, ER, Kleynhans AM. Edczak RM, eds. New York: Churchill Livingston. 2nd ed. 1985, pp 136–141.
55. Freitag FG. Osteopathic manipulative treatment of migraine. J Am Osteop Assoc 1983; 11:254–258.
56. Schmidt IC. The etiology and treatment of headache. Osteopath Ann 1983;11(12):19–31.
57. Bouquet J, Moore N, Boismare F. Monnier JC. Vertigo in post-concussional and migraineous patients. Implication of the autonomic nervous system. Aggressologie 1983;24:235–236.
58. Graham JR In: Aronoff G, ed. Evaluation and treatment of chronic pain. Baltimore: Urban and Schwarzenberg, 1985.
59. Vernon H, Dhami MSI. Vertebrogenic migraine. J Can Chiro Assoc 1983;29(1):20–24.
60. Gallager RM. Headache and chronic pain. Osteopath Ann 1985;13(5):34, 39–46.
61. Sjaastad O, et al. "Cervicogenic headache: an hypothesis." Cephalalgia 1983;3:249–256.
62. Gillet H, ed. Belgian chiropractic research notes. 10th ed. Huntington, CA: Motion Palpation Institute, 1973.
63. Ng SY. Upper cervical vertebrae and occipital headache. J Manipulative Physiol Ther 1980;3(3):137–141.

64. Mannen EM. The use of cervical radiographic overlays to assess the response to manipulation. J Can Chiro Assoc 1980;24:108–111.
65. Vernon H. Manipulative therapy in the chiropractic treatment of headaches: a retrospective and prospective study. J Manipulative Physiol Ther 1982;5:109–112.
66. Schimek JJ, Mohr U. The importance of manual therapy in the treatment of chronic headache. Man Med 1984;22:41–45.
67. Miller B, Maxwell JL, DeBoer KF. Chiropratic treatment of tension headache; a case study. ACA J Chirop 1984;21:62–66.
68. Jirout J. Comments regarding the diagnosis and treatment of dysfunctions in the C2–C3 segment. Man Med 1985;2:16–17.
69. Edmeads J. Headaches and head pains associated with diseases of the cervical spine. Med Clin North Am 1978;62(3):533–541.
70. Wight JS. Migraine: a statistical analysis of chiropractic treatment. J Am Chiro Assoc 1978;12:363–67.
71. Ricci V, Santoni P. "La Vertigine Certicale." Nouvo Arch Ital Oto Suppl. 19;1979;7.
72. Rose P. Statistical analysis of chiropractic patients. Bull Eur Chiro Union 1973;22:22–23.
73. Parker GB, Tupling H, Pryor DS. A controlled trial of cervical manipulation for migraine. Aust NZ J Med 1978;8:589–93.
74. Commission of Inquiry into Chiropractic. Chiropractic in New Zealand. NZ PD Hasselberg, 1979.
75. Parker GB, Pryor DS, Tupling H. Why does migraine improve during a clinical trial? Further results from a trial of cervical manipulation for migraine. Aust NZ J Med 1980;10:192–198.
76. Sachse J, Eckhardt E, et al. Phenomenological investigation in migraine patients. Man Med 1982;20:59–64.
77. Feuerstein M, Bush C, Corbisiero R. Stress and chronic headache: a psychophysiological analysis of mechanisms. J Psychosom Res 1982;26:167–182.
78. Graham JR. Migraine headache: diagnosis and management. Headache 1979; 19(3):133–141.
79. Wyke BD. Articular neurology: a review. Physiotherapy 1972;58:94–99.
80. Gelb H (ed.) CLinical management of head, neck and TMJ pain and dysfunction: a multidisciplinary approah to diagnosis and treatment. Philadelphia: WB Saunders, 1977.
81. Gunn CC. "Prespondylosis" and some pain syndromes following denervation supersensitivity. Spine 1980;5(2):185–192.
82. Melzack R. Myofascial trigger points: relation to acupuncture and mechanisms of pain. Arch Phys Med Rehabil 1981;62:114–117.
83. Simons CJ, Day E, Goodell H, Wolff HG. Experimental studies on headache: muscles of the scalp and neck as sources of pain. Proc Assoc Res Nerv Dis 1943;23:228–244.
84. Simons DG. Myofascial trigger points: a need for understanding. Arch Phys Med Rehab 1981;62:97–99.
85. Tilscher H, Wessely P, Eder M. The typical relations between facial pain and suboccipital maximal points. Man Med 1982;20:127–130.
86. Chambers WR. Posterior rhizotomy of the second and third cervical nerves for occipital pain. J Am Med Assoc 1954;155(4):431–432.
87. Chouret EE. The greater occipital neuralgia headache. Headache, April 1967;7:33–34.
88. Bogduk N, Engel R. The menisci of the lumbar zygopophyseal joints: a review of their anatomy and clinical significance. Spine 1984;9(5):454–460.
89. Haldeman S. Referred pain—extraspinal symptoms of spinal origin. J Aust Chiro Assoc 1974;Jan/March:14–17.
90. Feinstein B, Langton JNK, Jameson RM, Schiller F. Experiments on pain referred from deep somatic tissues. J Bone Joint Surg 1954:36A:981–997.
91. Kellgren JH. On the distribution of pain arising from deep somatic structures with charts of segmental pain areas. Clin Sci 1939;4:35.
92. Luttges MW, Gerren RA. Nerve compression: nerves and roots. In: Haldeman S, ed. Modern developments in the principles and practice of chiropractic. New York: Appleton-Century-Crofts, 1979.
93. Triano JJ, Luttges MW. Nerve irritation: a possible model of sciatic neuritis. Spine 1982;7(2):129–136.
94. Melzack R, Wall PD. Pain mechanisms: a new theory. Science 1965;150:971–979.
95. Korr IM. Somatic dysfunction, osteopathic manipulative treatment and the nervous system: a few facts, some theories, many questions. J Am Osteopath Assoc 1986;86(2):109–113.
96. Korr IM. The neural basis of the osteopathic lesion. J Am Osteop Assoc 1947;47:191–95.
97. Korr IM. Propioceptors and the behavior of lesioned segments. Presented at: 71st Clinical Conference of the New York Academy of Osteopathy, New York, 1974.
98. Denslow J, Korr IM, Drems AD. Quantitative studies of chronic facilitation in human motoneuron pools. Am J Physiol 1947;150:229–238.
99. Carella A. Slight anomalies of the atlas: their pathogenetic meaning. Neuroradiology 1972;3:224–227.
100. Rosenblum WI. Cerebral microcirculation: a review emphasizing the interrelationship of local blood flow and neuronal function. Angiology 1965;16:485.
101. Krog J. Autonomic nervous control of the cerebral blood flow in man. J Oslo City Hosp 1964;14:25.
102. Edvinsson L, Nielsen KC, Owman CH, West KA. Adrenergic influence on brain vessels. Abstract Panminerva Med 1971;13:175.
103. Falck B, Nielsen KC, Owman C. Adrenergic innervation of the pial circulation. Abstract Scan J Clin Lab Invest Suppl 1968;102.
104. Nielsen KC, Owman C, Sporrong B. Ultrastructure of the autonomic innervation apparatus in the main pial arteries of rats and cats. Brain Res 1971;27:25–32.
105. Nielsen KC, Owman C. Contractile response and amine receptor mechanism in isolated middle cerebral artery of cat. Brain Res 1971;27:33–42.

106. Owman CH, Edvinsson L, Nielsen KC. Autonomic neuro-receptor mechanisms in brain vessels. In: Dynamics of regeneration and growth in neurons. Fuxe K, Olson L, Zotterman Y, eds. New York: Pergamon Press, 1974, pp. 535–560.
107. Wei EP, Raper AJ, Konstos HA, Patterson JL. Determinants of response of pial arteries to norepinephrine and sympathetic nerve stimulation. Stroke 1975;6:654–658.
108. Kobayashi S, Waltz AG, Rhoton AL. Effects of stimulation of cervical sympathetic nerves on cortical blood flow and vascular reactivity. Neurology 1971;21:297–302.
109. Rubin LS, Graham D, Pasker R, Calhoun W. Autonomic nervous system dysfunction in common migraine. Headache 1985;25:40–48.
110. Meyer JS, Yoshida K, Sakamoto D. Autonomic control of cerebral blood flow measured by electromagnetic flow meters. Neurology 1967;17:638–648.
111. Deshinvkh SR, Meyer JS. Cyclic changes in platelet dynamics and the pathogenesis and prophylaxis of migraine. Headache 1975;17:101–108.
112. Hinoki M, Niki H. Neurotological studies on the role of the sympathetic nervous system in the formation of traumatic vertigo of cervical origin. Acta Otolaryngol Suppl 1975;330:185–196.
113. Lance JW, Lambert GA, Goadsby PJ, Duckworth JW. Brainstem influences on the cephalic circulation: experimental evidence from cat and monkey of relevance to the mechanism of migraine. Headache 1983;23:258–265.
114. Bates D, Weinshilboum RM, Campbell RJ, Sundt M Jr. The effects of lesions in the locus ceruleus on the physiological responses of the cerebral vessels in cats. Brain Res 1977;136:431–443.
115. De La Torre JC, Surgeon JW, Walker RH. Effects of locus ceruleus stimulation on cerebral blood flow in selected brain regions. Acta Neurol Scand Suppl 1977;64,56:104–105.
116. Ad Hoc Committee on the classification of headache. J Am Med Assoc 1962,179:717 718.
117. Oleson J, Larsen B, Lauritzen A. Focal hyperemia followed by spreading oligemia and impaired activation of ,CBF in classical migraine. Ann Neurol 1981;9:344–352.
118. Oleson J. Migraine and regional cerebral blood flow. Trends Neurosci 1985;July:318–321.
119. Rose FC. The pathogenesis of a migraine attack. Trends Neurosci 1983;July:247–248.
120. Featherstone HJ. Migraine and muscle contraction headaches: a continuum Headache 1985;25:194–198.
121. Ramirez JJ. A critical analysis of the traditional tension headache model. Headache 1985;25:337–339.
122. Phillips C. Tension headache: theoretical problems. Behav Res Ther 1978;16:248–261.
123. Roy CS, Sherrington CS. On the regulation of the blood supply of the brain. J Physiol 1890;11:85–108.
124. Bill A, Linder J. Sympathetic control of cerebral blood flow in acute arterial hypertension. Acta Physiol Scand 1976;96:114–121.
125. Appenzeller O. Reflex vasomotor function: clinical and experimental studies in migraine. Res Clin Stud Headache 1978;6:160–166.
126. Figar S, Krausova L. A plethysmographic study of the effects of chiropratic treatment in vertebrogenic syndromes. Rev Czech Med 1965;84–86.
127. Figar S, Stary O, et al. Changes in vasomotor reflexes in painful vertebrogenic syndromes. Rev Czech Med 1964;10(4):238–246.
128. Denny-Brown D, Yanigasawa N. The function of the descending root of the fifth nerve. Brain 1973;96:783–814.
129. Parkinson D, Johnston J, Chaudhuri A. Sympathetic connections to the fifth and sixth cranial nerves. Anat Rec 1978;19(?):221–226.
130. Wilkinson M, Blau JN. Are classical and common migraine different entities? Headache 1985; 25:211–212.
131. Pikoff H. Is the muscular model of headache still viable? A review of conflicting data. Headache 1984;24:186–198.
132. Khurana RK, Nirankari VS. Bilateral sympathetic dysfunction in posttraumatic headaches. Headache 1986;26:183–188.
133. Neuwirth E. The vertebral nerve in the posterior cervical syndrome. Letter. NY State J Med 1955;55:1380.
134. Pressman AH. The neurobiology of migraine. J Chiropractic 1979;19:309–321.
135. Pearce JMS. Migraine: a cerebral disorder. Lanet 1984;July:86–89.
136. Wolff HG. Headache and other head pain. New York: Oxford University Press, 1963, pp 227–386.
137. Tunis MM, Wolff HG. Cranial artery vasoconstriction and muscle contraction headache. Arch Neurol Psychiatry 1980;2:135–141.
138. Kayfetz DO. Whiplash injury and other ligamentous headache—its management with prolotherapy. Headache 1963;3:21.
139. Schlesinger E. Treatment of head and neck pain associated with disorders of the neck and cervical spine. In: Friedman AP, ed. Modern treatment (Symposium on the treatment of headache). Vol 6. New York: Harper & Row, 1964, pp 1404–1411.
140. Blumenthal LS. Injury to the cervical spine as a cause of headache. Postgrad Med 1974;56:147–153.
141. Grieve GP. Manipulation therapy for neck pain. Physiotherapy 1979;65(5):136–144.
142. Robinson DA. Cervical spondylosis and muscle contraction headaches. In: Dalessio DJ, ed. Wolff's headache and other head pain. 4th ed. New York: Oxford, 1980.
143. Tfelt-Hansen P, Lou I, Oleson J. Prevalence and significance of muscle tenderness during common migraine attacks. Headache 1981;21:49–54.
144. Ehni G. Cervical arthrosis: diseases of the cervical motion segments. Chicago: Yearbook Medical Publ, 1984, p. 186.
145. Hussar CJ, Retzlaff EW, Mitchell FL, Kalbfell JJ, Briner BJ. Combined osteopathic and dental

treatment of cephalgia. Abstract. J Am Osteopath Assoc 1986;86(10):605–606.
146. Schafer RC, ed. Chiropractic physical and spinal diagnosis. 1st ed. Oklahoma City: Associated Chiropractic Academic Press, Oklahoma 1980, pp. VIII-26-27.
147. Travell JG, Simons DG. Myofascial pain and dysfunction. The trigger point manual. Baltimore: Williams & Wilkins, 1983.
148. Elvidge AR, Choh-Luh L. Central protrusion of cervical intervertebral disc involving the descending trigeminal tract. Arch Neurol Psychiatry 1950;63:455–466.
149. Graff-Radford SB, Reeves JL, Jaeger B. Management of chronic head and neck pain: effectiveness of altering factors perpetuating myofascial pain. Headache 1987; 27:186–190.
150. Turk Z, Ratkolb O. Mobilization of the cervical spine in chronic headaches. Man Med 1987;3:15–17.

10 Autonomic Nervous System Disturbances of Cervical Origin Including Disorders of Equilibrium

David J. Brunarski, B.Sc., D.C., F.C.C.S.

Like pain, autonomic dysfunction and disturbances of equilibrium are uniquely subjective perceptual phenomena. As clinicians we see the effects of these disturbances, but we continue to experience great difficulty in establishing indisputable evidence for our clinical impressions. For example, the term dizziness is imprecise and should be avoided in our clinical vocabulary. What is known is that human equilibrium exists as a perception of appropriate orientation of the body in space (1). This state is maintained and dependent upon the harmonious integration of afferent sensory impulses arriving from the labyrinths, myofascial proprioceptors, and eyes via the vestibular nuclei of the brainstem (2). Figure 10.1 illustrates the hierarchy of reflex pathways required to convey both afferent and efferent signals within the vestibular network. A normal person is still able to remain nearly motionless while standing with feet together and eyes closed (Romberg test) because there are two separate reflex controls of posture that supervene when the visual apparatus is eliminated. Gravity-dependent fluid compartments of the inner ear alert the vestibular nuclei about instantaneous changes of position. Reflex eye movements and reactions by the proprioceptive righting reflexes within the joints and soft tissues of the neck try to maintain orientation of the head. Signals may even be generated in the limbs if it is necessary to control gross body movements and stabilize posture(3, 4).

All three of the reflex mechanisms are interdependent and complementary. Therefore, any disharmony in neural responsiveness may cause aberrations of impulse that, in turn, manifst as clinical conditions (Table 10.1).

AUTONOMIC NERVOUS SYSTEM DYSFUNCTION

The autonomic nervous system serves as the functional arbiter of efferent peripheral signals. In the posterior cervical sympathetic syndrome of Barre-Lieou(5), dysfunction of the posterior joints of the cervical vertebrae produce entrapment effects on the spinal nerves and vertebral arteries. In this instance, somatosympathetic reflexes are initiated by musculoskeletal lesions(6). A vicious cycle of noxious inputs produce lowered thresholds to pain, increased muscle hypertonicity, decreased local blood flow (ischemia), negative neurotrophic consequences, and a central excitatory state (facilitation)(7). Apparently, mechanical derangements at the first through third cervical vertebrae produce the most extensive disturbances(8). The muscles most typically implicated in sustaining this suboccipital lesion complex (chiropractic subluxation) are the rectus

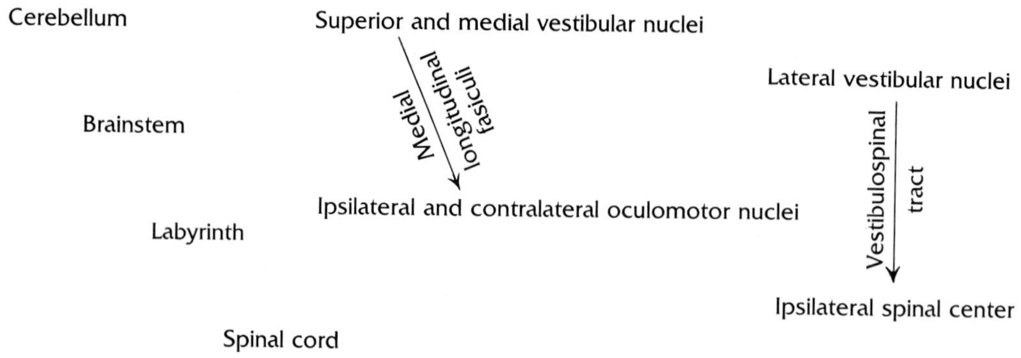

Figure 10.1. Integration of impulses in the maintenance of human equilibrium.

capitis posterior major, rectus capitis posterior minor, obliquus capitis superior, obliquus capitus inferior, rectus capitis anterior, and rectus capitis lateralis. These muscles all receive their nerve supply from the muscular branches of the first and/or second cervical nerves. Their blood supply is predominantly the muscular branches of the vertebral artery. Forward flexion of the neck and rotational movements of the head on the neck are compromised and painful(9). There may be coexisting symptoms of lightheadedness, nystagmus, and vertigo. A history of whiplash is characteristic, and cervical manipulation by a chiropractor is often relieving.

Disequilibrium

Disequilibrium implies that there is a problem with movement, particularly gait. The affected individual complains of unsteadiness and apprehension when attempting to alter positions. Coordination and balance seem to be impaired. The geriatric population is particularly vulnerable to the combined effects of several sensory deficits including alcohol or drug reactions, diminished visual acuity, osteoarthritis, and nerve degeneration(4, 10).

The doctor of chiropractic is uniquely trained to be able to distinguish and correct neuromuscular problems(11–13). Intervention is designed to restore normal ambulation and prevent recurrence. A functionally short leg with or without asymmetry of lumbopelvic movement (sacroiliac syndrome) is a significant predisposing cause of disequilibrium. Faulty biomechanical control of muscles and joints impoverish kinesthetic awareness and produce compensatory distortions in the spine(14).

Lightheadedness

This is the most common disorder of equilibrium. It is a manifestation of a decreased partial pressure of dissolved carbon dioxide in the arterial plasma (hypocapnia) and extracellular alkalosis. The most frequent cause is hyperventilation. The arterial response is a fall in blood pressure, systemic venoconstriction, and diminished cerebral blood flow. An individual might also complain of tingling in the hands and feet. Some patients report these symptoms before or after a chiropractic treatment. The mechanism here could be attributed to faulty breathing techniques, anxiety, orthostatic hypotension, or cerebrovascular ischemia. The treatment of lightheadedness greatly depends upon the ability to stabilize and predict the arterial response. It is important to ensure that the patient is comfortable and relaxed during treatment.

It is also probably more important to minimize negative reactions. An adequate examination should have ruled out conditions such as anemia, bulemia (metabolic alkalosis), hypoglycemia, pneumonia, pregnancy, salicylate toxicity, and vertebral artery syndrome.

Chiropractic techniques utilizing electrotherapy, soft tissue masage, and manipulation serve to reduce tension and reeducate respiratory movements of the

Table 10.1
Primary Disorders of Equilibrium

Disorder	Definition	Etiological Considerations
Disequilibrium	Unsteadiness and apprehension when attempting to alter body position	Alcoholism Cerebellar tumors Drugs (barbiturates, sedatives, tranquilizers) Gait disturbances Hyperventilation syndrome Hypoglycemia Hypothyroidism Low back pain Osteoarthritis Parkinson's disease Peripheral neuropathy Short leg syndrome Trauma Visual impairment
Lightheadedness	Vague nondefinition; described in exclusionary terms (i.e., absence of other differentiating characteristics)	Anemia Bulemia Cerebrovascular ischemia Hyperventilation syndrome Hypoglycemia Orthostatic hypotension Pneumonia Pregnancy Salicylate toxicity Vertebral artery syndrome
Syncope	Transient loss of consciousness	Cardiac arrythmias Carotid sinus syndrome Hyperventilation syndrome Hypoglycemia Organic heart disease Transient ischemic attacks Trauma Vasovagal hypotension
Vertigo	Illusion of body or environmental motion	Autonomic nervous system dysfunction Brainstem ischemia Cerebrovascular malformations Cervicogenic vertigo Demyelination Inflammation/fever Intramedullary neoplasia Toxicity Trauma

diaphragm and ribs. Overly vigorous treatments could provoke vasovagal reactions and respiratory distress(15).

Ménière's Disease

Also known as paroxysmal labyrinthine vertigo or endolymphatic hydrops, this condition is most commonly referred to as inner ear disease. There is an oversecretion of potassium-rich endolymph with resultant distention of the superior section of the membranous labyrinth(16).

Afferent discharge activity may be inhibited in one vestibular nerve, and nystagmus, if present, changes direction during different stages of the attack(16). Other clinical findings include progressive neurological deafness, continuous tinnitus, vertigo, and autonomic dysfunction in the form of increased sweating, pallor, nausea, and vomiting(17).

The etiology is unknown, but viral invasion is a likely causative agent(16).

Zerrillo and Lynch(18) also suggest that mechanical and osteoarthritic irritations localized to the cervical vertebrae predispose the individual to otovestibular disorders. In these cases, alleviation of the disturbed vertebral biomechanics could provide some relief, if not a cure.

Nystagmus

Under normal, healthy circumstances, the human eyes are capable of remaining fixated on a stationary object even while the head turns away. This is so because the neural tonus to the bilaterally matched extraocular muscles is continually balanced along the vestibular portions of the eighth cranial nerve(19).

Rotation of the head (spinning chair test) or irrigation of the ear (caloric test) temporarily imbalances endolymphatic flow. A normal physiological disturbance is produced. A slow conjugate eye movement is observed to move away from the direction of rotation or cold water irrigation followed by a quick, reflex, compensatory return eye movement (normal nystagmus). The cortex perceives an illusion of body or environmental motion (vertigo), and the medulla initiates nausea. The individual may fall toward the direction of rotation or cold caloric stimulation.

A delay in the signal along one peripheral vestibular nerve is pathological. Eye deviation is exerted by the dominant side even when the person is motionless and nystagmus occurs spontaneously(20).

In a diagnostic sense, atypical nystagmus is clear evidence that there is neurological damage somewhere along the course of the vestibular portion of cranial nerve eight. Lesions could originate in the cerebellum, brain stem, nuclei, peripheral nerve, or labyrinth. Brain tumors, cervical spondylosis, vascular defects, demyelinating disorders, and infectious diseases comprise the majority of causes(21).

Until the type of defect is identified or adequately ruled out, chiropractic manipulation is contraindicated(22).

Syncope

Loss of consciousness is always dramatic! In the case of isolated syncope, there is transient loss of consciousness but no evidence of neurologic or cardiovascular disease(23).

Sympathetic hyperactivity has been linked to the prodromal (presyncopal) response (24, 25). Following this initiation, a cascade of parasympathetic conservation reactions ensue. Bradycardia leads to decreased myocardial contractility, diminished cardiac output, a drop in blood pressure, and inadequate cerebral blood flow(24).

Of the various contributing factors in the evolution of syncope, the vasovagal faint and acutely reduced cerebral blood flow account for more than 75% of all pathological explanations(23). Therefore, chiropractic correction of biomechanical instability and attention to myofascial tension and pain patterns will mitigate against inordinate sympathetic expression(26–28).

Vertigo

The illusion of body or environmental motion is pathognomonic of vertigo. The brain reacts to this false perception because the delicate symmetry of incoming information has been upset. The labyrinths account for the most important peripheral vestibular cues but also fail in their task most often(1).

Cervical proprioceptive input tends to overcompensate via somatosensory projection(2, 29–32). This means that cervicogenic vertigo is both a cause and effect of autonomic dysfunction. So even if the primary cause of vertigo is brainstem ischemia, inflammatory disease, toxicity, or trauma, the doctor of chiropratic should be consulted to manage the cervicogenic components(33, 34).

SUMMARY

The four primary disorders of equilibrium, disequilibrium, lightheadedness, syncope, and vertigo, all express features of autonomic nervous system dysfunction. The cervical vertebrae, along with their myofascial structures, nerves, and blood vessels appear to be the most susceptible to malfunction. Interventions that are of low invasiveness and can restore neuromuscular integrity quickly are the hallmark of chiropractic practice. Herein lie the paths to successful clinical decision making: the application of knowledgeable judgments about diagnosis and treatment(35).

References

1. Bannister R. Brain's clinical neurology, 4th ed. London: Oxford University Press, 1975, pp 54–55.
2. Fitz-Ritzon D. Neural mechanisms involved in the control of the eye-head-neck co-ordinated movement: a review of literature with an emphasis on future directions for the chiropractic profession. J Manipulative Physiol Ther 7:1984;251–260.
3. Hinoki M. Role of the visceral brain in body equilibrium. Acta Otolaryngol (Stockh) Suppl 419:1985;30–52.
4. Wyke B. Cervical articular contributions to posture and gait: their relation to senile disequilibrium. Age Ageing 8:1979;251–258.
5. Gayral L, Neuwirth E. Oto-neuro-ophthalmologic manifestations of cervical origin: posterior cervical sympathetic syndrome of Barre-Lieou. NY State J Med July:1954;1920–1926.
6. Brunarski DJ. Functional considerations of spinal manipulative therapy. ACA J Chiro 14:1980;63–68.
7. Korr IM. Neurochemical and neurotrophic consequences of nerve deformation: clinical implications in relation to spinal manipulation. J Am Osteopath Assoc 5:1978;409–414.
8. Hinoki M. Vertigo due to whiplash injury: a neurological approach. Acta Otolaryngol (Stockh) Suppl 419:1985;9–29.
9. Cassidy JD, Diakow PRP, DeKorompay VL, Munkacsi I, Yong-Hing K. Treatment of neck-tongue syndrome by spinal manipulation: a report of three cases. Pain Clin 1:1986;41–46.
10. Venna N. Dizziness, falling and fainting: differential diagnosis in the aged (part 1). Geriatrics 41:1986;30–42.
11. Brunarski DJ. Chiropractic biomechanical evaluations: validity in myofascial low back pain. J Manipulative Physiol Ther 5:1982;155–161.
12. Brunarski DJ. Chiropractic clinical decision making and low back pain. ACA J Chiro 20:1983;55–67.
13. Brunarski DJ. Clinical trials of spinal manipulation: a critical appraisal and review of the literature. J Manipulative Physiol Ther 7:1984;243–249.
14. Hulse M. Disequilibrium, caused by a functional disturbance of the upper cervical spine: clinical aspects and differential diagnosis. Man Med 1:1983;18–23.
15. Kleynhans AM, Terrett AGJ. The prevention of complications from spinal manipulative therapy. In: Glasgow EF, Twomey CT, Scull ER, Kleynhans AM, eds. Aspects of manipulative therapy. 2nd ed. Melbourne: Churchill Livingstone, 1985, pp 161–175.
16. Rutka JA, Barber HO. Recurrent vestibulopathy: third review. J Otolaryngol 1975;15:105–107.
17. Henderson DJ. Significance of vertebral dyskinesia in relation to the cervical syndrome. J Manipulative Physiol Ther 2:1979;3–15.
18. Zerillo G, Lynch M. Importance of chiropractic in oto-vestibular pathology. In: Mazzarelli JR, ed. Chiropractic interprofessional Research. Milon: Offset Olona, 1983, pp 69–75.
19. Barrows HS. Guide to neurological assessment. Toronto: JB Lippincott, 1980.
20. Matsunoga T, Yamamoto K, Kubo T. Directional preponderance of nystagmus and excitement of autonomic nervous system. Acta Otolaryngol (Stockh) 99:1985;459–465.
21. Mayer B, Rieden K, Menda U. The importance of the general roentgenogram of the cervical spine for vertigo and pathological proprioceptive nystagmus. Laryngol Rhinol Otol Ihre Grenzgeb 64:1985;300–303.
22. Terrett AGJ, Webb MN. Vertebrobasilar accidents (VA) following cervical spine adjustment manipulation. J Aust Chiro Assoc 12:1982;24–27.
23. Savage DD, Corwin L, McGee DC, Kannel WB, Wolf PA. Epidemiologic features of isolated syncope: the Framingham study. Stroke 16:1985; 626–629.
24. McGrady AV, Bernal GAA. Relaxation based treatment of stress induced syncope. J. Behav Ther Exp Psychiatry 17:1986;23–27.
25. Shafar J. The syndromes of the third neurone of the cervical sympathetic system. Am J Med 40:1966;97–109.
26. Fitz-Ritson D. The direct connections of the C2 dorsal root ganglion in the macaca irus monkey: relevance to chiropractic. J Manipulative Physiol Ther 8:1985;147–156.
27. Hix EL. Reflex viscerosomatic reference phenomena. Osteopath Ann Dec:1976;496–502.
28. Sato A, Swenson RS. Sympathetic nervous system response to mechanical stress of the spinal column in rats. J Manipulative Physiol Ther 7:1984;141–147.
29. Boquet J, Moore N, Boismore F, Monnier JC. Vertigo in post-concussional and migrainous patients: implication of the autonomic nervous system. Aggressologie 24:1981;235–236.
30. Elies W. Cervicogenic disorders of the cochleo-vestibular system. H N O (Hals-Nasen-Ohrenheilk D) 32:1984;485–493.
31. Mohr U, Schimek JJ. Fusion disturbances in the eye in consequence of vertebragenic dysfunctions in the upper head joint area. Man Med 22:1984;2–4.
32. Reker U. Quantitative measurements of the intensity of cervico-ocular reflex. H N O (Hals-Nasen-Ohrenheilk D) 33:1985;426–429.
33. Lewit K, Berger M. Cervical pattern in vertigo patients. Man Med 21:1983;15–19.
34. Lewit K. The craniocervical junction and disturbance of equilibrium. Man Med 24:1986;26–29.
35. Sackett DL, Haynes RB, Tugwell P. Clinical epidemiology: a basic science for clinical medicine. Boston: Little, Brown and Company, 1985.

11 Vertebral Artery Syndrome

Part A: Vertebrobasilar Vascular Accidents Associated with Cervical Manipulation

Donald J. Henderson B.Sc., D.C., F.C.C.S., D.A.C.B.R., F.C.C.R., F.I.C.C.

J. David Cassidy D.C., B.Sc., F.C.C.S., M.Sc.

Spontaneous occlusion of a branch of the vertebral artery was first described as the posterior inferior cerebellar syndrome by Wallenberg in 1895(1). This branch of the vertebrobasilar arterial system supplies the cerebellum and is very susceptible to decreased blood flow following vertebral artery injury. Vertebral artery occlusion and stroke (VAS) associated with cervical manipulation has been documented in the literature since 1947(2). This serious and complex clinical entity is receiving further attention as manipulation is becoming more widely practiced by health professions other than chiropractic and osteopathy.

The vertebrobasilar insufficiency syndrome(3–14) is the result of transient, partial, or complete occlusion of one of the vertebral arteries or its branches. Compression is associated with hyperextension and rotation of the neck. With the cervical spine positioned in this manner, vertebral artery flow may be expected to decrease by 10–20% in the vertebral artery opposite the direction of rotation. This mechanical compression occurs most often at the atlantoaxial junction(15–18). Other levels within the cervical column may also be compromised contributing in some degree to arterial occlusion(19–21). Transient or subclinical occlusion can become more critical if the vessels are diseased, anomalous, or absent, or if the patient has a condition leading to hypoxia(22–27). Adequate collateral supply to the hind brain and cord from the opposite vertebral artery would normally sustain the needs of the central nervous system. Consider, however, a hypoplastic collateral vessel in which the dominant artery is significantly compressed. Excessive extension and rotation of the neck, whether sustained or instantly forceful, may likely result in vertebral artery occlusion with risk of VAS.

Within a certain accustomed range of motion, the cervical vertebral segments and adjoining supportive tissue will not normally exert sufficient pressure on the accompanying vertebral arteries to produce risk of harm. However, manipulative maneuvers that use excessive cervical extension and rotation in patients at risk threaten the extra insult necessary to produce the clinical syndrome of vertebral artery occlusion.

Clinical indications of VAS following manipulation(28–36) include postural collapse with or without loss of consciousness (drop attack), vertigo, ataxia, dysarthria, visual disturbances including diplopia, paresis, blurred vision, and nystagmus, suboccipital headache, and paresis of a limb or limbs. In some cases, death has resulted within hours or days following occlusion of one of the vertebral arteries or its branches. The clinical picture of VAS following manipulation is a consequence of cord, brainstem, and cerebellar ischemia or infarction.

The purpose of this report is to present cases in which varying degrees of vertebral artery compromise is thought to have occurred in susceptible individuals as a consequence of cervical manipulation. The last case presented did not have dramatic signs of VAS. However, to ignore possible effects of subtle vertebral artery compromise invites more serious harm if subsequent manipulative maneuvers are performed on the same patient—harm that can be avoided.

Case One

A 64-year-old man, H.F., consulted a chiropractor for a "cramping" pain over the upper right shoulder area and neck. This had been of gradual onset a few days earlier, and he had consulted his family physician. Tylenol with codeine and clinoril were prescribed. X-rays of the neck and chest were taken, but results were not known to his physician. As his family doctor left for vacation, another physician continued managing the case. The patient was instructed to rest with a heating pad as required.

As the patient had formerly seen a chiropractor with success 2 years previously, he decided to seek chiropractic assistance. Upon presentation, the patient was in acute distress but without remarkable antalgic list of the neck or back. The intermittent cramping pain had largely subsided, but he was left with a vague but intense ache in the right lower neck. He had never experienced this type of ache before; he had been worked up by his physician to exclude a heart condition. Claiming good health except for "telangiectasis," for which he took iron pills, he could not relate any reason for his present complaint. Any jarring movements such as going down steps would bring on an acute attack of pain.

Flexion, right rotation, and left lateral bending of the neck were moderately provocative of pain. Vital signs were normal and pulses in both arms were equal in rhythm, rate, and magnitude. Sensation, motor power, and reflexes were unremarkable. C5-6 was blocked to articular challenge on the right and C4-5 on the left. Moderate spasm was noted over the right levator scapula, trapezius, and scalene muscles.

Light mobilizing adjustments (manipulations) were given to the fixated segments. Electrotherapy was also used at a comfortable setting. He was instructed to use hot moist packs at home and a soft collar only when necessary. He was seen the following day and was slightly better. Light trigger point pressure was used over the muscles involved and slightly heavier adjustments were given. By the third and fourth days of treatment, he was about 50% better. On the fifth visit, the treating chiropractor was not available, and an associate treated Mr. H.F.

About an hour after this fifth treatment Mr. H.F.'s wife called the associate chiropractor to say that when her husband had arrived home, he had had difficulty standing, his speech had been slurred, and he had experienced dizziness. The chiropractor told her to take Mr. H.F. to the hospital immediately. The physician was contacted.

Upon arrival at the hospital, Mr. H.F. was semiconscious. Subsequent examinations revealed an upper motor neuron lesion with paralysis of the lower limbs. The patient was conscious, but the speech was slurred. Approximately 4 weeks later, the patient died. The physician reported to the family that multiple areas of hemorrhage were found in the brain stem and cerebellum, most likely the consequence of an occult bleeding disorder he had had for some time.

Clinical Comment

Patients with hemorrhagic diathesis should be evaluated carefully prior to a decision to use cervical manipulation. Medications known to inhibit clotting or otherwise increase the likelihood of bleeding in susceptible individuals increase the risk of complications. This includes women taking birth control pills. This patient had an occult bleeding disorder that may have been the initial cause for his nonspecific neck pain. His wife recalled that an afternoon of waterskiing preceded his neck discomfort. The last manipulation seems to have aggravated the brainstem and cerebellar bleeding and provoked an ischemic attack.

Case file notes should have reflected better any reservations the initial treating practitioner had before continued care was provided by an associate. In particular, the force, level, and direction of adjustive thrust should have been emphasized.

Case Two

Mrs. M.A., a healthy 31-year-old public school teacher, was referred for chiropractic care by her general practitioner. She presented with right-sided midcervical pain with radiation into the suboccipital and frontal regions of the head. This trouble began 3 weeks prior to consultation, when she awoke one morning with a stiff neck. The pain was described as a dull ache, worse in the morning, aggravated by twisting the neck, and relieved by massage and aspirin. There was no history of pain or numbness in the arms, impairment of vision or balance, or past history of neck pain. She was healthy otherwise, and her past medical history was noncontributory.

On examination, she had a normal range of motion in her cervical spine with the exception of left rotation and lateral flexion, which "pulled" on the right side of the neck. Her cranial nerve and brachial plexus examination was normal. She experienced no difficulty hyperextending and rotating her neck. Motion palpation disclosed a tender fixation at the C3-4-5 level on the right side of the neck. Pressure over the articular pillars at these levels reproduced her symptoms.

A diagnosis of midcervical joint dysfunction was made, and x-rays were not considered necessary. The patient received one right midcervical neck manipulation that day with no ill effects. She was seen 4 days later, was 100% improved, and was discharged from active care. The patient returned 6 months later with the same complaint and was again manipulated at the C5 level on the right with excellent results.

One year later, Mrs. M.A. presented again with right-sided neck pain with no radiation into the head. Her examination findings were similar to those of her first presentation, except that the level of joint dysfunction had changed to C2 on the right. She had been asymptomatic during the past year.

A diagnosis of right-sided C2 joint dysfunction was made, and the patient was given a right-sided C2 rotatory cervical manipulation. Immediately after the treatment, the patient developed right-sided nystagmus and vomited. She became quickly disoriented and was taken to the hospital immediately by ambulance. On route to the hospital, her blood pressure was 125/100 and her pulse was 96 beats/min. In the emergency department, the patient remained severely ataxic and disoriented and displayed an intention tremor and periodic bouts of right-sided nystagmus. She was admitted to the neurology ward.

In-hospital investigations included plain radiographs of the cervical spine, a computed tomography (CT) scan, and an aortic arch angiogram. The plain radiographs showed a small osteophyte at the anteroinferior corner of the body of C4 but were otherwise considered normal (Fig. 11.1). A CT scan of the brain was done from the base to the vertex of the skull without contrast (Fig. 11.2). The posterior fossa was found to contain a large well-defined, low-density lesion occupying a large portion of the right cerebellum. This finding was thought to be compatible with a diagnosis of right cerebellar infarct. The aortic arch angiogram showed that the right vertebral artery was absent (Fig. 11.3).

A clinical diagnosis of right cerebellar infarct was made, and the patient was kept in the hospital for 2 months for observation. At the time of discharge, she was no longer ataxic and was fortunate to have made a full recovery.

Clinical Comment

This patient had previously experienced neck pain that had responded well to specific manipulative treatments. A subsequent neck problem was evaluated with different segmental findings requiring manipulation at a higher level. A rotary manipulation at the level of axis resulted in a vascular accident. Absence of the vertebral artery on the right made this patient most susceptible to vascular compromise.

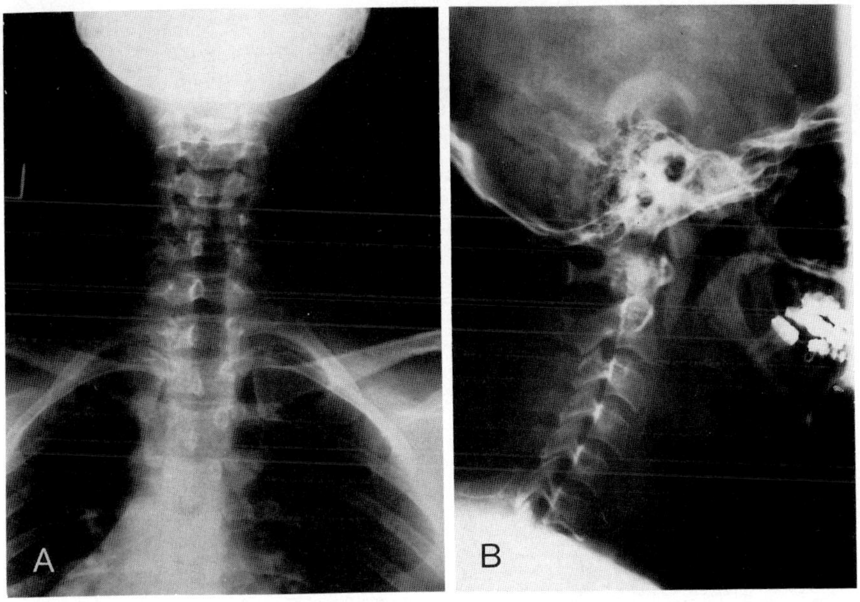

Figure 11.1. Anteroposterior **(A)** and lateral **(B)** x-rays of the cervical spine.

This case demonstrates the specificity of the level of the manipulative thrust and the fine difference between beneficial and catastrophic results. It also shows the wisdom in performing, on a routine basis, one or more of the available functional tests for vertebral artery insufficiency. The decision to arrange immediate hospital care was important in minimizing complications.

Case Three

Mr. H.H., a retired 65-year-old man, presented with acute lower back pain of 4

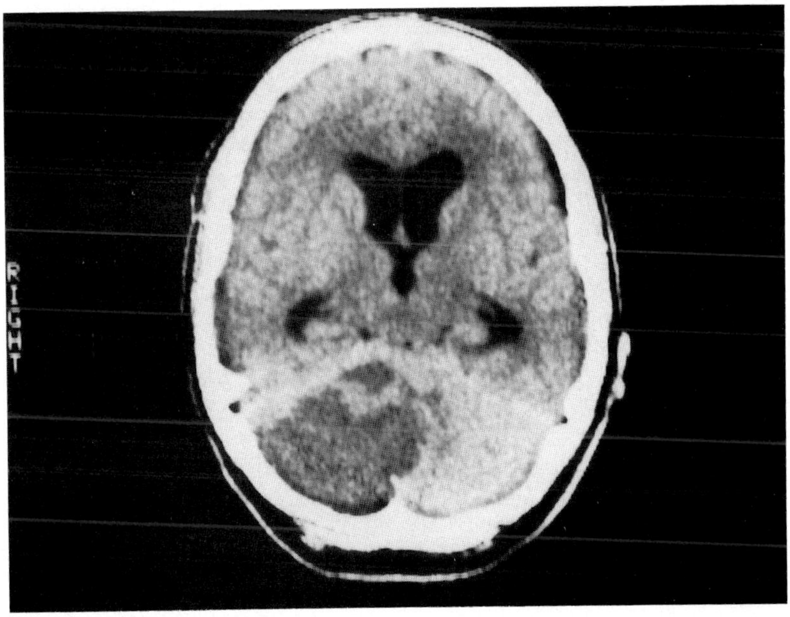

Figure 11.2. CT scan of brain.

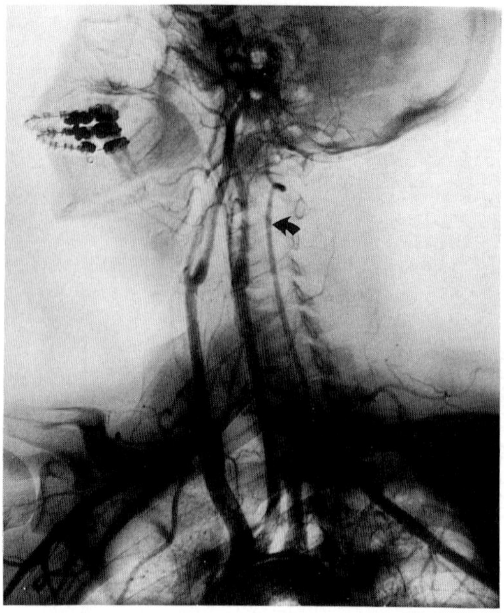

Figure 11.3. Aortic arch angiogram.

days duration. Onset occurred one morning as he was bending over to wash his face. History and examination were typical and consistent with a diagnosis of sacroiliac dysfunction. He responded well to manipulation and was essentially free of low back symptoms in about four visits.

During the spinal examination, it was noted that C1-2 was fixed on the right side. He recalled "passing out" 7 years previously. This, he stated, had started as a kink in his neck and had subsequently produced left arm pain. On a hospital examination, he was told that the problem had arisen from a calcium deposit in his neck.

On the third visit, the neck was adjusted also (C1-2 on the right) as part of a full spine treatment for his lower back pain. The neck was asymptomatic at the time. The patient returned for his fourth visit reporting that his lower back was excellent but that for 2 days, he had felt a persistent dizzy feeling aggravated by neck extension. He felt very disoriented. His memory and visual perception were slightly disturbed. Upon reaching for an object, he would reach past it before accurately judging the distance. It was believed that the patient's symptoms were neurovascular in origin.

A standing extension-rotation test for the vertebral artery was performed. Upon left rotation with extension, the patient lost his balance and dropped into the arms of the examiner. After about 10 seconds, he became more alert and noticed an unusual "sinking" feeling. The patient's neck was immobilized with a collar. He was instructed to rest for 10–15 minutes. Blood pressure was 140–150/95 mm Hg bilaterally in the supine position. Pulses were bilaterally equal in rate, rhythm, and magnitude at 66 beats per minute. By the time he left the office, he was feeling fine and resisted advice to see a vascular specialist.

The patient was seen on three further occasions over a 4-week period for lumbar spinal assessment and manipulation. No further adjustments of the neck were performed because of the initial reaction. The patient was discharged and advised that he should avoid any postures requiring prolonged extension or rotation of the neck and, more particularly, should avoid neck manipulation unless his condition was more thoroughly investigated.

Clinical Comment

In this case, the patient presented with a complaint related to the lumbar spine and had responded well to specific manipulation. However, when extending manipulation to other spinal areas remote from the original site of discomfort, equal diagnostic information should be sought. A more thorough history and examination including provocative tests for vertebral artery insufficiency may have revealed the potential for harm. Treatment of asymptomatic spinal areas can produce undesirable iatrogenic effects.

This patient's "drop attack," dizziness, dysmetria, and dystaxia, although mild, were thought to have originated from occlusion of the vertebral artery after a rotary adjustment to the atlantoaxial segment.

DISCUSSION

A review of the literature on VAS indicates that the presenting signs and symptoms of patients who sought and received manipulative care were usually benign(6, 37–40, 65). The chief complaint is frequently "upper neck pain," "headaches," "neck stiffness," "crick in my neck," and "lightheadedness." Patients with these complaints often respond well to manipulation and their symptoms are not generally relevant to the prodromata of VAS. A great number of patients seek chiropractic care for such conditions(41–44).

It is difficult to say whether, in some isolated cases, patients who seek chiropractic care do so because of early or subtle signs of VAS or, in fact, do so for manipulation-related problems that ordinarily fare well with this form of treatment. Specificity of history or physical tests to the condition are lacking. A clinical evaluation that may be considered in suspect patients is included in Table 11.1.

The influence of proprioceptive factors as the result of functional disturbances of the upper cervical spine, as well as irritation of the posterior recurrent autonomic chain (vertebral nerve), make the diagnosis of VAS equivocal. This is especially true in patients presenting with a subtle symptom picture. It is stressed that the clinician should assume the strong possibility of a vascular origin especially when a treatment regime of cervical manipulation is contemplated. Other data on this topic may be helpful in the differential diagnosis(25, 45–48).

A major misconception regarding VAS is that it is primarily a problem of the elderly (Habib, CC, Chairman, Neurology Section, Manitoba Medical Association, 1983, personal communication). The average age reported in the literature is 37.9, the youngest and oldest being 7 and 63, respectively. Female patients outnumber male almost two to one(6, 37, 39). Younger patients lack the degenerative changes that lead to progressive articular fixation. Since the range of possible motion is ordinarily greater in younger patients, the possibility of challenging the anatomical integrity of the vertebral artery fixed within the intertransverse foramen, particularly at the atlantoaxial level, becomes greater. In the older patient, degenerative changes modify and limit motion segment behavior and therefore pro-

Table 11.1
Manipulation-induced Vertebral Artery Syndrome: Identification of Potential Patient at Risk

Incidence
- Over 50 well-documented cases since 1947. Over 12 deaths.
- Mean age, 37.9. Female patients nearly 2:1

Past History
- Transient ischemic attack, subclavian steal syndrome, hyperlipidemia, hypercholesterolemia, arteriosclerosis, hypertension, medications with stroke risk, oral contraceptive, heavy smoking, postpartum or bleeding disorders, neck trauma, compression fractures, hypermobility syndromes or congenital instabilities, os odontoideum, atlantodental interval incompetency, autonomic instability, advanced spondyloarthrosis of cervical spine

Recent History
Cervical trauma, motor vehicle accident, unexplained torticollis
- Presenting signs and symptoms of vertigo, drop attacks (syncope), visual disturbances, nystagmus, dystaxia, nausea, vomiting, intense suboccipital headaches
- Neck position or neck, shoulder arm activity that accompanies above, especially vertigo, visual disturbances, near syncope, loss of balance (result of hind brain ischemia)

Physical Tests
- Bruit over carotid bifurcation, subclavian vessels
- Fundoscopy to evaluate state of retinal vessels
- Brachial anisosphygmia (systolic pressure difference greater than 10–20 mm Hg)
- Brachial anisopiesis suggests occlusive arterial disorder
- Standing cervical extension-rotation, eyes open then closed (30 seconds each side). Balance test is more sensitive than tests done sitting or recumbent. See text for explanation and variations.
- Test of manipulation: positioning of neck preparatory to adjustment when joint laxity taken up to determine patient tolerance or symptomatology

Radiographic Exam
- To rule out cervical pathology (structure) and hypermobility and/or instabilities (function)

Specialized Procedures
- Angiography, Doppler ultrasound, CT scan, oculoplethysmography, Electroencephalography in position of provocation

Medical Treatment
- Anticoagulation, antiplatelet therapy to prevent further thrombosis and embolization

Emergency Care
- In the event of VAS, moniter vital signs, arrange for immediate hospital transportation, cardiopulmonary resuscitation if necessary. Do not remanipulate, immobilize with cervical collar.

vide an inherent protection to mechanical insult. However, disc thinning and architectural remodeling of the vertebrae shorten the cervical column, with the result that the vertebral arteries assume a more tortuous path. Compression in this case may be just as likely. Degenerative osteophytic encroachment of the vertebral vessels can also compromise arterial flow(27, 49). Arterial disease further complicates the problem.

While this chapter concerns itself with VAS following manipulation, certain procedures used in medicine may similarly compromise vertebral artery flow. For example, in the field of neuro-otolaryngology, use of the positional nystagmus test(50, 51) used to assess vestibular function requires that the seated patient be rapidly supinated with cervical extension and rotation. This maneuver, designed to test whether the inner ear is causing vertigo or nystagmus, might well aggravate those symptoms by causing vertebral artery compression.

Intubation, resuscitation, and patient positioning in surgery where hyperextension and partial rotation are required may similarly compress the vertebral artery(52–55). One such case report of VAS describes a patient undergoing a left stellate ganglionectomy. The patient's head and neck were maintained in right rotation.

Infant delivery may also produce prolonged extension and rotation of the neck, and the presence of an anomalous vertebral artery may be made manifest first by ischemic brain injury. A study conducted by Yates(52) pursues the possible link between vertebral artery hemorrhage or thrombosis and birth trauma. One author (53) on the subject goes so far as to comment that "transient or permanent impairment of the vertebral blood supply to the brainstem or cervical cord may be the cause of acute craniocerebral injury that, at autopsy, presents no apparent pathological cause for death." Upper cervical trauma or subluxation causing compression of the cord or adjacent carotid-vertebral arteries may occur at the time of birth. This, in turn, may produce signs and symptoms that, in the early stages, resemble those seen in cerebral birth palsy(54). While VAS is a condition currently associated most readily with manipulative procedures, its occurrence and role in CNS diseases is not well understood and warrants further study.

Incidence of VAS following Manipulation

There are approximately 40,000 licensed chiropractors in the world. Over 85% practice in North America. Surveys(56 and 57) suggest that the average number of chiropractic treatments per practitioner is in the order of 4,000 per annum. Assuming half of these treatments included cervical manipulation specifically, then, as a minimum, over 70 million cervical manipulations are performed by chiropractors in North America each year. Livingston's(58) estimate in the early 1970s was 75 million cervical manipulations per year. The former estimate would not include other professions practising spinal manipulation, such as osteopaths, physicians, and physiotherapists, whose numbers probably exceed 10,000 internationally. It would not be unreasonable to suggest 100 million cervical manipulations world wide per annum. In the 38 years since Pratt-Thomas and Bergers'(2) 1947 description of VAS related to manipulation, less than 100 new cases have been reported. (There are 52 well-documented cases up to 1981)(59, 60). One hundred cases represent an incidence of one in 38 million.

Jaskoviak(37) reports that in the period of 1965 to 1980, an estimated 5 million treatments were given at the National College of Chiropractic clinics without a single case of VAS associated with manipulation. In a survey at the Canadian Memorial Chiropractic College outpatient clinic, more than half a million treatments were given over a 9-year period, again without incident. Maigne(61) reports less than one death in several tens of millions of manipulations, while Gutmann(62) and Dvorak(63) estimate that two or three more-or-less serious incidents concerning the vertebrobasilar system occur per million manipulative treatments of the upper cervical spine. Haldeman(64) agrees that there is less than one chance per million.

Daneshmend et al(59) and Robertson(60) suspect that the incidence of stroke arising from manipulation is under-reported. This is likely to be true as included case reports indicate, but Robertson's estimate of 360 additional cases is not supported by any acceptable evidence. One third of the 360 cases had carotid artery infarction. Carotid artery compression is anatomically less likely to receive direct mechanical insult during cervical manipulation. No mention was made of any patient damaged by manipulation.

Few, if any, of the reports since 1947(2) deal with the prior injury (a possible prelude to stroke) that brought the patient to the manipulator. Few, if any, adequately deal with the nature of the manipulative procedure as it relates to the vertebral artery injury site.

These authors(59, 60) tend to agree that VAS following manipulation is more common than the well-documented literature reports, but the incidence is still slight—probably about one in 10 million. To place this in perspective, the same result can occur with motor vehicle accidents, falls, ceiling painting, shaving, yoga, gymnastics, infant delivery, archery, surgical positioning, simple head turning, or any other activity of daily life(6, 13, 30, 37). The literature fails to collate these causes. Most cases of arterial thrombosis and infarction in other areas of the body are unrelated to trauma. There is no doubt that manipulation can and does have stroke as an iatrogenic effect, but in all probability, only in those patients who already have an underlying anomalous or pathological problem.

This complication should be taken very seriously, nonetheless, because of the severity of VAS when it does arise. All those who practise spinal manipulation should be cognizant of the well-documented reports found in the literature. Such serious potential harm from cervical manipulation is one of many reasons why a practitioner should want to have a thorough education in the field of manipulation before attempting it on a patient. It should be emphasized that the complication of stroke is a possibility no matter who the manipulator is. Manipulation is no different than any other therapeutic procedure in which there is risk of harm. It is hoped that political motives do not hinder cooperative efforts between professions in an effort to further discuss and understand methods of detection and prevention of VAS.

As a last comment on the matter of incidence, if it is accepted that manipulation can result in vertebral artery injury, by the same token, manipulation can be a corrective therapy in those whose injuries have already compromised blood flow. Cervical manipulation can alleviate the mechanical dysfunction that renders the vertebral arteries susceptible to further trauma.

Legal Considerations

Claims of malpractice with respect to VAS following manipulation have emerged in many jurisdictions. In Canada, statements of claim preparatory to litigation allege negligence, the particulars of which include the following: (1) failure to take a proper history, examination, and radiographs; (2) failure to read or interpret the details of the history, examination, and radiographs; (3) failure to arrive at an accurate diagnosis or to safely administer or use proper or proven techniques; (4) failure to obtain proper and informed consent prior to manipulative treatment; (5) application of excessive force or improper direction of the manipulation with the patient in an unsafe position; (6) failure to take proper, effective, or timely measures to remedy the injurious manipulation.

Claims are seldom for modest amounts. Some decisions seem to suggest a philosophy of absolute liability. A recent court decision now under appeal(64) accepted the chiropractic procedure as well as the performance of the procedure (manipulation) but ruled negligence on the part of the defendent for not informing the patient that in rare instances neck manipulation can cause stroke. Informed of this, the patient, it is reasoned, may have declined treatment and avoided potential injury.

A noted medical expert in the field of manipulation, Gutmann(62), feels that given the remarkably low incidence of VAS following manipulation, there is no legal obligation to instruct the patient in advance about such an unlikely possibility. It appears that the practitioner must decide whether advance warning is necessary. As each incident is evaluated separately, court decisions may vary from case to case in different jurisdictions(66). Common sense prevailing, if signs and symptoms as well as tests of provocation suggest risk, informed consent should be sought. With or without consent, litigation is more than likely to be pursued if an unfortunate coincidental accident does occur.

The following safeguards lessen the likelihood of accident and hence litigation (39): (1) careful appraisal of the patient; (2) development of a resumé to be given to the patient outlining the findings with explanation of the manipulative adjustment and possible reactions to the treatment; (3) good doctor-patient rapport; (4) exercising good clinical judgment at all times; (5) careful and gradual introduction to the manipulative technique; (6) prompt and appropriate personal response to the patient's complaints; and (7) careful documentation of records.

Detection and Prevention of VAS

As a matter of principle, the practitioner must recognize that VAS associated with manipulation does occur. Precautions can then be taken to evaluate the risk of injury (25, 45–47). Starting with the history, signs, and symptoms of dizziness, visual disturbances, loss of balance, fainting, nausea and vomiting, weakness of limb(s), and suboccipital headache, suggest that a patient is at risk. Other important features of past history are found in Table 11.1. With the information from the history, it is important to connect any sign or symptom with neck pain and, more especially, a specific neck position or movement.

Tests including detection of vascular bruit and asymmetrical systolic blood pressure and pulses suggest the possibility of arterial abnormality regardless of the patient's age. Fundoscopic examination, although not specific, helps in the evaluation of the condition of the small arteries and veins elsewhere in the body.

Ask the patient if he or she can reproduce the presenting complaint(s) by any maneuver or position. If so, this fact should be recorded and suggests the posture to avoid when considering manual treatment.

Instruct the patient to perform neck circumduction in one direction, then in the other as a general screening test. Follow this by rapid arm circumduction, the head and neck held stationary. This may trigger symptomatology by producing cervicobrachial neurovascular distraction or symptoms of the subclavian steal syndrome.

Use a balancing test to check the integrity of the equilibrium mechanism by asking the patient to close their eyes and stand perfectly still with arms outstretched in the supinated position. Ask the patient to open their eyes and extend the neck for approximately 20–40 seconds. Then instruct the patient to close eyes to eliminate visual righting cues. Repeat this for extension and rotation to left and right for the same time period with eyes closed. Ensure that you or an assistant is close by in the event of postural collapse. Note any deviation of side stray or pronation of the outstretched supinated arms. Variations of these cervical rotation and extension screening tests are known as the Hautant, Dekleijn, Underberger (marching in place) tests. Positive signs in addition to loss of balance include syncope, visual abnormalities, nystagmus, vertigo, nausea, and vomiting.

A supine test in which the head is gently rotated and extended can be performed. Suppression of arterial flow at the upper cervical level on the contralateral side, or ipsilateral side at lower levels (by hypertrophic spurs), may occur. This position should be held for a minimum of 45 seconds. If nystagmus, vertigo, visual disturbances, or near syncope ensue, the test should be stopped. This position of provocation is usually unilateral and suggests the direction in which an adjustment is contraindicated. Vertebrobasilar insufficiency is the most possible cause. Appropriate referral to a neurologist or vascular specialist may be necessary. Although the clinical manifestation described above can be influenced, to a lesser degree, by proprioceptive disturbances in the upper cervical spine as well as irritation to the sympathetic vertebral nerve, the clinician should assume the vascular origin as the preferred diagnosis, especially if manipulation is contemplated(25, 45).

If, after specific motion palpation, no fixation is evident but symptoms prevail, consider the cause of the patient's complaint to be nonvertebrogenic. If segmental dysfunction is present, manipulation should not be delivered in a direction that will exacerbate the symptoms, nor should the manipulation be delivered until the joint slack is taken up (test of manipulation). This assures that the patient is reasonably comfortable in the premanipulative position. If the patient is uncomfortable, consider an other technique that will bring about the same result. For instance, joint mobilization or gentle muscle stretching maneuvers may prove effective in the early stages of an acute problem(68).

If the practitioner does decide to embark on a trial of manipulative therapy for functional disturbances related to the neck, initial treatments should be light and never unduly forceful. It is better to work up to the required adjustive thrust gradually than to risk an adverse reaction. Record the findings and patient progress as these notes may be helpful in the future if recurrences are likely. Avoid extension of the neck when manipulating in the supine position. With the head rest up, the neck is partially flexed, avoiding vertebral artery compromise.

Radiographic screening(68) is important to rule out instabilities or anomalies of the upper cervical complex such as atlantodental interval widening, block vertebrae, canal stenosis, subluxation, arterial pressure erosions, and excessive degenerative spurring. Functional stress radiographs taken at the extremes of flexion and extension are useful in assessing cervical spine stability(69, 70) (see Table 11.2).

It should be emphasized that even after having taken these precautions, VAS may still occur as a spontaneous event. Even the diagnostic tests of provocation may result in infarction.

Finally, in the event that VAS does occur, it is important that the treatment *not be repeated* in the hope that it will reverse the problem. Cervical immobilization and immediate consideration for hospital transportation cannot be overstressed. Anticoagulant therapy may be the only emergency measure taken to lessen the complication of ischemia to vital central nervous tissues.

Table 11.2
Radiographic Conditions that May Be Associated with Vertebral Artery Insufficiency

Exuberant hypertrophic changes in the apophyseal and the uncovertebral joints of Luschka
Congenital anomalies
Os odontoideum
Atlantal assimilation
Condylar hypoplasia
Transverse ligament defects (Down's syndrome)
Aplasia of posterior atlantal arch (clefting anomalies)
Basilar impression (achondroplasia)
Klippel-Feil syndrome
Acquired disorders
Occipitocervical dysplasia (Paget's disease, osteomalacia)
Infection (Grisel's syndrome, tuberculous involvement about the transverse ligament)
Rheumatoid involvement at the atlantodental joint (RA, SLE, psoriasis)
Trauma
Odontoid fracture
Rupture of transverse ligament (widened atlantodental interspace)
Hypermobility at the craniocervical junction
"Whiplash" injuries
Tumors

Monitoring vital signs of blood pressure, pulses, respiratory rate, and pupillary response to light are necessary. Cardiopulmonary resuscitation must be performed in the event of an arrest. In the unlikely event of a vascular accident, the practitioner should be prepared to take charge until the patient is transported to the emergency department. The neck should be immobilized using a cervical collar.

Kleynhans(39) and others(35, 36) have reviewed the factors in practitioner-related complications arising from manipulation. Iatrogenic risk depends on the level of knowledge of the practitioner in arriving at a proper diagnosis, evaluating treatment precautions, and applying the proper manipulation. Lack of skill in the performance of the manipulative adjustment is probably as important as the former consideration. One may demonstrate excellent diagnostic capabilities but if unskilled in the delivery of the technique, serious damage can result. Medical personnel should be prepared to spend at least 1 full year of postgraduate training before performing spinal manipulative therapy. One cannot expect that a few weekend courses will provide the unqualified practitioner with the necessary training and skill to start manipulating patients in their offices the following week. An analogy might be a chiropractor taking a weekend course to learn the skills necessary to remove a diseased appendix. Board certified specialties in medicine already demonstrate the need for selective expertise in providing quality health care.

Dvorak(71) conducted a 5-month educational tour of osteopathic and chiropractic colleges in 1981. In considering the increase in popularity of manipulative medicine, he concluded that "as seen with osteopathic physicians and chiropractors, it is obvious that . . . extensive training (in medicine) is necessary to teach the fundamentals of diagnosis and therapy of the locomotor system."

Both osteopathy and chiropractic have been instrumental in setting standards that give solid foundation and knowledge in disease states of the locomotor system similar to other fields taught in medical school. The 1979 New Zealand Commission of Inquiry into Chiropractic (72) supports this need both in expert testimony and in the document's conclusions.

CONCLUSION

From a review of the literature, it is apparent that

(1) VAS is a related complication of cervical manipulative therapy.

(2) Mechanical compression or injury to the vertebral artery is more likely with the head and neck in a position of extension and rotation preparatory to instantly forceful manipulation.

(3) VAS following manipulation may be under-reported or escape unnoticed. Well-documented unbiased reports are necessary to determine the true extent of the problem.

(4) Notwithstanding the foregoing comment, from the literature on reports of occurrence, the documented incidence of serious VAS complications related to manipulation appears to be in the order of 1 in 10 million. Other activities of daily living may also spontaneously cause insufficiency within the vertebrobasilar artery.

(5) Individuals at risk are difficult to isolate and their presenting symptom(s) may represent a subtle prelude to stroke. Anatomical variation or pathological changes within the vertebral arterial system or upper cervical complex render the vertebral arteries more susceptible to injury.

(6) A few physical tests combined with a careful review of the patient's history and radiographic screening may be helpful in identifying patients at risk.

(7) A new wave of interest surrounds this syndrome, and this may very well be reflected in litigation and political controversy for the chiropractic profession even though many other groups perform manipulation and in spite of the extremely low incidence.

(8) There is a definite need to control or limit manipulation performed by any member of the health care team who does not demonstrate adequate training and continuous practical experience necessary for the safe and effective application of spinal manipulative therapy.

(9) Manipulation can alleviate the segmental dysfunction that may render the vertebral artery susceptible to mechanical injury. Properly administered manipulation is a safe procedure. However, once symptoms consistent with VAS have occurred, no attempt should be made to remanipulate in an effort to reverse the complication.

(10) Finally, cooperation between professions would be helpful in elucidating the cause and effect relationship between manipulation and VAS, as well as evaluating methods of detection and prevention.

References

1. Wallenberg A. Acute bulbaraffection. Arch Psychiat. Nervenkr 1895;27:504–540.
2. Pratt-Thomas HR, Berger KE. Cerebellar and spinal injuries after chiropractic manipulation. JAMA 1947;133:600–603.
3. Fazekas JF, Alman RW, Sullivan JF. Vertebral-basilar insufficiency. Arch Neurol 1963;8:115–120.
4. Ford FR. Syncope, vertigo and disturbances of

vision resulting from intermittent obstruction of the vertebral arteries due to defect in the odontoid process and excessive mobility of the second cervical vertebra. Bull Johns Hopkins Hosp 1952;91:168–173.
5. Milne E. Giddiness in vertebro-basilar arterial insufficiency. Med J Aust 1968;Aug:417–418.
6. Krueger BR, Okazaki H. Vertebral basilar distribution infarction following chiropractic cervical manipulation. Mayo Clin Proc 1980;55:322–332.
7. Powers SR, Drislane TM, Nevins S. Intermittent vertebral artery compression: a new syndrome. Surgery 1961;49:257–264.
8. Lewis RC, Coburn DF. The vertebral artery. Missouri Med 1956;53:1059–1063.
9. Latchaw RE, Seeger JF, Gabrielsen TO. Vertebrobasilar arterial occlusions in children. Neuroradiology 1974;8:141–147.
10. Parkin PJ, Wallis WE, Wilson JL. Vertebral artery occlusion following manipulation of the neck. NS Med J 1978;88:441–443.
11. Zauel D, Carlow TJ. Internuclear ophthalmoplegia following cervical manipulation (letter). Ann Neurol 1977;1:308.
12. Miller RG, Burton R. Stroke following chiropractic manipulation of the spine. JAMA 1974;229:189–190.
13. Okawara S, Nibbelink D. Vertebral artery occlusion following hyperextension and rotation of the head. Stroke 1974;5:640–642.
14. Schwartz GA, Geiger JK, Spano AV. Posterior inferior cerebellar artery syndrome of Wallenberg after chiropractic manipulation. Arch Int Med 1956;97:352–354.
15. deKleyn A, Nieuwenhuyse P. Schwindelanfalle und nystagmus dei einer bestimmten stellung des kopfes. Acta Otolaryng. 1927;11:155 157.
16. Horn SW. The "locked in" syndrome following chiropractic manipulation of the cervical spine. Am Emerg Med 1983;12:648–650.
17. Schellhas KP, Latchaw RE, Wendling LR, Gold LHA. Vertebrobasilar injuries following cervical manipulation. JAMA 1980;224:1450–1453.
18. Tissington-Tatlow WF, Bammer HG. Syndrome of vertebral artery compression. Neurology 1957;7:331–340.
19. Selecki BR. The effects of rotation of the atlas on the axis: experimental work. Med J Aust 1969;May:1012–1015.
20. Toole JF, Tucker SH. Influence of head position upon cerebral circulation. AMA Arch Neurol 1960;2:616–622.
21. Hutchinson EC, Yates PO. The cervical position of the vertebral artery; a clinico-pathological study. Brain 1956;79:319–331.
22. Rogers RL, Myer JS, Shaw TG, Mortel KF, Mardenberg JP, Zaid RR. Cigarette smoking decreases cerebral blood flow suggesting increased risk of stroke. JAMA 1983;250:2796–2800.
23. Ask-Upmark E, Bickerstaff ER. Vertebral artery occlusion and oral contraceptives. Br Med J 1976;1:487–488.
24. Ryan RE. A controlled study of the effect of oral contraceptives on migraine. Headache 1978;Jan:250–252.
25. Henderson DJ. Significance of vertebral dyskinesia in relation to the cervical syndrome. J Manipulative Physiol Ther 1979;2:3–15.
26. Carpenter S. Injury of neck as a cause of vertebral artery thrombosis. J Neurosurg 1961;849–853.
27. Sheehan S, Bauer RB, Meyer JS. Vertebral artery compression in cervical spondylosis. Neurology 1960;10:968–986.
28. Mehalic T, Farhat SM. Vertebral artery injury from chiropractic manipulation of the neck. Surg Neurol 1974;2:125–129.
29. Green D, Joynt RJ. Vascular accidents to the brain stem associated with neck manipulation. JAMA 1959;170:522–524.
30. Sherman DG, Hart RG, Easton JD. Abrupt change in head position and cerebral infarction. Stroke 1981;12:2–6.
31. Braun IF, Pinto RS, DeFilipp GJ, Lieberman A, Pasternack P, Zimmerman RD. Brain stem infarction due to chiropractic manipulation of the cervical spine. South Med J 1983;76:1199–1201.
32. Simmons KC, Soo YS, Walker G, Harvey P. Trauma to the vertebral artery related to neck manipulation. Med J Aust 1982;1:187–188.
33. Bose B, Northrup BE, Osterholm JL. Delayed vertebro-basilar insufficiency following cervical spine injury. Spine 1985;10:108–110.
34. Crawford JP, Hwang BY, Asselbergs PJ, Hickson GS. Vascular ischaemia of the cervical spine: a review of relationship to therapeutic manipulation. J Manipulative Physiol Ther 1984;4:149–155.
35. Ladermann SP. Accidents of spinal manipulation. Ann Swiss Chiro Ass 1981;7:161–208.
36. Gatterman MI. Contraindications and complications of spinal manipulative therapy. ACA J Chirop 1981;15:75–86.
37. Jaskoviak PA. Complications arising from manipulation of the cervical spine. J Manipulative Physiol Ther 1980;3:213–219.
38. Gotlib AC, Thiel H. A selected annotated bibliography of core biomedical literature pertaining to stroke, cervical spine, manipulation and head/neck movement. J Can Chiro Ass 1985;29:80–89.
39. Kleynhans AM. Complications and contraindications to spinal manipulative therapy. In: Haldeman S ed, Modern developments in the principles and practice of chiropractic. New York: Appleton-Century-Crofts, 1980, pp 359–384.
40. Kleynhans AM. The prevention of complications from spinal manipulative therapy. In Idezak (ed): Aspects of Manipulative Therapy. Melbourne, Lincoln Institute of Health Sciences, 1980, p 133–141.
41. Breen AC. Chiropractors and the treatment of back pain. Rheumatol Rehabil 1977;16:46.
42. Vear HJ. A study into the complaints of patients seeking chiropractic care. J Can Chiro Ass 1972;16:9.
43. Kelner M, Hall O, Coulter I. Chiropractors—do they help? Toronto: Fitzhenry & Whiteside, 1980, pp 28–31, 134–139.
44. Sherman RA. A statistical investigation of 500 patients. J Clin Chiro 1974;34–40.
45. Hulse M. Disequilibrium caused by functional disturbance of the upper cervical spine: clinical as-

pects and differential diagnosis. Man Med 1983;18–23.
46. Giles LGF. Vertebro-basilar artery insufficiency. J Can Chiro Ass 1977;21:112–117.
47. Lewit K. The contribution of clinical observation to neurobiological mechanisms in manipulative therapy. In: Korr IM ed, The neurobiologic mechanisms in manipulative therapy. New York: Plenum Press, 1978, pp 3–25.
48. Stevens AJJE. Doppler sonography and neck rotation. Man Med 1984;1:49–53.
49. Hadley LA. Anatomico-roentgenographic studies of the spine. Springfield, IL: Charles C Thomas, 1973, pp 160–170.
50. Dix MR, Hallpike CS: The pathology, symptomatology and diagnosis of certain common disorders of the vestibular system. Proc Roy Soc Med 1952;45:341.
51. Wolfson RJ, Myers D, Schlosser WD, Winchester RA. Vertigo. Clinical Symposia, Ciba Corporation, 1965.
52. Yates PO. Birth trauma to the vertebral arteries. Arch Dis Child 1959;34:426–431.
53. Schneider RC, Schemm GW. Vertebral artery insufficiency in acute and chronic spinal trauma. J Neurosurg 1961;18:348–360.
54. Keggi KJ, Granger DP, Southwick WO. Vertebral artery insufficiency secondary to trauma and osteoarthritis of the cervical spine. Yale J Biol Med 1966;38:471–478.
55. Alexander E, Misland R, Harris C. Anterior dislocation of the first cervical vertebra simulating cerebral birth injury in infancy. Am J Dis Child 1953;85:173–181.
56. Phillips RB, Butler R. Survey of chiropractic in Dade County, FLorida. J Manipulative Physiol Ther 1982;5:83–89.
57. Phillips RB. A survey of Utah chiropractic patients. ACA J Chiro 1981;18:113–123.
58. Livingston MC. Spinal manipulation causing injury; a three year study. Clin Orthop 1971;81:82–6.
59. Daneshmend TK, Hewer RL, Bradshaw JR. Acute brain stem stroke during neck manipulation. Br Med J 1984;287:189.
60. Robertson JT. Neck manipulation as a cause of stroke. Stroke 1982;13:260–1.
61. Maigne R. Manipulations vertebrales et les thromboses vertebro basilaires. Angeiologie 1969;21:287.
62. Gutmann G. Verletzungen der arteria vertebralis durch manuelle therapie. Man Med 1983;21:2–14.
63. Dvorak J, Orelli F. How dangerous is manipulation to the cervical spine? Man Med 1985;2:1–4.
64. Mason H vs Forgie D. December 1984, Judicial district of Saint John, New Brunswick. S/C/1569/82. Haldeman S. Testimony.
65. Hildebrandt RW. Vertebral artery syndrome resulting from manipulation of the cervical spine. J Manipulative Physiol Ther 1979;2:77–78.
66. Kellsey DC. The anatomy of orthopaedic malpractice: a survey of 250 cases. J Bone Joint Surg 1975;57-a:1013–1018.
67. Mierau DR, Cassidy JD. Degenerative spondylothesis in the cervical spine: a report of a case. J Can Chiro Ass 1984;28:368–370.
68. Henderson DJ, Korbelas PA. Fracture dislocation at the atlanto-axial junction: a case report to demonstrate the importance of radiographic examination in chiropractic practice. J Can Chiro Ass 1980;24:157–160.
69. Henderson DJ, Dormon TM. Functional roentgenometric evaluation of the cervical spine in the sagittal plane. J Manipulative Physiol Ther 1985;8:219–227.
70. Yochum TR, Rowe LJ. Arthrotides of the upper cervical complex. ACA J Chiro 1981;15:1–10.
71. Dvorak J. Manual medicine in the United States and Europe in the year 1982. Man Med 1983;1:3–9.
72. Chiropractic In New Zealand—Report of the Commission of Inquiry, Government Printer, Wellington, New Zealand, 1979, pp 308–316.

Part B: Annotated Literature Review*

Allan C. Gotlib B.Sc., D.C.*
Haymo Thiel, D.C.

Our bibliography is an initial attempt to construct a temporal sequential shared paradigm of the literature surrounding our subject matter. By so doing, we place parameters on the past knowledge base to better define particular information. With definition and classification comes a succinct grasp of information trends or shifts. Succeeding clinical and pathological studies will ultimately shift our information core, and we will attempt to maintain our depth and currency of knowledge by continual revision.

We have chosen the decade as a temporal parameter having regard to ease of future discussion. Manuscripts were selected for their relevancy to the core. Not all references relating to our topic are included either because the information is superfluous or has not yet come to our obvious attention. Searching the literature is by no means an easy task. Information retrieval can never be absolutely complete. However, thoroughness and persistence will capture the essence of a particular subject matter. We have scanned both the indexed (i.e., Index Medicus, CRAC) and the non indexed literature, an exceptionally time-consuming task.

No analysis of our proposed paradigm is intended or offered since much of the data is subject to interpretation, and the reader should fully understand this. Certain trends, however, are clear:

(1) The complications to cervical spinal manipulation are being more fully recognized and reported with increasing frequency.
(2) A cause and effect relationship between cervical spine manipulation and stroke has yet to be established. Manipulation is but one of many factors to be considered in this relationship.
(3) A screening mechanism that is firstly reliable, secondly valid and thirdly reasonable, needs to be established as a standard of chiropractic practice.
(4) There is a need to establish an international registry of incidents that occur related to our subject matter.
(5) Cervical spine manipulation performed by a qualified competent clinician is a relatively safe procedure.

*Modified from Gotlib AC, Thiel H. A selected annotated bibliography of the core biomedical literature pertaining to stroke, cervical spine, manipulation and head/neck movement. J Can Chiro Assoc 1985;29(2):80–89.

1800–1899

1. Taylor H. Embolism of the left vertebral artery: paralysis of the glosso pharyngeal nerve: death from starvation. Br Med J 1871;2:527.

Earliest description relating vertebral artery to traumatic embolic occlusion, stroke, and cranial nerve palsy.

2. Wallenberg A. Acute bulbaraffection (embolie der art cerebellar post. inf sinistre). Archiv Fur Psychiatric 1895;27:504–40.

Single case study, detailed 2 year clinical observation of 30 year old male with sudden onset of progressive dizziness, dysphagia and other symptoms. Speculates on occlusion of cerebellar artery associated with certain signs and symptoms.

1900–1909

1. Roberts JB. Fracture dislocation of the atlas without symptoms of spinal cord injury. Ann Surg 1907;45:632–5.

   Describes a case report of traumatically induced fracture of odontoid process and forward displacement of atlas but no cord injury. Subsequent inappropriate manipulation by osteopath.
2. Corner EM. The physiology of the lateral atlanto-axial joints. J Anat 1907;41:149–54.

   Gives a description of the mechanics of upper cervical movement. Describes case reports of atlas dislocations and atlas subluxation as related to neck rotation. Actually describes a motion palpation procedure for analyzing atlas movement.

1910–1919

1. Jonas AF. Dislocation of the first cervical vertebra, unilateral and backward, produced by manipulation. Trans Am Surg Assoc 1961;34:466–72.

   Discussion regarding cervical spine dislocations and relates to varying degrees of spinal cord injury. Detailed case report of dislocation without fracture (C1) and without cord lesion, produced by manipulative effort (osteopath) used with therapeutic intent.
2. Stopford JSB. The arteries of the pons and medulla oblongata. J Anat Physiol 1916;50:131–64.

   In depth analysis of 150 brains to determine distribution of arteries (vertebral, basilar, internal carotid, circle of Willis) and branches to hindbrain. Cites statistics of anomalies and variations. Vertebral artery size inequality in 92% of sample. Posterior inferior cerebellar artery in 15% of sample.

1920–1929

1. Ramsbottom A, Stopford JSB. Occlusion of the posterior inferior cerebellar artery. Br Med J 1924;1:364–5.

   Discusses the symptom complex and examination findings associated with occlusion.
2. Blaine ES. Manipulative (chiropractic) dislocations of the atlas. JAMA 1925;85(18):1356–9.

   Anatomical description followed by 3 case reports of atlas dislocation, one with fracture, all induced by chiropractic manipulation (age 6, 18, 29), with one eventual death. Cited are 9 other cases (one death) but these are considered anecdotal.
3. Grinker RR, Guy CC. Sprain of cervical spine causing thrombosis of anterior spinal artery. JAMA 1927;88:1140–42.

   Detailed case report (15 year old male) of self induced flexion sprain after vigorous muscular movements, producing anterior spinal arterial occlusion at C5 segment with eventual death. The anterior spinal arteries arise from the vertebral arteries.
4. deKleyn A, Nieuwenhuyse P. Schwindelanfalle and Nystagmas bei einer bestimmten Stellung des Kopfes. Acta Oto-Laryngolica 1927;11:155–7.

   Brief discussion relating head position with vertebral artery occlusion and nystagmus and vertigo (Ger.)

1930–1939

1. Society proceedings. Malpractice: death resulting from chiropractic treatment for headache. JAMA 1934;103:1260.

   Report of stroke from chiropractic manipulation to cervical spine with eventual death. Possibly the first recorded stroke related death in the English literature associated with chiropractic manipulation.
2. Hall AJ, Eaves EC. Posterior inferior cerebellar thrombosis with unusual features. Lancet 1934;227:975–9.

   Detailed case report of 33 year old male complaining of headache and epistaxis who incures thrombosis. Relates to small size of left posterior inferior cerebellar artery and symptoms and signs attributed to occlusion.
3. Society proceedings. Malpractice: cerebral hemorrhage attributed to chiro-

practic adjustment. JAMA 1935;105: 1714.

Further discussion pertaining to reference 1.

4. Diggle FH, Stopford JSB. Posterior inferior cerebellar and vertebral thrombosis. Lancet 1935;1:1214–5.

Discussion of a case of thrombosis following long standing atheroma in 76 year old male and nature of lesion.

5. Sheehan D, Smyth GE. A study of the anatomy of vertebral thrombosis. Lancet 1937;2:614–8.

Literature review of retro-olivary syndrome (24 cases) from 1924 to 1937. Detailed description of 2 cases. Refers to occlusion confined to the posterior inferior cerebellar artery as Wallenburg's syndrome, and occlusion confined to the vertebral artery as Babinski-Nageotte syndrome.

6. Society proceedings. Malpractice: death resulting from chiropractic treatment for headache. JAMA 1937;109–3:233–4.

Further discussion pertaining to reference 1.

1940–1949

1. Kubik C, Adams R. Occlusion of the basilar artery—a clinical and pathological study. Brain 1946;69:73–121.

Detailed case reports of 18 deaths (11 thrombic, 7 embolic) attributed to sudden onset basilar occlusion (autopsy), not proceded by tangible causal factors. Age range 32 to 82. Death ensues 32 hours to 35 days later. Symptoms include headache, dizziness, confusion, dysarthria, paraesthesia. Findings include ocular movement disorders, hemiplegia, cranial nerve palsy and pupillary abnormalities.

2. Pratt-Thomas HR, Berger KE. Cerebellar and spinal injuries after chiropractic manipulation. JAMA 1947;133(9):600–3.

Detailed case descriptions of deaths (age 31, 32, 35) related to chiropractic neck manipulation. Two cases show thrombosis in 3 vessels of vertebrobasilar system. Authors speculate on mechanism involved.

1950–1959

1. Ford FR. Syncope, vertigo and disturbances of vision resulting from intermittent obstruction of the vertebral arteries due to defect in the odontoid process and excessive mobility of the second cervical vertebra. Bull Johns Hopkins Hosp 1952;91:168–73.

Detailed case report on 17 year old male with attacks of syncope. Absent odontoid (chiropractic diagnosis) and excessive mobility of C2, causing presumed intermittent arterial compromise. Mentions 2 additional cases of brainstem infarction after chiropractic manipulation (anecdotal).

2. Kunkle EC, Muller JC, Odom GL. Traumatic brainstem thrombosis: report of a case and analysis of the mechanism of injury. Ann Int Med 1952;36:1329–35.

Detailed case report of brainstem infarction induced by chiropractic manipulation in 35 year old male with rheumatoid spondylitis. No angiography. Author speculates on mechanism of vascular compromise.

3. Ford FR, Clark D. Thrombosis of the basilar artery with softenings in the cerebellum and brainstem due to manipulation of the neck. Bull Johns Hopkins Hosp. 1956;98:37–42.

Discusses 2 case reports of head rotation related to thrombosis. Death from layman manipulation in 37 year old male. Thrombosis in 41 year old male following chiropractic manipulation. Also makes anecdotal mention of a fatal case following chiropractic manipulation. Speculates on mechanism of injury.

4. Schwartz GA, Geiger JK, Spano AV. Posterior inferior cerebellar artery syndrome of Wallenberg after chiropractic manipulation. Ann Int Med 1956;97:352–4.

Case report of Wallenberg syndrome in 28 year old female following chiropractic manipulation.

5. Tissington-Tatlow WF, Bammer HG. Syndrome of vertebral artery compression. Neurology 1957;7–5: 331–40.

Three case reports relating neurologic signs and symptoms (especially dizziness) to changes in head position (particularly rotation). Describes clinical investigation to demonstrate relationship. Single cadaver study shows vertebral artery narrowing with rotation.

6. Green D, Joynt RJ. Vascular accidents of the brain stem associated with neck manipulation. JAMA 1959;170:522–4.

Presents 2 case reports (female—31, male—55) of signs and symptoms suggestive of brainstem vascular accident after chiropractic neck manipulation. Offers reasonable speculation as to mechanism.

7. Boldrey E, Maass L, Miller E. The role of atlantoid compression in the etiology of internal carotid thrombosis. J Neurosurg 1956;13(2):127–39.

Clinical review of 24 cases of angiographically demonstrated occlusion of the internal carotid artery assumed in all to be caused by thrombosis. Discusses compression of internal carotid artery by lateral process of atlas in 6 cases. Suggests age 40 rather than 50 be associated with non-hemorrhagic stroke.

8. Medical legal abstracts. Chiropractors: rupture of brain tumor following adjustment. JAMA 1952;148(8):669.

Discussion of injuries arising from chiropractic manipulation to neck and judgement in favor of plaintiff (state of Montana).

9. Medicolegal abstracts. Chiropractors: injury to spinal meninges during adjustment. JAMA 1955;159(8):809.

Death resulting from chiropractic neck manipulation (state of Missouri).

10. Boshes L. Vascular accidents associated with neck manipulation (letter). JAMA 1959;171(11):1602.

Anecdotal mention of 3 cases of intermittent paralysis from chiropractic manipulation.

11. Hutchinson E, Yates P. The cervical portion of the vertebral artery—a clinicopathological study. Brain 1956; 79:319–31.

Examines the cervical portion of the vertebral artery, the incidence of atheroma and its relationship to carotid artery disease of the neck.

12. Gutmann G, Tiwisina T. Zum problem der irritation der arteria vertebralis. Stuttgart: Hippokrates-Verlag GmbH. 1959(15).

Mechanical irritation of the vertebral artery and nerve is described in relation to cervical spine spondylosis. Vasospasm produced leads to vascular insufficiencies in the posterior aspects of the brain. Rotation movements of head and neck may irritate the vertebral artery and nerve.

13. Kovacs A. Subluxation and deformation of the cervical apophyseal joints. Acta Radiologica 1955;43:1–16.

Discusses subluxation of small joints resulting in circulatory disturbance in the vertebral artery and impaired function of the sympathetic plexus. Relates superior articular process topography to arterial compromise.

14. Neuwirth E. The vertebral nerve in the posterior cervical syndrome (letter). NY State J Med 1955;55:1380.

Describes the vertebral nerve briefly.

15. Lewis R, Coburn D. The vertebral artery. J Missouri St Med Assoc 1956;53(12):1059–63.

Describes 11 cases (ages 23 to 52) of vertebral artery circulatory interference with postural head changes demonstrated angiographically.

16. Schneider R, Lemmen L. Traumatic internal carotid artery thrombosis secondary to non-penetrating injuries to the neck. J Neurosurg 1952;9:495–507.

Reviews 5 previous cases (1872, 1935, 1941, 1943, 1944) and presents 2 additional cases of thrombosis related to trauma history.

17. Suechting R, French L. Posterior inferior cerebellar artery syndrome. J Neurosurg 1955;312:187–9.

Single case report of fracture dislocation of 5th on the 6th cervical vertebra in 29 year old male in whom a posterior inferior cerebellar artery syndrome developed following skeletal head traction.

18. Murray D. Post-traumatic thrombosis of the internal carotid and vertebral

arteries after non-penetrating injuries of the neck. Br J Surg 1957;44:556–61.

Literature review of 9 previous cases of internal carotid artery thrombosis following non-penetrating neck injury. Adds one further case and also a case of traumatic thrombosis of the vertebral artery in a 16 year old male.

1960–1969

1. Sheehan S, Bauer RB, Meyer JS. Vertebral artery compression in cervical spondylosis. Neurology 1960;10:968–86.

Defines the syndrome of vertebral artery compression due to cervical spondylosis, or a combination of spondylosis and cerebrovascular atherosclerosis. Presents 26 cases of cervical spondylosis with vertebral artery compression (arteriography). Compares films before and after neck rotation.

2. Stewart DY. Current concepts of the Barre syndrome or the posterior cervical sympathetic syndrome. Clin Orth 1962;24:40–8.

Discusses the relationship between the cervical sympathetic system and the vertebral artery.

3. Smith RA, Estridge MN. Neurologic complications of head and neck manipulations. JAMA 1962;182:130–3.

Two cases of vascular accident of the brain stem subsequent to neck manipulation presented. Death in 33 year old female after chiropractic manipulation. Wallenberg syndrome in a 48 year old female after osteopathic manipulation. Speculates on mechanism.

4. Simeone FA, Goldberg HI. Thrombosis of the vertebral artery from hyperextension injury to the neck. J Neurosurg 1968;29:540–4.

Describes post traumatic delayed occlusion of the cervical vertebral artery following hyperextension injury to the neck (single case study). Bony foramen transversarium of C6 acts as fulcrum for arterial stretching.

5. Selecki BR. The effect of rotation of the atlas on the axis: experimental work. Med J Austr 1969;56:1012–15.

Studies of 4 cadaveric cervical spine show rotation to 30° produces kinking of contralateral vertebral artery at C2 transverse foramen. Rotation of 45° to 150° affects both vertebral arteries. Describes lateral displacement of upper cord and medulla away from direction of rotation, with indentation of anterior dural sac and anterior spinal artery by the protruding tip of odontoid process.

6. Milne E. Giddiness in vertebrobasilar arterial insufficiency. Med J Aust (letter) 1968;2:417–8.

Anecdotal discussion regarding cervical subluxation and ischaemia.

7. Bauer R, Wechsler N, Meyer J. Carotid compression and rotation of head in occlusive vertebral artery disease. Ann Int Med 1961;55(2):283–91.

Clinical study to determine if patients with vertebrobasilar insufficiency (proved angiographically) were susceptible to EEG abnormalities by rotation of head after digital carotid compression. Mechanisms are postulated.

8. Bauer S, Sheehan S, Meyer J. Arteriographic study of cerebrovascular disease. Arch Neuro 1961;4:119–31.

Tortuosity and kinking of at least one major cerebral vessel (with stenosis and reduction of blood flow through involved vessel) during rotation of head noted angiographically in 1/4 of 71 cases with cerebrovascular disease.

9. Toole J, Tucker S. Influence of head position upon cerebral circulation. Arch Neuro 1960;2:616–23.

Study of 20 autopsy specimens to determine how much influence position of head has in altering blood flow through vertebral and carotid arteries. Motions of rotation, flexion, extension and tilt and combinations are examined. Results indicate that side of vessel occlusion can not be predicted.

10. Faris A, Poser C, Wilmore D, Agnew C. Radiologic visualization of neck vessels in healthy men. Neurol 1963;13(5):386–96.

Arteriographic study of 43 selected

healthy males demonstrates that a majority of healthy asymptomatic individuals have significant arterial abnormalities in the neck vessels.

11. Keggi K, Granger D, Southwick W. Vertebral artery insufficiency secondary to trauma and osteoarthritis of cervical spine. Yale J Biol Med 1966;38:471–8.

Case report of osteophyte obstructing vertebral artery (C5–6) in 51 year old male and neurologic signs and symptoms. Speculates about vertebral artery injury and cerebral palsy.

12. Coburn D. Vertebral artery involvement in cervical trauma. Clin Orth 1962;24:61–2.

Describes how sympathetic fibers in the walls of the vertebral artery may cause vasospasm, particularly in the region of the suboccipital triangle.

13. Brain L. Some unsolved problems of cervical spondylosis. Br Med J 1963:Mar 23:771–7.

Reviews cervical spondylosis, vertebrobasilar ischaemia, effects of head movement on cerebral circulation.

14. Cramer A. Zur chirotherapie des cervical syndrome. Plysik Med U Rehab 1967;8:63–66.

Discussion regarding indications and contraindications to manual therapy for cervical syndrome.

15. Roesner J. Beobachtungen zur Frage der funktionellen Durchblutungsstorungen im Arteria-vertebralis-Bereich und therapeutische Konsequenzen. Manuelle Medizin 1969;1:1–6.

Discusses functional spasm of the vertebral artery (angiography) related to morphological changes of the cervical spine.

16. Chrast B, Korbicka J. Die Beeinflussung der stromungsverhaltnisse in der Arteria vertebralis durch verschiedene Kopf und Halshaltungen. Deutsche Zeitschrift fur Nevenheilkunde 1962;183:426–48.

Study of 20 cadavers analyzing flow rate in the vertebral arteries with various head and neck movements, and combination of movements.

17. Gutmann G. Halswirbelsaule und durchblutungsstorungen in der vertebralis-basilaris-strombahn. In: . . . Die wirbelsaule in forschung und praxis. Stuttgart: Hippokrates, 1962(25):138–55.

Presents 6 case reports regarding cervical spine and vertebrobasilar insufficiency. Discusses sensitization of vertebral artery via mechanical stimuli (tension, compression, shearing, coupled with fixed motion segments).

18. Husni E, Bell H, Storer J. Mechanical occlusion of the vertebral artery. JAMA 1966;196(6):101–4.

Angiographic analysis of 20 symptomatic subjects (age 27–66) in both AP and rotational projections. Head rotation produced vertebral artery occlusion at level of C6 vertebra. Relates mechanism of occlusion to scalenus anticus and longus colli muscle attachments. Surgical resection restores normal flow.

19. Husni E, Storer J. The syndrome of mechanical occlusion of the vertebral artery. Angiology 1967;18(2):106–116.

Arteriography of 67 patients in AP and lateral projections demonstrating total occlusion (23 patients) of a normal vertebral artery at level of C6 produced by neck muscles (longus colli, scalenus anticus, medius) when head turned to one side. Mean age 40.

20. Fields W, Ratinoy G, Weibel J, Campos R. Survival following basilar artery occlusion. Arch Neurol 1966;15:463–471.

Arteriographic studies in 8 patients with vertebrobasilar insufficiency showed abnormality of vertebral arterial circulation extracranially or intracranially as a result of congenital variation (hypoplasia of vertebral artery, asymmetrical Circle of Willis).

21. Hardin C, Williamson W, Steegman T. Vertebral artery insufficiency produced by cervical osteoarthritic spurs. Neurology 1960;10:855–8.

Single case study of 50 year old male with basilar artery insufficiency due to congenital absence of one vertebral artery and compression of the opposite vertebral artery by osteoarthritic spur.

22. Foutz C. Functional vascular changes affecting the posterior inferior cerebellar artery. J Nat Chiro Assoc 1960:March:13–14.

Anecdotal discussion.

23. Powers S, Drislane T, Nevins S. Intermittent vertebral artery compression—a new syndrome. Surgery 1961;49(2):257–264.

Congenital anomalous anatomic variation of subclavian vertebral axis causing intermittent arterial insufficiency (angiographically) in 28 cases. Compression of vertebral artery by scalenus anticus, thyrocervical trunk or subclavian artery related to vertigo.

24. Fasekas J, Alman R, Sullivan J. Vertebrobasilar insufficiency. Arch Neur 1963;8:215–20.

Detailed analysis of 26 cases (ages 37–80) of vertebrobasilar insufficiency and the influence of anticoagulant therapy.

25. Grossiord A. Les accidents neurologiques des manipulation cervicales. Ann Med Phys 1966;9:283–98.

Reviews 17 cases of complications arising from manipulation of cervical spine.

26. Husni E, Storer J. The syndrome of mechanical occlusion of the vertebral artery—further observations. Angiology 1967;18:106–16.

A study of 67 cases of basilar insufficiency (angiographically). Mechanical occlusion of a normal vertebral artery is produced by the action of longus colli, scalenus anticus and medius muscles with head rotation.

27. Eadie M. Paroxysmal positional giddiness. Med J Aust 1967;54:1169–73.

Suggests that some instances of positional giddiness may be related to disturbed cervical muscle contraction.

28. Currier R, Giles C, DeJong R. Some comments on Wallenberg's lateral medullary syndrome. Neurology 1961;11:778–91.

Clinical detailed analysis (without pathologic correlation) of symptomatology in relation to presumed infarct location in medulla.

29. Carpenter S. Injury of neck as a cause of vertebral artery thrombosis. J Neurosurg 1961;18:849–53.

Single case report (42 year old male) of vertebral artery thrombosis following trauma.

30. Hardesty W, Roberts B, Toole J, Royster H. Studies on carotid artery flow. Surgery 1961;49:251–6.

Clinical study (15 patients) analyzing flow rate. Mean internal carotid flow 364 ml. per minute. Turning of head to opposite side reduces flow through internal carotid artery.

31. Hardin C. Cerebral ischaemia due to extracranial vertebral occlusion. Surgery 1962;52:627–31.

Reports on 23 cases of intermittent vertebral artery compression due to extraluminal fascial bands, bony spurs and kinking, and surgical correction.

32. Hardesty W, Whitacre W, Toole J, Randall P, Royster H. Studies on vertebral artery blood flow in man. Surg Gyn Obs 1963;116:662–4.

Clinical study (8 patients) of vertebral artery flow rate. Mean flow 45 ml. per minute (10 to 87 ml). Vertebral artery contributes 11% of cerebral blood flow. Head rotation decreases flow rate.

33. Gurdjian E, Hardy W, Lindner D, Thomas L. Closed cervical cranial trauma associated with involvement of carotid and vertebral arteris. J Neurosurg 1963;20:418–27.

Closed impacts to head and neck (5 patients) cause intimal and medial tears to carotid and vertebral arteries with occlusive thrombosis.

1970–1979

1. Dabbert O, Freeman DG, Weir AJ. Spinal meningeal hematoma, therapy and chiropractic adjustment. JAMA 1970;214:2058.

Single case report of spinal hemorrhage following chiropractic manipulation in a 54 year old female on anticoagulant therapy.

2. Livingston MCP. Spinal manipulation causing injury. Clin Orthop Rel Res 1971;81:82–6.

Retrospective study 676 patients that received spinal manipulation. Presents case reports of injuries.

3. Hargrave-Wilson W. The cervical syndrome. Austr J Physio 1972;18:144–7.
   Describes symptoms of cervical syndrome and includes vertebrobasilar ischaemia.
4. Livingston M. Spinal manipulation causing injury. BC Med J 1972;14–3:78–81.
   Same study as reference 2.
5. Marks RL, Freed MM. Nonpenetrating injuries of the neck and cerebrovascular accident. Arch Neurol 1973;28:412–14.
   Single case report of bilateral vertebral artery occlusion following fracture dislocation of cervical vertebrae (16 year old male). Discusses a slow progression of thrombosis.
6. Latchaw RE, Seeger JF, Gabrielson TD. Vertebrobasilar arterial occlusions in children. Neuroradiology 1974;8:141–7.
   Reports 3 cases of vertebrobasilar occlusion (ages 7, 11, 12) demonstrated angiographically. Reviews literature of 10 previous cases of angiographically confirmed sudden thrombosis in children under age of 18 years.
7. Mehalic T, Farhat SM. Vertebral artery injury from chiropractic manipulation of the neck. Surg Neurol 1974;2:125–9.
   Presents 2 cases (male 40, male 30) of vertebral artery occlusion demonstrated angiographically following chiropractic manipulation.
8. Miller RG, Burton R. Stroke following chiropractic manipulation of the spine. JAMA 1974;229–2:189–90.
   Presents 2 case reports (female 52, male 35) of vascular occlusion (angiography in one case) following chiropractic manipulation. Partial review of literature.
9. Lyness SS, Wagman AD. Neurologic deficit following cervical manipulation. Surg Neurol 1974;2:121–4.
   Single case report (female 20) of cerebrovascular compromise (angiography) after osteopathic manipulation.
10. Kramer KH. Wallenberg-syndrom nach manueller behandlung. Manuelle Medizin 1974;4:88–9.
   Single case report (female 35) of Wallenberg syndrome following manipulation (physician) demonstrated angiographically.
11. Davidson KC, Weiford EC, Dixon DG. Traumatic vertebral artery pseudoaneurysm following chiropractic manipulation. Radiology 1975;115:651–2.
   Single case report of vertebral artery pseudoaneurysm (female 42) shown angiographically with neurological deficit.
12. Mueller S, Sahs AL. Brainstem dysfunction related to cervical manipulation. Neurology 1976;26:547–50.
   Reports 3 cases (female 43, female 28, male 38) of vertebrobasilar ischaemia with neurologic deficit following manipulation (one with hemorrhagic infarction).
13. Beatty RA. Dissecting hematoma of the internal carotid artery following chiropractic cervical manipulation. J Trauma 1977;17–3:248–9.
   Single case report (male 37) of hematoma and occlusion of internal carotid artery following chiropractic manipulation, demonstrated angiographically.
14. Easton JD, Sherman DG. Cervical manipulation and stroke. Stroke 1977; 8:594–7.
   Presents 3 case reports (female 38, female 48, female 44) of vertebrobasilar infarction associated with manipulation (2 chiropractic, 1 spontaneous head rotation with eventual death), demonstrated angiographically in 2 cases.
15. Zimmerman AW, Kumar AJ, Gadoth N, Hodges FJ. Traumatic vertebrobasilar occlusive disease in childhood. Neurology 1978;28:185–8.
   Single case report (male 7) of vertebral artery occlusion following gymnastics and chiropractic manipulation, demonstrated angiographically.

16. Parkin PJ, Wallis WE, Wilson JL. Vertebral artery occlusion following manipulation of the neck. NZ Med J 1978;88:441–3.

Single case report of (female 23) brainstem infarction after physiotherapist manipulation, demonstrated angiographically.

17. Schmitt HP. Manuelle therapie der halswirbelsaule. Manuelle Medizin 1978;4:71–77.

Extensive literature review regarding vertebral artery occlusion and manipulation. Adds 2 cases of occlusion following manipulation (1 death), one demonstrated angiographically.

18. Wolff HD. Komplikationen bei manueller therapie der halswirbelsaule. Manuel Medizin 1978;4:77–81.

Discussion regarding manual therapy and qualifications of manipulator. Most deaths occur between 30–50 years of age.

19. Hildebrandt RW. Vertebral artery syndrome resulting from manipulation of the cervical spine (editorial) J Manip Physiol Therap 1978;2–2:77–8.

Discussion regarding provocation test of vertebral artery insufficiency.

20. Carella A. Slight anomalies of the atlas: their pathogenetic meaning. Neuroradiology 1972;3:224–7.

Retrospective atlas x-ray analysis in 51 cases. Attempts to relate headache and symptoms of vertebrobasilar insufficiency to bone anomaly.

21. Barton JW, Margolis MT. Rotational obstruction of the vertebral artery at the atlantoaxial joint. Neuroradiology 1975;9:117–20.

Presents 2 case reports (male 48, male 52) of vertebrobasilar ischaemia in whom angiography demonstrated obstruction of vertebral artery upon rotation of head.

22. Sorenson BF. Bow hunter's stroke. Neurosurg 1978;2(3):259–61.

Single case report (male 39) of vertebral artery ischaemia following head rotation (angiography).

23. Gorman RF. Cardiac arrest after cervical spine mobilization. Med J Aust 1978;2:169–70.

Single case report (male 38) of cardiorespiratory arrest following neck rotation.

24. Gorman RF. Vertebral artery occlusion following manipulation of the neck. NZ Med J (letter) 1979;90(640):76.

Discussion regarding use of manipulation to treat vertebrobasilar ischaemia.

25. Kanshepolsky J. Danielson H, Flynn RE. Vertebral artery insufficiency and cerebellar infarct due to manipulation of the neck. Bull Los Angeles Neurol Soc 1972;37(2):62–6.

Single case report (female 39) of neurologic deficit with cerebellar infarction after chiropractic manipulation (angiography, ventriculography).

26. Anderson R, Carleson R, Nylen O. Vertebral artery insufficiency and rotational obstruction. Acta Med Scand 1970;188:475–77.

Single case report (male 38) of intermittent vertebrobasilar insufficiency from rotational obstruction. Hypoplastic right vertebral artery with anomalous origin of left (angiography).

27. Nagler W. Vertebral artery obstruction by hyperextension of the neck: report of the three cases. Arch Phys Med Rehabil 1973;54:237–40.

Presents 3 case reports (male 18, male 55, female 28) of neurologic deficit following hyperextension of neck during gymnastics, calisthenics and yoga. Quadraplegia in 2 cases from anterior spinal artery ischaemia.

28. Fraser RAR, Zimbler SM. Hindbrain stroke in children caused by extracranial vertebral artery trauma. Stroke 1975;6(2):153–9.

Vertebrobasilar stroke in 6 year old male resulting from atlantoaxial subluxation and nonfusion of odontoid process demonstrated angiographically.

29. Okawara S, Nibbelink D. Vertebral artery occlusion following hyperextension and rotation of the head. Stroke 1974;5(5):640–2.

Lateral medullary syndrome of Wallenberg following vertebral artery occlusion precipitated by hyperextension, rotation and lateral flexion of head within physiologic limits in 43 year old male (angiography).

30. Klein RA, Snyder RD, Schwarz HJ. Lateral medullary syndrome in a child—arteriographic confirmation of vertebral artery occlusion. JAMA 1976;235(9):940–1.

Lateral medullary syndrome of Wallenberg demonstrated angiographically in 8 year old male.

31. Hanus SH, Homer TD, Harter DH. Vertebral artery occlusion complicating yoga exercises. Arch Neurol 1977;34:574–5.

Single case report of vertebrobasilar stroke in 25 year old male demonstrated angiographically following sustained rotation and extension of neck.

32. Nyberg-Hansen R, Loken AC, Tenstad O. Brainstem lesion with coma for five years, following manipulation of the cervical spine. J Neurol 1978;218(2): 97–105.

Case report of eventual death (female 38) after neck manipulation (physician) resulting from temporary vertebrobasilar occlusion and subsequent infarction.

33. Nagashima C, Iwama K, Sakata E, Miki Y. Effects of temporary occlusion of a vertebral artery on the human vestibular system. J Neurosurg 1970;33: 388–94.

Vestibular responses elicited by temporary occlusion of one vertebral artery were observed in 25 cases of intermittent vertebral artery compression during surgical treatment by periarterial denervation of an isolated vertebral artery.

34. Gow PJ. Vertebral artery occlusion following manipulation of the neck. NZ Med J (letter) 1979;89(638):493.

Vertebrobasilar insufficiency considered a contraindication to manipulative treatment.

35. Gorman RF. Vertebral artery occlusion following manipulation of the neck. NZ Med J (letter) 1979;89(635):362.

Vertebrobasilar insufficiency considered an indication for manipulative treatment.

36. Fisk JW. Neck manipulation. NZ Med J (letter) 1979;89(628):61. Discussion regarding provocative test of extensive and rotation.

37. Goodbody RA. Proceedings: Fatal post traumatic vertebrobasilar ischaemia. Clin Pathol 1976;29(1):86–7.

Case report of death following osteopathic manipulation (23 year old male).

38. Jones MW, Kaufman JCE. Vertebrobasilar artery insufficiency in rheumatoid atlantoaxial subluxation. J Neurol Neurosurg Psych 1976;39(2):122–8.

Present 2 case reports (female 45, male 74) of vertebral artery intermittent compression from neck movement, one with eventual death.

39. Rinsky L, Reynolds G, Jameson R, Hamilton R. A cervical spinal cord injury following chiropractic manipulation. Paraplegia 1976;13(4):223–7.

Single case report (male 44) of permanent C4 tetraplegia following chiropractic manipulation of a patient with ankylosing spondylitis.

40. Brust J, Plank C, Healton E, Sanchez G. The pathology of drop attacks: a case report. Neurology 1979;29:786–90.

Literature review of drop attacks with single case report (male 65) demonstrating vertebrobasilar insufficiency.

41. Ueda K, Toole J, McHenry L. Carotid and vertebrobasilar transient ischemic attacks: clinical and angiographic correlation. Neurology 1979;29:1094–1101.

Study attempts to correlate clinical phenomena with angiographic findings to evaluate relationship of bruits and lesions and to ascertain whether risk factors differ in vertebrobasilar and carotid TIA's.

42. LaBan M, Meerschaert J, Johnstone K. Carotid bruits: their significance in the cervical radicular syndrome. Arch Phys Med Rehabil 1977;58:491–4.

During routine evaluation of 600 patients with neck shoulder pain associated with cervical radiculopathy, 11 patients had cervical artery bruits.

43. Heyden S. Extrakranialer thrombotischer Arterienverschluss als Folge von Kopf und Halsverletzung. Mat Med Nordm 1971;23:24–32.

Presents 3 cases of extracranial thrombotic artery occlusion following injuries to head and neck (male 65, male 39, female 29). Vertebral artery thrombosis in 29 year old female following chiropractic manipulation.

44. Jung A, Kehr P. Das zerviko-enzephale syndrom bei arthrosen und nach traumen der Halswirbelsaule. Manuelle Medizin 1972;5:97–103.

45. Jung A, Kehr P. Das zerviko-enzephale syndrom bei arthrosen und nach traumen der Halswirbelsaule. Manuelle Medizin 1972;6:127–33.

Literature review with discussion of hemodynamics of vertebrobasilar systems, angiography and symptoms.

46. Gutmann G. Durchblutungsstorungen der arteria vertebralis im zusammenhang mit Halswirbelsaulenverletzungen. Manuelle Medizin 1971;5:112–116.

Discussion regarding secondary changes following injuries to the cervical spine and provocation of transitory circulatory disturbances with dizziness up to syncope by continuously recurring low grade mechanical irritation to the vertebral artery.

47. Giles L. Vertebral-basilar artery insufficiency. JCCA 1977;21:112–117.

Brief review of vertebrobasilar insufficiency. Describes a test of provocation.

48. Schmitt HP. Rupturen und thrombosen der arteria vertebralis nach gedeckten mechanischen insulten. Schweizer Arch Fuer Neurlogie Psychiatrie 1976;119(2):363–79.

Review 5 cases of vertebral artery thrombosis following various insults (manipulation, motor vehicle accident, gymnastics) with one death.

49. Hensell V. Neurologische schaden nach repositions massnahmen an der wirbelsaule. Med Welt 1976;27(14):656–58.

Single case report of 52 year old female with Wallenburg syndrome following neck manipulation (physician) with eventual death.

50. Dtsch Gesellsch Man Med (1979) Memorandum. Zur verhutung von zwischenfallen bei gezielter handgrifftherapie an der halswirbelsaule. Manuelle Medizin 1979;17:53–58.

Literature review. Discusses diagnostic tests to be used in manual therapy.

51. Peiffer J, Haas H, Boellaard JW. Basilaris-vertebralis-aneurysmen als ursache scheinbarer halswirbelsaulensyndrome. Klinische und morphologische untersuchungen an funf klinisch nicht diagnostizierten fallen. Dtsch Med Wschr 1978; 103:331–35.

Reviews 5 cases of vertebrobasilar aneurysm and discusses the symptoms involved as compared to a cervical syndrome.

52. Kunert W. Halswirbelsaule und durchblutungsstorungen im vertebralis-basilaris-stromgebiet und ihre klinischen erscheinungen. In: Trostdorf E, Stender H. Wirbelsaule und nervensystem. Stuttgart: Thieme, 1970:62–68.

Discussion regarding predisposition of vertebral artery to circulatory disturbances due to functional and mechanical relationship to cervical spine.

53. Lorenz R, Vogelsang HG. Thrombose der arteria basilaris nach chiropraktischen manipulationen an der halswirbelsaule. Dtsch Med Wschr 1972;97:36–43.

Single case report (female 29) of basilar artery thrombosis after chiropractic manipulation with eventual death (angiography).

54. Lewit K. Komplikationen nach chiropraktischen manipulationen (letter). Dtsch Med Wschr 1972;97:784.

55. Lorenz R, Vogelsang H. Komplikationen nach chiropraktischen manipulationeen (letter). Dtsch Med Wschr 1972;97:784.

56. Kipp W. Todlicher hirnstamminfarkt nach HWS-manipulation [Dissertation]. Tubingen: Eberhard Karls Universitat. 1975. 39p.

Single case report (female 34) of

brainstem infarction after cervical spine manipulation with eventual death. Discusses similar reported cases.

57. Singer W, Haller J, Wolpert S. Occlusive vertebrobasilar artery disease associated with cervical spine anomaly. AM J Dis Child 1975;129:492–495.

A case study of a six year old boy relating (a) non-union of odontoid process, (b) repeated arterial trauma, and (c) stretching and tearing of the intima of vertebral arteries to vertebrobasilar thromboembolic occlusion.

58. Castaigne P, Lhermitte F, Gautier J, et al. Arterial occlusions in the vertebrobasilar system. Brain 1973;96:133–154.

A study of 44 patients with postmortem data examining occlusion of the vertebrobasilar system related to atherosclerosis. Vertebral artery occlusion may or may not result in medullary and/or cerebellar infarction. Cardiac embolism (9.1%) is a source of vertebrobasilar occlusion. Also suggests some patients with single vertebral artery occlusion may be asymptomatic if contralateral artery is of adequate size.

59. Harwood-Nash D, Mcdonald P, Argent W. Cerebral arterial disease in children. Am J Roentgenol 1971;3(4):672–86.

An angiographic study of 40 cases regarding sudden hemiplegia in children. Discusses a direct relationship between nasopharyngeal infection and acute hemiplegia in some children. Considers concept of undue sensitivity of arteries, arteritis, thrombus and arterial trauma.

60. Buscaglia L, Crowhurst H. Vertebral artery trauma. Am J Surg 1979;138:269–72.

Five case studies report the relationship of vertebral arteriovenous fistulas and the findings pulsatile tinnitus and bruit in the cervical region.

61. Shaw C, Alvord C. Injury of the basilar artery associated with close head trauma. J Neurol Neurosurg Psych 1972;35:247–57.

One of 3 cases presented discussed delayed rupture of the basilar artery occurring 3–4 weeks after an injury, which caused aneurysmal formation. The suggested mechanism is sudden overstretching or torsion of the artery causing intimal tears which remain silent until the damaged arterial wall serves as a locus minoris resistentiae for development of focal atheroma.

62. Ouvrier R, Hopkins I. Occlusive disease of the vertebrobasilar arterial system in childhood. Develop Med Child Neurol 1970;12:186–92.

Three examples of vertebro-basilar insufficiency in children (ages 4, 9, 14) documented by arteriography are described. The causes of occlusion were arteritis, embolic bacterial endocarditis or unknown.

63. DeVivo D, Farrell F. Vertebrobasilar occlusive disease in children. Arch Neurol 1972;26:278–81.

Single case study in 10 year old boy, inferring vertebral artery tortuousity predisposes to intermittent occlusion depending on neck position.

64. Kleynhans A. Vascular changes occurring in the cervical musculoskeletal system. JCCA 1970;14(4):19–21.

Discussion regarding vertebral artery and cervical musculoskeletal venous plexuses.

65. Houle J. Assessing hemodynamics of the vertebrobasilar complex through angiothlopsis. Digest Chiro Econo 1972;15(2):14–15.

Reviews briefly the vertebrobasilar complex and discusses a provovation test before manipulation.

66. Marks R, Freed M. Nonpenetrating injuries of the neck and cerebrovascular accident. Arch Neurol 1973;28:412–14.

Single case report (male 16) of bilateral vertebral artery occlusion following closed trauma. Fracture dislocation with quadriplegia (angiography).

67. Hyyppa S, Laasonen E, Halonen V. Erosion of cervical vertebrae caused by elongated and tortuous vertebral arteries. Neuroradiology 1974;7:49–51.

Present 9 cases of vertebral artery loops (ages 34–74). A tortuous vertebral artery sometimes produces symptoms provoked by nerve root compression (angiography).

68. Barratt J. Enlargement of cervical intervertebral foramina by coiling of the vertebral artery. Austr Radiol 1974;18(2):171–4.
Single case report (male 48) with review of previous 3 cases (angiography).

69. Zauel D, Carlow T. Internuclear ophthalmoplegia following cervical manipulation (letter). Ann Neurol 1977;1(3):308.
Single case report (female 47) of internuclear ophthalmoplegia following chiropractic manipulation.

1980–1984

1. Krueger BR, Obazaki H. Vertebrobasilar distribution infarction following chiropractic cervical manipulation. Mayo Clin Proc 1980;55:322–32.
Extensive literature review. Presents 10 cases of vertebrobasilar occlusion (average age 38) following chiropractic manipulation, one with death resulting (angiography).

2. Jaskoviak PA. Complications arising from manipulation of the cervical spine. J Manip Physiol Therap 1980;3(4): 213–20.
Extensive literature review. Suggests a routine screening procedure before manipulation.

3. Schellhas KP, Latchaw RE, Wendling LR, Gold L. Vertebrobasilar injuries following cervical manipulation. JAMA 1980;244:1450–3.
Presents 4 cases of brainstem stroke (age 36, 31, 32, 20) following chiropractic manipulation in 3 cases and self performed manipulation in one case (angiography).

4. Kleynhans AM. Complications of and contraindications to spinal manipulative therapy. In: Haldeman S, ed. Modern developments in the principles and practice of chiropractic. New York: Appleton-Century-Crofts, 1980: 359–84.
Extensive literature review.

5. Gatterman MI. Contraindications and complications of spinal manipulative therapy. ACA J Chiro 1981;15:75–86.
General discussion of contraindications and complications. Outlines diagnostic procedures to identify high risk patients.

6. Laderman JP. Accidents of spinal manipulation. Ann Swiss Chiro Assoc 1981;7:161–208.
Extensive literature review (French, English, German) of 140 accidents attributed to vertebrotherapy (54 with vascular/neurological lesions).

7. Hosek RS, Schram SB, Silverman H, Myers JB, Williams SE. Cervical manipulation (letter). JAMA 1981;245:922.
Discussion relating vertebrobasilar injury from cervical manipulation as one in 1 million chances.

8. Robertson JT. Neck manipulation as a cause of stroke (editorial). Stroke 1981;12:1.
Discussion regarding manipulation and stroke. Calls for liaison with Stroke Council of American Heart Association.

9. Sherman DG, Hart RG, Easton JD. Abrupt change in head position and cerebral infarction. Stroke 1981;12:2–6.
Presents 8 cases of vertebrobasilar artery infarction (2 deaths) following chiropractic manipulation (6) or spontaneous head turning (2) (angiography).

10. Fraser DM. Neck manipulation as a cause of stroke (letter). Stroke 1982;13:260.
Discussion regarding reference 9. Selection of patients excludes risk of stroke.

11. Sherman DG, Hart RG, Easton JD. Neck manipulation as a cause of stroke (letter in reply). Stroke 1982;13:260.
Discussion regarding reference 9. It is not possible to predict patients likely to develop stroke as a consequence of neck manipulation or spontaneous head turning.

12. Robertson JT. Neck manipulation as a cause of stroke (letter in reply). Stroke 1982;13:260–1.
Discussion regarding German Society of Manipulative Medicine and

Stroke registry Committee, also Stroke Council of American Heart Association. Injury is not rare.

13. Dvorak J, Orelli F. How dangerous is manipulation of the cervical spine? Manuelle Medizin 1982;20:44–8.

Single case report (female 35) of tetraplegia following chiropractic manipulation. Inquiry among Swiss medical group for manual medicine reports slight neurological complications observed in 1 of 40,000 cases and one important complication observed in 1 of 400,000 manipulations.

14. Simmons KC, Soo, Y, Walker G, Harvey P. Trauma to the vertebral artery related to neck manipulation. Med J. Austr 1982;1:187–8.

Single case report (male 41) of brainstem ischaemia related to neck manipulation (angiography).

15. Meyermann R. Possibilities of injury to the artery vertebralis. Manuelle Medizin 1982;20:105–14.

Single case report of death in 36 year old female following manipulation (physician). Discusses the possibilities of injury to vertebral artery.

16. Chakera T, Anderson J, Edis R. Atlantoaxial dislocation and vertebral artery aneurysm. Br J Rad 1982;55:863–4.

Single case report (male 20) of brainstem stroke relating vertebral artery aneurysm caused by chronic arterial trauma due to excessive movement at the C1/C2 level (angiography).

17. Saternus K, Fuchs V. Is the artery vertebralis endangered in resuscitation: Manuelle Medizin 1982·20:101–4.

Postmortem angiographic study of 35 nontraumatic deaths after emergency intubation. Found 2 cases of circumscribed perivascular hemorrhage. Must consider traction and hyperextension of neck during intubation.

18. Schmitt HP. Axis fracture after chiropractic manipulation on spondylosis carcinomatosis. Manuelle Medizin 1982;20:123–5.

Single case report (male 67) of pathological fracture following chiropractic manipulation.

19. Kewalramani LS, Kewalramani DL, Krebs M, Saleem A. Myelopathy following cervical spine manipulation. AM J Phys Med 1982;61:165–75.

Presents 3 case reports (male 46, female 23, male 62) of tetraplegia (myelopathy) associated with cervical spine manipulation (myelography). Myelopathy distinguished from vertebrobasilar occlusion.

20. Grossman RI, Davis KR. Positional occlusion of the vertebral artery: a rare cause of embolic stroke. Neuroradiology 1982;23:227–30.

Single case report (male 19) of embolic stroke demonstrated angiographically, following positional occlusion of vertebral artery. Stasis produces small thrombi and subsequent embolism.

21. Gutmann G. Injuries to the vertebral artery caused by manual therapy. Manuelle Medizin 1983;21:2–14.

Reports 7 cases of vertebral artery injury (1 death) following manual therapy. Some details lacking. Discusses patients at higher risk. Estimates 2–3 serious incidents concerning the vertebrobasilar system occur in 1 million manipulations to the upper cervical spine.

22. Ziv I, Rang M, Hoffman HJ. Paraplegia in osteogenesis imperfecta. J Bone Joint Surg 1983;65(B):184–5.

Single case report of paraplegia in 12 year old girl with osteogenesis imperfecta after chiropractic manipulation.

23. Horn SW. The locked-in syndrome following chiropractic manipulation of the cervical spine. Ann Emerg Med 1983;12:648–50.

Single case report (male 34) of tetraplegia and basilar artery occlusion following chiropractic manipulation (angiography).

24. Braun IF, Pinto RS, Defilipp GJ, Lieberman A, Pasternack P, Zimmerman RD. Brainstem infarction due to chiropractic manipulation of the cervical spine. South Med J 1983;76(9):1199–1201.

Single case report of brainstem infarction caused by vertebral artery occlusion after chiropractic manipulation in 47 year old male (angiography).

25. Hulse M. Disequilibrium caused by a functional disturbance of the upper cervical spine. Manuelle Medizin 1983;1:18–23.

Discussion—dysequilibrium caused by functional proprioceptive disturbance not always attributed to blood flow disturbance of vertebral artery.

26. Dhamoon SK, Iqbal J, Collins GH. Ipsilateral hemiplegia and the Wallenberg syndrome. Arch Neurol 1984; 41:179–80.

Single case report (male 78) documenting anatomic basis for hemiplegia occurring on same side of body as the lateral medullary infarction (autopsy).

27. Daneshmend TK, Hewer RL, Bradshaw JR. Acute brainstem stroke during neck manipulation. Br Med J 1984;288: 189.

Single case report (male 31) of vertebral artery occlusion following osteopathic neck manipulation (angiography).

28. George PE, Silverstein HT, Wallace H, Marshall M. Identification of the high risk pre-stroke patient. ACA J Chiro 1981;15:26–8.

Proposes a screening procedure for presence of cerebral ischaemia.

29. Weintraub M. Dormant foramen magnum meningioma activated by chiropractic manipulation. NY State J Med 1983;83:1039–40.

Single case report (male 40) of quadraplegia associated with meningioma, vertebral artery and chiropractic manipulation.

30. Wolff H. Kontra-Indikationen gezielter Handgrifftherapie an der Wirbelsaule. Manuelle Medizin 1980;3:39–49.

Discussion regarding contraindications of manual spinal therapy.

31. Sulkava R, Kovanen J. Locked-in syndrome with rapid recovery: a manifestation of basilar artery migraine? Headache 1983;23:238–9.

Single case report (female 29) suggesting that transitory brainstem ischaemia be considered as a possible complication of vertebrobasilar migraine.

32. Cote R, Battista R. Asymptomatic cervical bruits. Can Med Assoc J 1984;130:997–1000.

Literature review regarding carotid and vertebral artery bruits and related stroke risk.

33. D'Alton J, Norris J. Carotid doppler evaluation in cerebrovascular disease. Can Med Assoc J 1983;129:1184–9.

Reviews doppler technique in 246 examinations and compares angiographic findings in same patients. Doppler is not a substitute for angiography. It poorly evaluates the posterior vertebrobasilar circulation.

34. McGregor M, Sheldon H, Dwyer D, et al. The role of intimal hyperplasia in arterial spasm. Can Med Assoc J 1984;131:329–30.

Animal study demonstrating arterial spasm experimentally induced did not produce greater reduction in arterial lumen diameter in artery with intimal hyperplasia.

35. Schmidley J, Koch T. The noncerebrovascular complications of chiropractic manipulation. Neurology 1984;34: 684–5.

Single case report (male 52) of cervical cord myelography from osteophytic spur in patients with ankylosing spondylitis exacerbated by chiropractic manipulation.

36. Crawford J, Hwang B, Asselbergs P, Hickson G. Vascular ischemia of the cervical spine: a review of relationship to therapeutic manipulation. J Manip Physiol Ther 1984;4:;149–55.

Extensive literature review.

37. Levien L, Fritz V, Lurie D, Cooke P, Hertzanu Y. Fibromuscular dysplasia of the extracranial carotid arteries. S Afr Med J 1984;65:261–5.

Presents 7 cases of fibromuscular dysplasia of carotid artery. Characteristically affects vessel at level of C2. Important cause of cerebrovascular disease in younger adult age group. Associated with high incidence of intracranial aneurysm (angiography).

38. Grundy D, McSweeney T, Jones H. Cranial nerve palsies in cervical injuries. Spine 1984;9(4):339–43.

Presents 8 cases (mean age 30) of cranial nerve palsies in cervical injuries related to brainstem ischaemia due to vertebral artery spasm, compression or thrombosis.

39. Keller H, Turina M, Imhof H, Valavanis A. Ultraschall doppler sonographie der halsgefasse und schwindel. Manuelle Medizin 1984;22:107–115.

Clinical study of 471 patients with vertigo or dizziness using ultrasound doppler and specific provocation maneuvres.

40. Hulse M. Die zervikalen gleichgewichtsstorungen. Berlin: Springer Verlag. 1983:4–9.

Extensive literature review and in depth discussion related to vertebral artery.

41. Schmitt HP. Zur inzidenz, pathomorphologie und pathomechanik der komplikationen bei der manualtherapie der halswirbelsaule. In: Odenbach E, Lauterbach H, Verheggen-Buschhaus H, eds. Jahrbuch 1983–84 Fortschritt und fortbildung inder medizin VII. Interdisziplinares forum der bandesarztekammer 12 bis 15 Januar 1983. Kiln: Deutscher Arzte-Verlag. 1983:461–71.

Extensive literature review and analysis, regarding incidence and pathomechanics of complications following manual therapy of cervical spine. Spiral motions of head and neck (rotation with extension with traction) are most dangerous.

42. Wolff HD. Vaskulare aspekte der manuellen medizin. Bemerkungen zu beziehungern zwischen funktionsstorungen des vaskularen systems und funktionsstorungen am achsenorgan. Manuelle Medizin 1983;21:100–106.

Discussion regarding vascular aspects in manual therapy, the relationship between functional disturbance of the circulatory system and functional disturbance of the axial skeleton.

43. Stevens A. Doppler sonography and neck rotation. Manuelle Medizin 1984;1:49–53.

A doppler investigation of the vertebral artery (19 subjects ages 20–30) analyzing flow with passive neck rotation. Mean obstruction angle for contralateral rotation 73° bilateral, while ipsilateral rotation is 77° left and 89° right. Mean critical angle contralateral rotation 56° bilateral, while ipsilateral rotation is 55° left and 71° right. Mechanism of occlusion relates arterial transmural pressure to elongation caused by rotation.

44. Terrett A, Webb M. Vertebrobasilar accidents following cervical spine adjustment manipulation. J Aust Chiro Assoc 1982;12(5):24–7.

Literature review of incidence, mechanics, provocation tests, signs and symptoms.

45. Terrett A. Importance and interpretation of tests designed to predict susceptibility to neurocirculatory accidents from manipulation. J Austr Chiro Assoc 1983;13(2):29–34.

Reviews a screening procedure prior to manipulation.

46. Gutman G, ed. Arteria vertebralis-traumatologie und funtionelle pathologie. Berlin/Heidelberg: Springer-Verlag, 1984.

Extensive literature review on functional anatomy, mechanics, injury mechanisms, clinical diagnosis and manual therapy.

12 Neck-Tongue Syndrome and Spinal Manipulative Therapy

Allan G. J. Terrett, Dip. App. Sc. (Hum Biol), B. App. Sc. (Chir)(PIT), Grad. Dip. Tert. Ed. (HIE); F.A.C.C.S.

HISTORY

The first description of the neck-tongue syndrome (NTS) as a distinct syndrome was in 1980 by Lance and Anthony(1), who described NTS as a syndrome of nuchal or occipital pain, with or without associated numbness, accompanied by transient ipsilateral numbness of the tongue brought on by turning the head. The pain is often ushered in by an "electric shock, heat or burning feeling" suggesting that the pain is at least, in part, neurogenic.

Cyriax(2) had previously described three cases of lingual paresthesia (Table 12.1, cases 1–3) and in the 1962 edition of his book(3), as mentioned by Lance and Anthony(1), described aggravation by neck rotation. Cyriax attributed the tongue numbness to involvement of the third cervical nerve root, as he did not consider that it could be due to involvement of the first or second cervical nerves at least in the young before the onset of occipitoatlantoaxial arthrosis since there is no cervical disc at the level of the upper two nerves. He believed that symptoms in the C1 and C2 nerves were produced by extrasegmental reference from the dura mater caused by disc lesions at lower levels(2). For additional background, see Table 12.1, which reviews 33 cases of NTS that have appeared in the literature(1–12).

CASE DESCRIPTIONS

It is not possible to determine the incidence of this syndrome, but since the previous description of cases A–D(13), the author has received a continual flow of reports from colleagues reporting similar favorable responses of this syndrome to spinal manipulative therapy (SMT), suggesting that it is not as rare as initially believed. Eight cases that presented to practitioners of spinal manipulative therapy are described.

Case A

A 29-year-old nurse was involved in a head-on motor car collision in December 1980. She first consulted the author 19 months later complaining of, among other things, difficulty with moving the neck, pain and stiffness in the neck, headaches, constant pain in the left shoulder, and difficulty in moving the left arm.

Premanipulative tests for possible signs of cerebral ischemia were conducted. While positioning the cervical spine in left rotation, right lateral flexion, and extension, the patient related that the right side of her tongue had "become numb, similar to that following a dental analgesic." To the author at that time, this suggested involvement of the trigeminal nerve, or of "strange" symptoms produced by brain stem ischemia induced by neck position. There were, however, no other signs to indicate vertebrobasilar ischemia.

Other possible etiologies were (1) vertebrobasilar or carotid artery pathology, but this would normally be expected to be associated with hemianesthesia of at least the face, if not the entire body; (2) hyper-

Table 12.1
Previously Described Cases of NTS

Case	Source	Sex (* = unknown)	Age	Symtoms
1	Cyriax J (2, 3)	Female	45	Paresthesia on half of the tongue and the posterior palate, with no muscular weakness.
2	Cyriax J (2, 3)	*	*	Paresthesia on half of the tongue, with no muscular weakness.
3	Cyriax J (2)	*	*	Paresthesia felt at the inferior surface of the tongue, as well as in both feet, abolished by cervical manipulation.
4	Lance JW, Anthony M (1)	Male	26	Transient numbness of the right side of the tongue and right 4th and 5th fingers, provoked by head rotation and present since a blow on the head when 8.
5	Lance JW, Anthony M (1)	Male	15	Transient tongue numbness and pain in the head and occipital region associated with a feeling of faintness produced by sharp neck rotation to either side. The tongue became numb and felt as if it were twisting in the mouth. Aggravated by swimming, softball, bowling, or swinging on parallel bars.
6	Lance JW, Anthony M (1)	Male	17	Intermittent occipital pain for 3 years and numbness on half the tongue for 10 months produced by turning the head, and associated with trasient tingling in the fingers.
7	Lance JW, Anthony M (1)	Female	15	Pain in the neck for 3 years, tongue, neck, and mastoid numbness began 9 months later, aggravated by neck turning. Relief was obtained by keeping the neck still, or tilting the head to the right.
8	Elisevich K et al (4)	Female	53	Patient with assimilation of the atlas to the occiput presented with a 6-year history of right-sided neck discomfort, which radiated to the back of her head, and a 1-year history of ipsilateral tongue paresthesia, aggravated by neck rotation. She also suffered a mild dysphagia, because of a feeling of muscle spasm in her throat. After being intermittent for several years, the symptoms became persistent and increasingly incapacitating. Partial relief after resection of fibrosed C2 ventral ramus.
9–11	Lance JW (5)	*	*	Three cases of neck-tongue syndrome that started in late childhood or adolescence.
12	Lance JW (5)	Female	19	This patient had no tongue paresthesia but had a 5-year history of paroxysmal pain in the left side of the neck on sudden neck turning accompanied by deviation of the tongue for 10 seconds, during which time she was unable to speak.
13	Lance JW (5)	Male	60	Episodes since the age of 10 years. He felt as though the tongue was cleaving to the roof of the mouth.
14	Webb et al (6)	Male	36	A patient with ankylosing spondylitis with anterior syndesmophytic bridging between C4 and C7 accidentally jarred his neck producing high cervical pain radiating to the left side of the tongue (like a dental anesthetic) that occurred several times a day lasting 1–3 minutes. Wearing a cervical collar and taking care to avoid sudden jolting virtually eliminated his symtoms.
15	Webb et al (6)	Female	65	Patient with degenerative spondylosis, after an active day, developed low back, cervicothoracic, suboccipital, and a left-sided head, jaw, and tongue pain (of a lancinating pseudoneuralgic

Table continues

Table 12.1 (*Continued*)

Case	Source	Sex (* = unknown)	Age	Symtoms
				quality, like a nail being driven into it). The sub-occipital, head, jaw, and tongue symptoms were induced by virtually any neck movement and lasted 30 seconds to several minutes. A program of postural control, isometric neck exercises, and use of a cervical collar controlled the patient's symptoms.
16	Webb et al (6)	Male	34	Left-sided neck pain radiating to the occiput, associated with ipsilateral aching and numbness of the tongue. Symptoms were "shock-like" in onset with a few seconds of pain followed by several minutes of numbness and paresthesia over the left occiput and tongue. The symptoms occurred during recently resumed competitive swimming (turning of the head for breathing). He remembered experiencing the same symptoms between 10 and 22 years old, when he was a competitive swimmer.
17	Noda A, Umezaki H (7)	Female	35	Patient developed symptoms of acute upper thoracic spinal cord transverse myelopathy at 23 years. She developed tonic seizures lasting about 60 seconds. About 20 seconds after beginning, the neck and occipital region on the left became numb, accompanied by simultaneous numbness of the left half of the tongue, lasting for 30–60 seconds. These attacks occurred about once an hour, and were suppressed by 400 mg of carbamazepine daily.
18–26	Bertoft ES, Westerberg C (8)	*	*	Nine cases of NTS, 6 with a complete syndrome, 3 with an incomplete form of the syndrome. One case (incomplete) was the son of a patient with the complete syndrome. Two cases had rheumatic disease (ankylosing and psoriatic arthritis) affecting the lateral atlantoaxial joints. Both of these had a complete NTS, and in one, symptoms were abolished after fusion of C1–C2.
27	Fortin CJ, Biller J (9)	Female	57	Numbness of the posterior right half of the tongue, posterolateral oropharynx, and the 4th and 5th fingers of her right hand with ipsilateral "ear pressure" and sharp pain along the border of the trapezius to the acromioclavicular joint and a pressure sensation in the occiput. This had insidiously progressed over 2 months, was precipitated by right neck rotation, persisted for 30 seconds with maximum intensity, and then slowly abated over several minutes. Remainder of the neurological examination was normal. Symptoms were nearly totally alleviated after wearing a cervical collar for several weeks and failed to return in the following 6 months.
28	Fortin CJ, Biller J (9)	Male	29	This radiologist had had two motorcycle accidents 6 and 7 years previously. Two years later he developed 2 groups of symptoms precipitated by cervical rotation or extension. That related to the NTS was ipsilateral (usually right) hemiglossal and facial "tingling" paresthesia, sharp occipital pain "shooting to the periorbital region, dysarthria, marked nasal congestion, sialorrhea, and paresthesia in both ulnar distributions. Symptoms were precipitated by neck

Table continues

Table 12.1 *(Continued)*

Case	Source	Sex (* = unknown)	Age	Symtoms
				rotation. This patient obtained significant relief by wearing a hard cervical collar, but symptoms return immediately when the collar is removed.
29	Cassidy JD et al (10)	Female	48	No recollection of previous trauma. Since childhood, rotation of the head to the right caused suboccipital pain with radiation to the vertex, and numbness on the right side of the tongue. On examination, the range of motion was limited in all directions except left rotation. She was given a 2-week course of daily manipulations directed toward mobilizing the upper and lower cervical spine on the right, after which she reported she was symptom free. Review at 3 months, 1 year, and 2 years after therapy revealed no further symptoms.
30	Cassidy JD et al (10)	Female	28	One-year history of left-sided suboccipital and neck pain, and left sided tongue numbness developed after a whiplash injury. Physiotherapy (hot and cold packs and traction) to the neck was of little benefit. Examination revealed that rotation of the neck to the left was reduced by 50% and provoked neck pain and tongue numbness. She experienced a decrease in light touch sensation on the left lateral border of the tongue during left neck rotation and pressure over the left atlantoaxial articulation. She was given a 2-week course of daily manipulations directed toward mobilizing the upper cervical spine. At the end of this treatment, the tongue numbness was gone and could not be provoked. Review at 2 weeks, 3 months, and 6 months after treatment revealed no further episodes of tongue numbness.
31	Cassidy JD et al (10)	Female	57	No history of trauma. A long history of recurrent left suboccipital pain radiating to the vertex. She also complained of a feeling of numbness and burning on the left side of the tongue. Both the neck pain and the tongue numbness were aggravated by left neck rotation and cold drafts. Pressure over the left atlantoaxial articulation provoked both the pain and the tongue numbness. This patient was given a 2-week course of daily manipulations directed toward the left side of the upper cervical spine. She reported no further episodes of neck pain or tongue numbness when reviewed after 2 and 6 months.
32	Lois I (11)	Female	54	Patient presented with temporomandibular joint, back, shoulder, and headache problems that were believed to be myogenic in origin due to inappropriate working posture. Two years previously she had consulted a chiropractor for the head and shoulder symptoms and following cervical manipulation, developed left-sided tongue numbness, a metallic taste, and a feeling that the head was falling backward. The metallic taste lasted a week, the head instability continued about a year, and the tongue numbness was still present 2 years later. A lingual speech disorder occurred sporadically when pronouncing words with the letter "L." A diag-

Table continues

Table 12.1 (*Continued*)

Case	Source	Sex	Age (* = unknown)	Symtoms
				nosis of hypermobility was made. Treatment was aimed at normalizing mandibular movement and stabilizing the postural muscles of the head. Review 10 months later revealed absence of headaches and infrequent tongue numbness when the patient unconsciously rotated the head suddenly.
33	Hankey GJ (12)	Female	14	Four month history of unilateral upper nuchal pain radiating to the ipsilateral side of the tongue upon ipsilateral neck rotation. The pain was intense, and followed by residual numbness over the posterolateral aspect of the upper neck and ipsilateral tongue for 3–5 minutes. Right sided symptoms occurred more frequently than left sided symptoms. There was no history of cervical trauma. Physical and x-ray examinations were normal. The patient was advised to be cautious during sporting activities. Was managed "conservatively" with success.

ventilation syndrome, but this would involve the lips and tongue bilaterally; (3) migraine, but there was no prodrome, eye pain, nausea, etc.; (4) intrinsic tongue pathology, of which there was no evidence.

Neurological examination of cranial nerves V, VII, IX, and XII and the lateral spinothalamic and spinocerebellar tracts was conducted. In view of normal findings, the author decided to proceed with SMT.

Following manipulation involving contacts on the second and seventh cervical vertebrae, paresthesia of the tongue could not be reinduced by the above-mentioned head position. On subsequent visits, over an 18-month period, this provocative testing position did not reinduce tongue numbness, but the patient did mention that the right side of her tongue sometimes felt numb on very cold winter mornings, the significance of which is unknown.

Case B

A 33-year-old typesetter, whose only history of major trauma was a waterskiing accident at age 18, presented in May 1983 to a colleague, complaining of neck, upper thoracic and trapezius pain, and suboccipital headaches. She also described that sharp rotation of the neck would paralyze her tongue for about 5 seconds, and that this had been present since age 26. She demonstrated this by sharply turning her head to the right.

She had no atrophy of the tongue. She stated that there might have been a numbness, but continued: "It definitely doesn't feel like a dental anesthetic, it feels swollen as if it fills the throat" and "as if there is a knife at the back of the tongue which holds it rigid, so that it cannot be moved."

In July 1984, 14 months and 12 visits after her initial visit, her other symptoms had responded to SMT, but not the tongue complaint, which she stated could still be produced by head rotation, either right or left.

This patient was afraid to rotate her cervical spine, so that if she wanted to look to either side, she turned her whole trunk. She had become annoyed when practitioners to whom she described her complaint appeared to disbelieve her symptoms or told her it was a manifestation of a migraine headache.

Case C

A 20-year-old female student described in July 1984 that when about 12 years of age, she had begun to suffer from low back pain, neck pain, and headaches. She related how on turning her head quickly to either side, it produced sharp pain in the neck and dysesthesia in the region of the right angle of the mandible and tongue. The feeling in the tongue was described as not being like a dental anesthetic, but of a "painful, burning, tingling sensation" that caused her to suddenly stop whatever she was doing for a few minutes. At that time, these attacks occurred up to four times a day. Initially she did not realize that this was anything abnormal and therefore did not become concerned or worried; as she believed this must also happen to other people, she did not try to avoid neck rotation.

When she was about 14 years old, her mother took her to consult a chiropractor for her backaches, headaches, and neck pain. Following SMT, her back pain, neck pain, and headache all responded favorably and a decrease in the NTS attacks was noticed. She described that during the next 8 years, subsequent NTS attacks have been relieved by SMT, with her last attack being 12 months previously.

Case D

In December 1983, a 30-year-old carpenter was struck by a motor vehicle, being flung over the hood and hitting his head on the windscreen. Five days later at work, he received a blow on the head by a length of timber. Two days later, the patient became aware of tongue numbness, which was reported as similar to that felt when he had received a local dental anesthetic. On examination, various x-rays and tests were performed with no apparent indication of cause for the symptoms. Rotation of the head to the left was somewhat limited, and the patient held his head to the right. He had pain and tenderness overlying the right mastoid region.

After two manipulations to the atlantoaxial joint, the patient's symptoms had totally disappeared. Four months after the first treatment, the patient was reexamined. The tongue complaint had not returned, and neck range of motion and other tests were normal at that time.

Case E

In January 1984, a 19-year-old shop assistant was involved in a rear-end car accident. She developed a constant "numbing ache" in the cervical and suboccipital region, headaches, a painful left shoulder, and a painful numbness of the right side of the tongue. The tongue symptoms could be aggravated by turning to either side, but usually to the left.

The pain ran from the neck to behind the right ear, and the tongue went very numb. The patient described the symptoms as a feeling of a very thick, heavy, swollen, numb tongue, which "takes up all the room in the mouth, can't move it, like it had a mind of its own, it doesn't do what I want it to do," resulting in a slurring of speech.

Treatment consisted of traction and soft tissue and SMT. Significant relief was obtained from the musculoskeletal pain. This treatment decreased the frequency but not the intensity of the NTS attacks. In January 1985, the patient was involved in a second vehicle accident. This reestablished the spinal musculoskeletal pain and headaches and aggravated the tongue numbness. Following the second accident, the NTS has been totally unresponsive to SMT.

Case F

A 46-year-old man was involved in a motor vehicle accident in December 1983. This produced severe neck and head pains, with almost complete loss of cervical range of motion, and numbness in the fingers. Head rotation especially to the left produced suboccipital pain.

He was treated subsequently by medication, physiotherapeutics, acupuncture, and spinal manipulation, all with limited benefit. He has had three attacks of NTS. The first was in November 1985. On all three occasions, he awoke with his neck twisted to the left. The tongue was numb and rigid, which produced slurred speech. Since beginning SMT, he has adopted the habit of "forever cracking" his neck for relief of pain. On these three occasions, he manipulated his own neck by rotating his head to the right. The tongue symptoms disappeared and he could speak again.

Case G

A 26-year-old female computer operator presented with cervical and left shoulder pain of 1-week duration that was associated with suboccipital, temporal, and retro-orbital headaches. The shoulder pain was aggravated by right rotation that sent a sharp pain to the left trapezius and suboccipital musculature. This was associated with an altered sensation on the left side of the tongue, described as "thick, as if I couldn't move my tongue." This had begun 12 months previously and was occurring 2–3 times a week, lasting up to 60 seconds. There was no history of trauma. Rotation to either side could induce the tongue symptoms but most frequently to the right.

Treatment consisted of SMT to the upper three spinal articulations, with complete relief of the headaches and suboccipital pain and marked reduction in trapezius tenderness and the tongue symptoms. The NTS has only been experienced twice in 3 months since treatment began, and the duration has markedly decreased to 1–2 seconds.

Case H

A 40-year-old man presented with a history of migraine headaches and cervical muscle tension, during which time if he turned his head to the right, the right side of his tongue would become numb, "like a dental anesthetic." When not having the headache and neck tension, rotation did not produce the tongue symptoms. Consequently he is hesitant to turn his neck when suffering headaches and neck tension, and the frequency is related to unguarded neck movements. The numbness has lasted for a few seconds up to a minute.

The patient had 3 rear-end motor vehicle accidents between 1979 and 1981, and he developed the tongue symptoms after the second accident. When driving his car, he is hesitant to look to his right side.

Manipulative treatment from several different practitioners produced the tongue "tingling and numbness," so that he had be come hesitant and had reservations about going to manual therapy practitioners. He has since found a practitioner who manipulates his neck, relieving the headache and neck tension without producing the tongue symptoms. "Now the numbness only lasts moments." He feels the difference in the practitioners is that the latter practitioner first massages his neck muscles and is not as forceful in his subsequent manipulation.

TONGUE PARESTHESIA

If sensation from the tongue were conveyed by only the lingual nerve (a branch of the trigeminal nerve), it would have been difficult to explain paresthesia of the tongue by the mechanism of cervical spine involvement or nerve compression because the lingual nerve has no relationship to the cervical spine. It was therefore enlightening to note the descriptions, studies, and explanation put forward by Lance(5). Evidence that proprioceptive fibers do not pass back to the CNS by the lingual nerve is easily demonstrated as; (1) human subjects retain position sense and control of tongue movement after analgesic blockade of the inferior alveolar and lingual nerves(14); and (2) afferent discharges have been recorded from the hypoglossal nerve during stretching of the tongue in cats and monkeys, but no proprioceptive impulses were found in the lingual nerve upon stretching or twisting the tongue(15).

Corbin and Harrison(15) found (*Macaca mulatta* monkey) degenerating proprioceptive fibers in the most peripheral portion of the hypoglossal nerve after removal of the C2 dorsal root ganglion, section of the ascending branch of C2 (Fig. 12.1*i*), and section of the descending branch of C2 (Fig. 12.1*ii*), which joins C3 to form the ansa cervicalis. A pathway to the C1 ventral ramus has also been described. Yee et al. (16) observed degenerating fibers in the hypoglossal nerve in the rabbit after removal of the C1 dorsal root ganglion.

Additional detailed neuroanatomical evidence was provided by Fitzgerald and Sachithanandan(17) by silver impregnation after nerve section on Cynamolgus monkeys. Lingual nerve section was without apparent effect on tongue proprioceptors. Distal hypoglossal nerve section (near its point of entry into the tongue) caused severe depletion of ipsilateral proprioceptors and fusimotor nerves; but more proximal hypoglossal section (at the skull base) caused degeneration of fusimotor but not

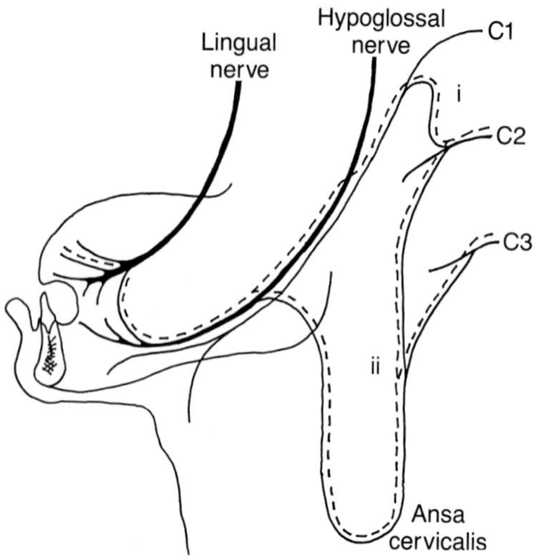

Figure 1. Proprioceptive fiber pathways *(broken lines)* from the lingual nerve to the hypoglossal nerve, to the C2–C3 ventral nerve roots (1) via a branch of C1 (which joins and travels with the hypoglossal nerve to supply the geniohyoid and thyrohyoid muscles) down the ascending branch of the second cervical ventral ramus, to the C2 ventral ramus (which, as described later, crosses the atlantoaxial joint); and (2) via the ramus descendens hypoglossi to the ansa cervicalis to the C2 and C3 ventral rami. Adapted from the following sources: Lance JW, Anthony M. Neck-tongue syndrome on sudden turning of the head. J Neurol Neurosurg Psychiatry 1980;43:97–101. Lance JW. Unusual syndromes in neurological practice. Med J Aust 1984;140(7):409–416. Corbin KB, Harrison F. The sensory innervation of the spinal accessory and tongue musculature in the rhesus monkey. Brain 1939;62:191–197. Fitzgerald MJT, Sachithanandan SR. The structure and source of lingual proprioceptors in the monkey. J Anat 1979;128(3):523–552.

proprioceptive nerves(17). Section of *i* (Fig. 1) C2 ventral ramus connection with the hypoglossal nerve together with section of *ii* (Fig. 1) the ramus descendens hypoglossi caused depletion of lingual proprioceptors, while procedures at *i* or *ii* alone had a lesser effect. It was concluded (in agreement with Corbin's earlier study) that lingual proprioceptive afferent fibers occupying the distal hypoglossal nerve leave it via two routes to reach the C2 and C3 cord levels (see Fig. 12.1).

These anatomical studies are further supported by experiments of Bowman and Combs(18) who described a pathway of proprioceptive fibers from the tongue to the cortex. Using monkeys (*M. mulatta,* after section of the lingual nerve), they demonstrated that stimulation of the distal hypoglossal nerve evoked potentials in the contralateral cerebral cortex. The cortical potentials evoked by a volley in the hypoglossal nerve disappeared completely after sectioning C2 dorsal root (in 50% of cases), C3 dorsal root (in 25% of cases), or both C2 and C3 dorsal roots (in 25% of cases). It is interesting to note that Sherrington, on discussing a human fetus with an extreme degree of spina bifida, commented that the hypoglossal nerve "seems to be almost exclusively formed by a branch from the second cervical ganglion and another from the vagus . . ."(19).

ANATOMY OF THE NECK-TONGUE SYNDROME

The C2 ventral root, ganglion, and spinal nerve are invested by fascia, which holds them against the capsule of the lateral atlantoaxial joint. Often the C2 ventral ramus courses transversely across the lateral atlantoaxial joint, gives articular branches to innervate the joint, and ultimately arches over the vertebral artery and enters the

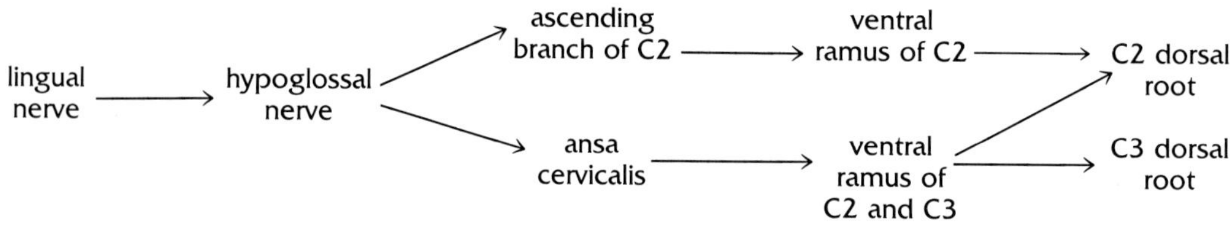

Figure 12.1a. Pathway of tongue proprioceptive fibers.

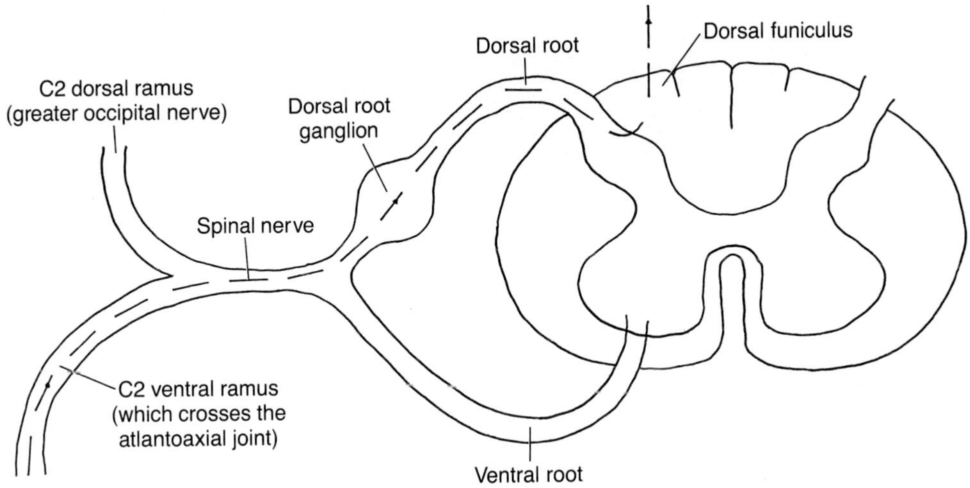

Figure 12.2. Proprioceptive fiber pathway *(broken line)* from C2 ventral ramus to the dorsal funiculus.

cervical plexus(20) (Fig. 12.3). The ventral root is also invested in a layer of strong fascia adherent to the undersurface of the inferior oblique muscle(10).

The above anatomy is not of mere arcane academic interest but has clinical application in the neck-tongue syndrome(5, 10, 20) and occipital neuralgia(21). There have been two theories proposed for the production of tongue numbness by head rotation(10, 20).

Bogduk(20), in 1981, following dissection of the C2 nerve roots and rami, concluded that the pathogenesis of the simul-

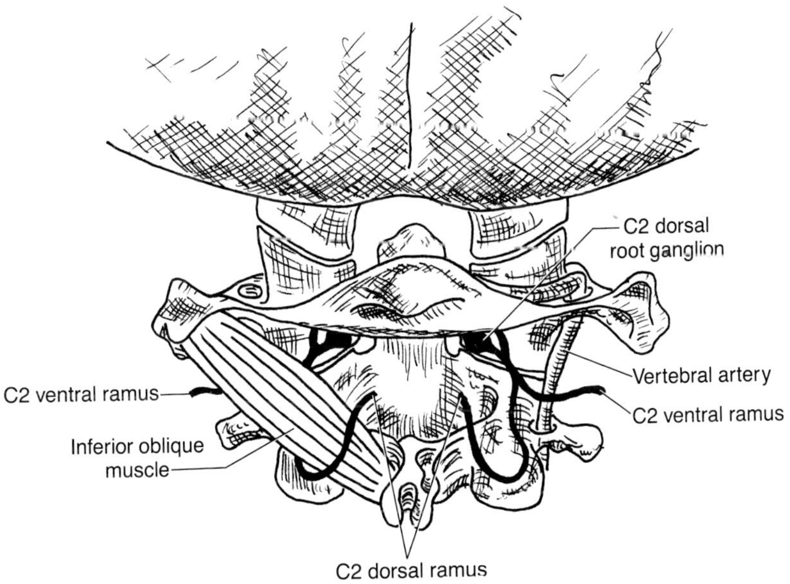

Figure 12.3. Posterior view of the occiput-atlas-axial region, showing the relationship of branches of C2 with the atlantoaxial joint and the inferior oblique muscle. Adapted from the following sources: Kapandji IA. The physiology of joints. Vol 3. 2nd ed. London: Churchill Livingstone 1974, p 191. Cassidy et al. Treatment of the neck-tongue syndrome by spinal manipulation: a report of three cases. Pain Clin 1986;1(1):41–46. Bogduk N. An anatomical basis for the neck-tongue syndrome. J Neurol Neurosurg Psychiatry 1981;44:202–208. Bogduk N. The anatomy of occipital neuralgia. Proc Aust Assoc Neurol 1981;17:167–184.

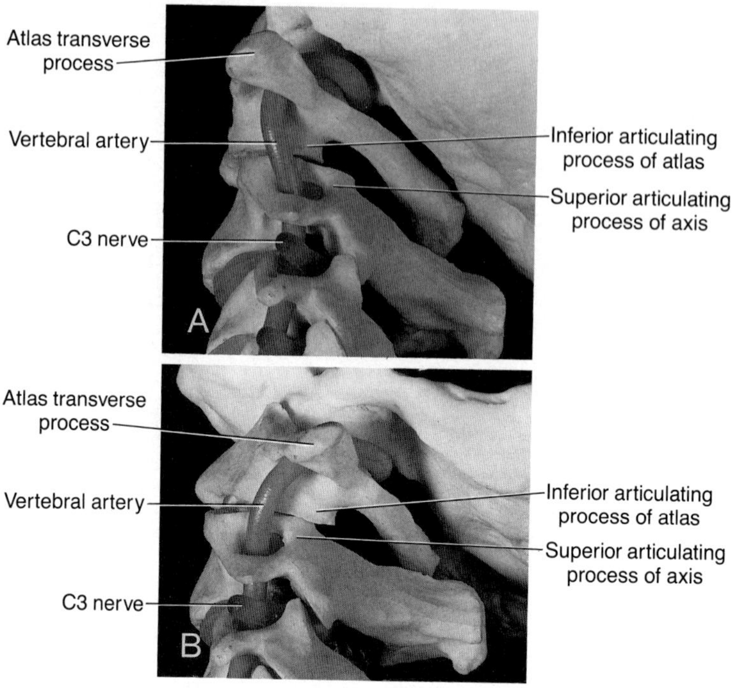

Figure 12.4A. Lateral view of the left side of the upper cervical spine. This depicts how, on turning the head to the right, the left lateral mass of the atlas moves anteriorly. In a case in which the C2 ventral ramus crosses the atlantoaxial joint, it can be seen how it will be drawn over the superior articular process of the axis. **B.** Lateral view of the left side of the upper cervical spine. This depicts how, on turning the head to the left, the left lateral mass of the atlas moves posteriorly. In a case in which the C2 ventral ramus crosses the atlantoaxial joint, it can be seen how it will be drawn over the inferior margin of the lateral mass of the atlas.

taneous occurrence of suboccipital pain and ipsilateral numbness of the tongue was most likely a subluxation of the lateral atlantoaxial joint with impaction of the C2 ventral ramus against the subluxated articular process. When turning the head to the right, the left lateral mass of the atlas, in company with the C2 root, moves anteriorly, and in a case where the C2 ventral ramus crosses the atlantoaxial joint, it will be drawn over the margin of the superior articular process of the axis, separated from it only by the capsule (Fig. 12.4A). When the head is turned to the left, the left lateral mass moves posteriorly and the C2 ventral ramus will be drawn over the inferior margin of the lateral mass of the atlas (Fig. 4B).

Cassidy et al(10), in 1986, proposed another mechanism, as they point out that there is no direct evidence that atlantoaxial instability or subluxation exists in this syndrome, and that this type of instability is usually associated with infection, trauma, or congenital anomalies and can result in more severe neurological deficits with cord compression. NTS patients have evidence of local muscle spasm and reduced mobility at the atlantoaxial joint. Relief and increased range of motion were achieved following SMT (Table 12.1, cases 29–31). If there was atlantoaxial instability in these cases, it was argued that SMT would have been expected to aggravate rather than relieve the symptoms. This theory argues that spasm of the inferior oblique muscle (Fig. 12.3) is responsible for both entrapment of the ventral ramus of C2 and the reduced range of cervical motion.

There has been only one case(4) in which the nerve/apophyseal joint relationship has been actually visualized in a NTS patient. In this case the right atlantoaxial process was more protuberant than the left, stretching the right C2 spinal nerve in a caudad direction. The ventral ramus passed directly over the joint capsule. Ventral and dorsal rami were tougher to palpation on the side of symptoms. Examination revealed loss of both myelinated and unmyelinated nerve fibers, fibrosis, and fibrohyaline thickening of many small blood vessels(4). The pathological changes demonstrated in the resected nerves(4) are likely to have been caused by repeated trauma and could be explained by either the Bogduk(20) or Cassidy(10) hypothesis.

The tongue paresthesia is therefore attributable to nerve compression, but the suboccipital pain is not(20). The suboccipital pain is due to a sprain of the atlantoaxial joint capsule(20). It has been demonstrated experimentally that intermittent compression of spinal roots, spinal nerves, or peripheral nerves produces paresthesia and/or paralysis but not pain(20–33). "Acute compression of the root or nerve does not produce more than several seconds of repetitive firing"(27). This was observed as early as 1797 by Felice Fontana, who noted that pressure on a nerve blocks conduction without causing stimulation(22).

Compression is known to produce morphological consequences in neural tissues and neural support tissues, but there is a good deal of suspicion that morphological alterations are neither necessary nor sufficient to produce pain(23). This is supported by a random autopsy study(33) in which it was found that 5 of 12 lateral femoral cutaneous nerves were suffering entrapment compromise severe enough to have initiated Wallerian degeneration and to have generated abnormal fibrotic changes in the collagen of the endoneurium and endoneurial arteries, yet the subjects had not had any clinical symptoms prior to death.

The tongue numbness without impaired touch and pain perception is similar to the facial numbness often experienced in patients with Bell's palsy. Disturbances of sensation in the face are usually due to trigeminal nerve involvement, but in Bell's palsy, the numbness is due to compression of proprioceptive fibers in the facial nerve with no disturbance in the trigeminal nerve.

DISCUSSION OF CASES

Analysis of the cases indicates the presence of findings other than merely transient tongue paresthesia triggered by neck rotation. The following observations are discussed.

(1) The relationship of this syndrome to trauma has not been addressed before. Cases 4, 14, 28, 30, A, D, E, F, and H appear to demonstrate a causal relationship to head/neck trauma, especially motor vehicle trauma. Of these, six were treated with SMT, and five responded well.

Trauma to joints may cause damage or attenuation to capsuloligamentous supporting structures, which produces a change in joint function, thus allowing a greater degree of mobility (hypermobile subluxation) of the atlantoaxial joint, possibly leading to the mechanism for NTS proposed by Bogduk(20), i.e., of mechanical compression of the C2 ventral ramus as it crosses the atlantoaxial joint. Similarly, following upper cervical trauma, protective muscle spasm is a common finding. This supports the Cassidy hypothesis(10) of possible C2 ventral ramus entrapment beneath the inferior oblique muscle.

(2) Cases 5, 12, 13, 32, B, E, F, and G suggest that reflex movement of the tongue may result from compression of proprioceptive fibers in the second cervical nerve root or that, in some instances, motor fibers to the tongue may traverse the second cervical root as previously noted by Lance(1). Case 8 developed a mild dysphagia because of a feeling of muscle spasm in her throat(4). This may have been due to globus hystericus, as this occurred when the head and right arm pain was severe; or it may have been due to involvement of glossopharyngeal branches, as such a neuronal circuit has been previously described(9) to explain the occurrence of oropharyngeal, palatal, and otic paresthesias in case

27(9), providing another neuroanatomical substrate for referred symptoms from the second cervical ventral ramus to the tongue.

(3) Four cases of the incomplete form of this syndrome have been described,(5, 8) i.e., lack of the paroxysmal numbness in the tongue, but their descriptions of the attacks are characteristic and indistinguishable from those with the complete syndrome(8). It is possible that these patients may at a later time develop the complete syndrome, as this has occurred in cases 5–8 and F in which the tongue numbness appeared 12 months, 18 months, 9 months, 5 years, and 2 years, respectively, after the onset of the incomplete syndrome.

(4) In cases B, C, and E, all described a similar frustration in that when they described their symptoms to medical and chiropractic practitioners, they were not believed; and in case B, the patient was told it was a manifestation of migraine in spite of the absence of other signs and symptoms.

(5) The frequency with which conditions predisposing to atlantoaxial instability are reported on in association with NTS is most likely more than coincidental. There were 2 cases of ankylosing spondylitis(6, 8), one case of psoriatic arthritis(8), and three cases with occipitalization of the atlas(1, 4, 5). Inflammatory laxity of the transverse ligament of the atlas with rheumatic disease is well known. Occipitalization of the atlas "implicates agenesis of the transverse ligament"(34). Both these conditions can therefore result in instability of the atlantoaxial joint. These conditions were found in 15% (6 of 40) of cases described in the available literature. In four of the cases of Bertoft and Westerberg(8), laxity of peripheral joints was found on examination, which most likely implicates spinal joints as well. The author believes that the various conditions accompanied by excessive laxity in 10 (or 25%) of the cases mentioned strengthens the "excessive mobility theory" of which trauma is an important possible cause.

(6) Cases B, E, 8, and 28 were unresponsive to conservative therapies including medication, collar, and manipulation. In two of these (cases 8 and 28), symptoms were almost constant; and in cases B and E, it was aggravated by neck motion. In case B, repeated trauma to the nerve over 7 years may have produced changes that made it nonresponsive to SMT.

Case E is interesting as prior to the second accident, she responded partially to SMT. Following the second vehicle accident, she was totally unresponsive. It is possible that a greater degree of joint mobility was possibly responsible for imparting a greater degree of physical trauma to the nerve resulting in degenerative changes similar to those reported by Elisevich et al. (4) and therefore requiring operative treatment for relief. It is also possible that the second accident increased the suboccipital muscle spasm so that it was no longer responsive to SMT.

(7) The appearance of NTS in early life has been suggested as being possibly related to a genetically determined laxity of ligaments and/or joint capsules(8). To support this, in five of the seven nonrheumatic cases of Bertoft and Westerberg(8), ligamentous laxity was also present in one relative (parent or sibling); and in four of these patients, laxity of peripheral joints was found on examination. Laxity of peripheral joints would suggest laxity of spinal supporting structures as well.

(8) Paresthesia in the fingers occurring simultaneously with NTS has been described in cases 4, 7, 8, 27, 28, 29, and F. These symptoms cannot be related to C2 ventral ramus compression, but Lance and Anthony suggest that it may be due to traction on the lower nerve roots by the dura mater during atlantoaxial subluxation(1). Paresthesia in the fingers was a symptom of atlantoaxial subluxation due to rheumatoid arthritis in six of 22 patients described by Robinson(35). There is no anatomic data to support the dural traction hypothesis(1).

(9) Cases 31 and A were aggravated by cold. The significance of this is unknown.

MEDICAL TREATMENT FOR THE NECK-TONGUE SYNDROME

Surgical treatment for NTS has been described by Elisevich et al(4) and Bertoft and Westerberg(8).

The case described by Elisevich et al. (case 8) did not respond to previous medication or a cervical collar. After surgery (resection of a fibrosed C2 ventral ramus), this patient experienced no tingling sensations in her tongue; but after a week, she reported a mild recurrence, which suggested a facilitation of residual proprioceptive fibers in the adjacent uninjured spinal roots(4). Elisevich et al stated that "greater amelioration of symptoms would have occurred if the C1 and C3 roots, which may also contain sensory fibers from the tongue, had been resected at the same time as the C2 roots"(4).

Bertoft and Westerberg described a patient with rheumatic disease of the cervical spine where symptoms were abolished after immobilization by fusion of C1–C2(8).

Cases 14, 15, 27, and 28 reported a favorable response to immobilization in a neck collar. A program of postural control and neck exercises was found beneficial in cases 15, which also included a collar, and 32. Relief by these means could be used to support either of the proposed theories of etiology.

In case 17 in which the NTS was associated with tonic seizures/spasm, 400 mg of carbamazepine daily suppressed the attacks(7).

SPINAL MANIPULATIVE THERAPY FOR THE NTS SYNDROME

A review of the literature suggests that this syndrome does not spontaneously disappear. In fact, it is usual to be present for years. The effectiveness of SMT has been documented previously(10, 13), and four additional cases (E–H) are presented here.

The favorable response to SMT of cases 29, 30, 31, A, C, D, F, G, and H and the temporary response of case E appear to indicate that SMT is a useful procedure in uncomplicated forms of this syndrome. Since it is hypothesized that this syndrome is due to either dysfunction of the atlantoaxial joint(20) or muscle spasm(10), it would appear that the treatment of choice should be musculoskeletal therapy.

It is recognized that joint manipulation increases joint mobility(36–48) and decreases muscle spasm(38, 46–50). The following therapeutic effects are suggested:

(1) Muscle relaxation. If there is a loss of motion due to muscle spasm in adjacent spinal motion segments producing a compensatory increase in atlantoaxial motion(6, 36, 37, 51), then manipulation to increase the mobility of those adjacent hypomobile joints would decrease the compensatory hypermobility and therefore reduce the intermittent subluxation at the atlantoaxial joint. If the symptoms were due to inferior oblique spasm, producing C2 ventral ramus entrapment, then the reflex relaxation effect on muscle hypertonus of SMT could explain the relief following SMT.

(2) Compensatory hypermobility. Webb et al noted that loss of motion in adjacent joints "places undue stress upon levels immediately above and below during spinal movement"(6); and Hviid, after studying the dynamics of spinal movement, stated that "hampered movement at one level gives rise to a compensatory increase in mobility at another"(36). Jirout, after performing "dynamic" examination of the spine on 1500 individuals, stated: "The functional deficit in one segment has to be compensated elsewhere. The compensation may usually be discovered in the nearest upper segment in which the motility of the vertebrae is increased; we have called this compensatory hypermotility" that produces "greater strain on the ligaments in the neighboring segments"(37). This may have been an aggravating factor in cases 4, 7, and 8 in which there was occipi-

talization of the atlas. Functional stress x-ray examination of the cervical spine usually involves flexion and extension views. Since the primary function of the atlantoaxial joint is rotation rather than flexion and extension, these views do not adequately or thoroughly evaluate atlantoaxial biomechanical motion characteristics, or the lack of ligamentous stability, other than severe transverse ligament compromise. To evaluate this joint in future cases of NTS to test the hypermobility theory(20), the technique described by Tasharski et al for evaluation of dynamic atlantoaxial abberation could be used(52).

(3) Meniscoid derangement. The atlantoaxial articulation on the side of symptoms may develop a degree of excessive mobility in compensation for a decrease in mobility of the adjacent spinal articulations or the contralateral atlantoaxial articulation. According to Dorr(53), the earliest mention of spinal apophyseal menisci was in 1855 by Henle, who described them as synovial folds, and in 1904 by Fick, who described them as "kapselfalten" or capsular folds(54). Intraarticular meniscoid bodies have been described in all spinal apophyseal joints and are true menisci as they are found at all ages from 70-mm embryos. The lack of synovial cells over the majority of the surface has suggested to various authors that these structures actually bear weight(53–65). Schmincke and Santo, in 1932(56), gave a clear description of structures in the cervical apophyseal joints that they considered to be true intraarticular discs. Many authors since have hypothesized that these structures can block gliding of the joint surfaces and create pain from tension on its capsular attachment with resultant pain and muscle spasm(54, 55, 66–9).

Spinal joint locking appears in the literature under a number of different labels: acute locked back(54, 55); "blocage vertebral"(58, 59); spinal joint stiffening(66); acute cervical joint lock(67, 68); vertebral locking(70); "wirbelblockierung"(71); locked facet (72); facet synovial impingement(73). It would appear that all of these terms are synonymous for one condition. In discussing the meniscoid entrapment theory, Bogduk and Engel stated "the logical treatment for this condition then is manipulation, in which the apposed articular cartilages are separated and the trapped apex released"(54). The author proposes that if the mechanism is related to joint hypermobility(20), then manipulation to adjacent fixated segments, or the atlantoaxial joint contralateral to the symptoms, would result in the total rotational movement of the segment(s) being more evenly shared, effectively decreasing the degree of intermittent atlantoaxial subluxation on the side of symptoms.

(4) Functional atlantooccipital block. In otherwise "normal" patients, a functional atlantooccipital block may be visualized on roentgenograms taken in the flexed and extended positions(51, 69). Normally, the posterior atlantooccipital space increases during flexion, whereas it remains unchanged when there is a functional block. This often follows trauma to the head and/or neck, or patients may be able to relate a particular neck movement or transient body posture from which the symptoms began(69). As it can be removed by manipulation(69), it represents either an extraarticular muscular or an intraarticular meniscoid fixation. Wackenheim states that this functional atlantooccipital block is compensated by atlantoaxial hypermobility"(51), and is an objective sign frequently seen in patients with cervico-occipital neuralgia(51, 69), which he attributed to stretching of the C2 nerve across the hypermobile atlantoaxial joints(51). As such a "blockage" is usually associated with suboccipital muscle spasm, it is also possible that this could be the mechanism to cause or aggravate cases of NTS, rather than compensatory hypermobility.

(5) Traumatic joint dysfunction. Why is this syndrome apparently seen so rarely in cases of neck trauma? Clinicians are well aware of referred pain in the area

of the second cervical nerve due to trauma or degenerative or inflammatory changes, and yet the tongue symptoms are usually not reported in cases of traumatic neuropathy of the second cervical nerves(74). If the tongue numbness is due to the mechanism described by Bogduk(20), it seems difficult to understand how in Robinson's(35) description of 22 patients with atlantoaxial subluxation due to rheumatoid arthritis, there was no mention of any patient with tongue numbness. Trauma may be similar to the discussion of Webb et al of this syndrome with cervical arthritis, in which they stated that the tongue symptoms may not be uncommon but may be submerged in the plethora of other symptoms(6).

CONCLUSION

The anatomy and clinical findings of the neck-tongue syndrome have been reviewed. Two theories as to the possible etiology have been described, and both may be operational in different cases. This condition is not a contraindication to spinal manipulative therapy, as illustrated by the beneficial response. Those cases that did not respond may be due to atlantoaxial joint subluxation as suggested by Bogduk(20).

It is suggested that NTS

(1) is more common than is currently acknowledged;
(2) has a causal relationship with neck trauma;
(3) In some cases, may respond to spinal manipulative therapy and that in such cases, a short trial may be beneficial;
(4) some cases will not respond to SMT and may require neck immobilization or surgery.

Acknowledgments

Thanks are extended to Dr. A. M. Kleynhans, Dr. N. Bogduk, Prof. J. W. Lance, and Dr. B. F. Walker for their help and suggestions in the preparation of this paper.

References

1. Lance JW, Anthony M. Neck-tongue syndrome on sudden turning of the head. J Neurol Neurosurg Psychiatry 1980;43:97–101.
2. Cyriax J. Textbook of orthopaedic medicine. Vol 1. Diagnosis of soft tissue lesions. 7th ed. London: Baillier Tindall, 1978, pp 114, 143.
3. Cyriax J. Textbook of orthopaedic medicine. Vol 1, 4th ed. London: Cassell, 1962, 158 (quoted by Lance and Anthony 1.)
4. Elisevich K, Stratford J, Bray G. Surgical management of the neck-tongue syndrome: case report. Can J Neurol Sci, 1982;9:283. (Also reported in: J Neurol Neurosurg Psychiatry. 1984;47:407–409.)
5. Lance JW. Unusual syndromes in neurological practice. Med J Aust 1984;140(7):409–16.
6. Webb J, March L, Tyndall A. The neck-tongue syndrome: occurrence with cervical arthritis as well as normals. J. Rheumatol. 1984;11(4):530–533.
7. Noda S, Umezaki H. Spinal neck-tongue syndrome. J Neurol Neurosurg Psychiatry 1984;47:751.
8. Bertoft EF, Westerberg C. Further observations on the neck-tongue syndrome. In: Olesen J, Tfelt-hansen P, Jensen K, eds. Precedings of the 2nd International Headache Congress. Copenhagen, (June 18–21, 1985 pp 312–313. (Also in: Cephalalgia 1985; Supp 3:312–3.)
9. Fortin JC, Biller J. Neck tongue syndrome. Headache. 1985;25:255–258.
10. Cassidy JD, Diakow PRP, DeKorompay VL, Munkacsi I, Yong-Hing K. Treatment of the neck-tongue syndrome by spinal manipulation: a report of three cases. Pain Clin 1986;1(1):41–6.
11. Lois I. The cervicolingual syndrome. Man Med 1987;3:63–6.
12. Hankey GJ Neck-tongue syndrome on sudden neck rotation. Aust NZ J Med 1988;18:181.
13. Terrett AGJ. The neck tongue syndrome. J Aust Chiro Assoc 1984;14(3):100–7.
14. Adatia AK, Gehring EN. Proprioceptive innervation of the tongue. J Anat 1971;110:215–20.
15. Corbin KB, Harrison F. The sensory innervation of the spinal accessory and tongue musculature in the rhesus monkey. Brain 1939;62:191–197.
16. Yee J, Harrison F, Corbin KB. The sensory innervation of the spinal accessory and tongue musculature in the rabbit. J Comp Neurol 1939;70:305–314.
17. Fitzgerald MJT, Sachithanandan SR. The structure and source of lingual proprioceptors in the monkey. J Anat 1979;128(3):523–552.
18. Bowman JP, Combs CM. The cerebrocortical projection of hypoglossal afferents. Exp Neurol 1969;23:291–301.
19. Sherrington CS. On the anatomical constitution of nerves of skeletal muscles: with remarks on recurrent fibres in the ventral spinal nerve root. J Physiol (Lond) 1894;17:211–58.
20. Bogduk N. An anatomical basis for the neck-tongue syndrome. J Neurol Neurosurg Psychiatry 1981;44:202–8.
21. Bogduk N. The anatomy of occipital neuralgia. Proc Aust Assoc Neurol 1981;17:167–84.

22. Fontana F (1797). Cited by: Meek WJ, Leaper WE. The effect of pressure on conductivity of nerve and muscle. Am J Physiol. 1911;27:308–22 (quoted by Sharpless SK, Ref 28).
23. Luttges MW, Gerren RA. Compression physiology: nerves and roots. In: Haldeman S, ed. Modern developments in the principles and practice of chiropractic. New York: Appleton-Century-Crofts, 1980: 65–92.
24. Macnab I. The mechanism of spondylogenic pain. In: Hirsch C, Zotterman Y, eds. Cervical pain. Oxford: Pergamon, 1972, pp 89–95.
25. MacKenzie RA, Burke D, Skuse NF, Lethlean AK. Fiber function and perception during cutaneous nerve block. J Neurol Neurosurg Psychiatry 1975;38:865–73.
26. Howe JF, Loeser JD, Calvin WH. Mechanosensitivity of dorsal root ganglia and chronically injured axons: a physiological basis for the radicular pain of nerve root compression. Pain 1977;3: 25–41.
27. Perl ER. Mode of action of nociceptors. In: Hirsch C, Zotterman Y, eds. Cervical pain. Wenner-Gren Centre International Symposia Series. Oxford: Pergamon. 1971;17:157–164.
28. Scham SM. Tension signs in lumbar disc prolapse. Clin Orthop 1971;75:195–204.
29. Sharpless SK. Susceptibility of spinal roots to compression block. In: Goldstein M, ed. The research status of spinal manipulative therapy. Bethesda: NINCDS Monograph No 15, 1975, pp 155–61.
30. Kelly M. Is pain due to pressure on nerves? Spinal tumors and the intervertebral disc. Neurology 1956;6:32–36.
31. Haldeman S. The importance of neurophysiological research into principles of spinal manipulation. In: Goldstein M, ed. The research status of spinal manipulative therapy. Bethesda: NINCDS Monograph No 15, 1975, pp 183–7.
32. Wall PD. The mechanisms of pain associated with cervical vertebral disease. In: Hirsch C, Zotterman Y, eds. Cervical pain. Wenner-Gren International Symposia Series. Oxford: Pergamon. 1971, pp 201–10.
33. Jefferson D, Eames RA. Subclinical entrapment of the lateral femoral cutaneous nerve: an autopsy study. Muscle Nerve 1979;2:145–154.
34. Wackenheim A. Radiodiagnosis of the vertebrae in adults. New York: Springer-Verlag, 1983, p 170.
35. Robinson HS. Rheumatoid arthritis—atlanto-axial subluxation and its clinical presentation. Can Med Assoc J 1966;94:470–477.
36. Hviid H. Functional radiography of the cervical spine. Ann Swiss Chiro Assoc 1965;3:37–65.
37. Jirout J. Studies in the dynamics of the spine. Acta Radiol 1956;46:55–60.
38. Lewit K. The contribution of clinical observation to neurobiological mechanisms in manipulative therapy. In: Korr IM, ed. The neurobiological mechanisms in manipulative therapy. New York: Plenum Press, 1978, pp 3–25.
39. Jirout J. The effect of mobilization of the segmental blockade on the sagittal component of the reaction on lateroflexion of the cervical spine. Neuroradiology 1972;3:210–215.
40. Paris SV. Gross spinal movements and their restriction as the basis of joint manipulation. Prog Phys Ther 1970;1:208–213.
41. Howe DH, Newcombe RG, Wade MT. Manipulation of the cervical spine—a pilot study. J Roy Coll Gen Pract 1983(Sept);33:574–579.
42. Carrick FR. Treatment of pathomechanics of the lumbar spine by manipulation. J Manipulative Physiol Ther 1981(Dec);4(4):173–178.
43. Nall SK. The role of specific manipulation towards alleviating abnormalities in spinal motion. J Manipulative Physiol Ther 1982;5(1):11–15.
44. Hviid H. The influence of the chiropractic treatment on the rotary mobility of the cervical spine. A kinesiometric and statistical study. Ann Swiss Chiro Assoc 1971;5:31–44.
45. Haldeman S. The pathophysiology of the spinal subluxation. In: Goldstein M, ed. The research status of spinal manipulative therapy. Bethesda: NINCDS monograph No. 15. DHEW Publication No. (NIH) 76-998. 1975, pp 217–26.
46. Wyke BD. Articular neurology and manipulative therapy. In: Glasgow EF et al, eds. Aspects of manipulative therapy. 2nd ed. London: Churchill-Livingstone, 1985, pp 72–77.
47. Haldeman S. Spinal manipulative therapy in the management of low back pain. In: Finneson BE, ed. Low back pain. 2nd ed. Philadelphia: JB Lippincott Co, 1980, pp 245–275.
48. Gitelman R. The treatment of pain by spinal manipulation. In: Goldstein M, ed. The research status of spinal manipulative therapy. Bethesda: NINCDS monograph No. 15. DHEW Publication No. (NIH) 76-998. 1975, pp 277–285.
49. England RW, Deibert PW. Electromyographic studies. Part 1: Consideration in the evaluation of osteopathic therapy. J Am Osteop Assoc 1972;72(2):221–3.
50. Grice AS. Muscle tonus change following manipulation. J Can Chiro Assoc 1974(Dec);18(4):29–31.
51. Wackenheim A. Functional atlanto-occipital block. Neuroradiology 1971;3:81–2.
52. Tasharski CC, Heinze WJ, Pugh JL. Dynamic atlanto-axial aberration: a case study and cinefluorographic approach to diagnosis. J Manipulative Physiol Ther 1981;4(2):65–8.
53. Dorr WM. Uber die anatomie der wirbelgelenke. Arch orthop unfallchir 1985;50:222–234.
54. Bogduk N, Engel R. The menisci of the lumbar apophyseal joints. A review of their anatomy and clinical significance. Spine 1984;9(5):454–60.
55. Bogduk N, Jull G. The theoretical pathology of acute locked back: a basis for manipulative therapy. Man Med 1985;1:78–82.
56. Schmincke A, Santo E. Zur normalen und pathologischen anatomie des halswirbelsaule. Z Allgem Pathol 1932;55:369.
57. Lewin T, Moffett B, Viidik A. The morphology of the lumbar synovial intervertebral joints. Acta Morphol Neerl Scand 1961;4:299–319.
58. Kos J, Wolf J. Die menisci der zwischenwirbelge-

lenke und ihre mogliche Rolle Lei Wirbelblockierung. Man Med 1972;10:105–114.
59. Kos J, Wolf J. Les menisques intervertebraux et leur role possible dans les blocages vertebraux. Ann Med Phys 1972;15:203–218.
60. Hadley LA. Anatomico-roentgenographic studies of the spine. Springfield, IL: Charles C Thomas. 1964; p 175.
61. Penning WL, Tondury G. Entstehung, bau und funktion der meniskoiden strukturen in den halswirbelgelenken. Z Orthop Grenzgeb 1963;98:1–14.
62. Tondury G. Beitragzur Kenntnis der kleinen wirbelgelenke. Z Anat entwicklungsgesch 1940;110:568–575.
63. Tondury G. Anatomie fonctionelle des petites articulations du rachis. Ann Med Phys 1972;15:173–191.
64. Putz R, Pomaroli A. Form und funktion der articulatio atlanto-axialis lateralis. Acta Anat 1972;83:333–345.
65. Mercer S. The menisci of the cervical synovial joints. In: Proceedings: fourth biennial conference, Manipulative Therapists Association of Australia (22–25 May 1985) pp 109–114.
66. Bourdillon JF. Spinal manipulation. 3rd ed. New York: Appleton-Century-Crofts, 1982, pp 27–28.
67. Maitland GD. Acute locking of the cervical spine. Aust J Physiol 1978;24(3):103–109.
68. Spraque RB. The acute cervical joint lock. Phys Ther 1983;63(9):1439–1444.
69. Grieve GP. Common vertebral joint problems. London: Churchill-Livingstone, 1981, pp 206–209, 253, 306.
70. Stoddard A. Manual of osteopathic practice. New York: Harper & Row, 1969; p 81.
71. Tager KH. Wirbelmeniskus oder synovialfortsatz. Z Orthop Grenzgeb 1965;99:439.
72. Wood L. Acute locked facet syndrome and its treatment under local periarticular anesthesia—Part 1. Clinical perspective and pilot study proposal. J Manipulative Physiol Ther 1984;7(4):211–7.
73. Kraft GL, Levinthal DH. Facet synovial impingement. Surg Gynec Obst 1951;93:439–443.
74. Behram S. Traumatic neuropathy of second cervical spinal nerves. Br Med J 1983;1:1312–1313.

Index